footapsy

faggot

Go to Page
38

BEING

HEALTHY

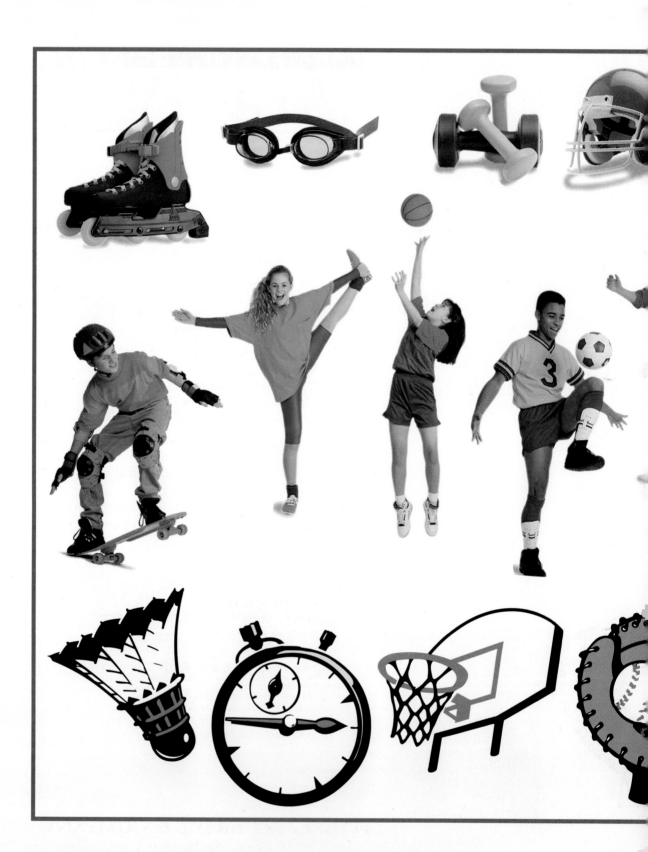

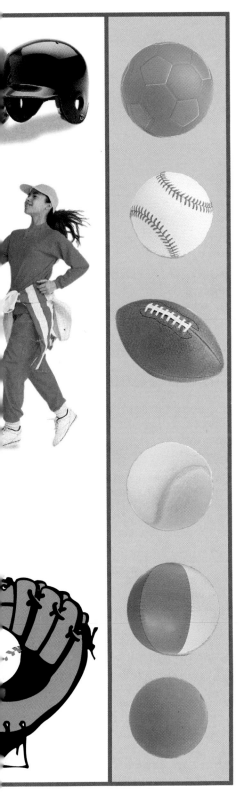

B E I N G.
HEALTHY

Larry K. Olsen
Professor of Health Education
The Pennsylvania State University
University Park, Pennsylvania

Richard W. St. Pierre
Professor and Head
Department of Health Education
The Pennsylvania State University
University Park, Pennsylvania

Jan M. Ozias, Ph.D., R.N.
Coordinator of Health Services
Austin Independent School District
Austin, Texas

SENIOR EDITORIAL ADVISORS

Ernest D. Buck, M.D.
Pediatrician
Corpus Christi, Texas

Barbara A. Galpin
Teacher of Health and Physical Education
Islip Public Schools
Islip, New York

Howard L. Taras, M.D., F.R.C.P.C.
Assistant Professor of Pediatrics
University of California, San Diego
   and District Medical Consultant
San Diego Unified School District
San Diego, California

HARCOURT BRACE & COMPANY
Orlando   Atlanta   Austin   Boston   San Francisco   Chicago   Dallas   New York
Toronto   London

ACKNOWLEDGMENTS

CONTENT ADVISORY BOARD

MENTAL HEALTH

Sharon Smith Brady, Ph.D.
Licensed Psychologist
Lawton, Oklahoma

Charlotte P. Ross
President and Executive Director
Youth Suicide National Center
Burlingame, California

HUMAN GROWTH AND DEVELOPMENT, DISEASES AND DISORDERS, AND PUBLIC HEALTH

Thomas Blevins, M.D.
American Diabetes Association,
   Texas Affiliate, Inc.
Austin, Texas

Ernest D. Buck, M.D.
Pediatrician
Corpus Christi, Texas

Linda A. Fisher, M.D.
Chief Medical Officer
St. Louis County Department
   of Health
St. Louis, Missouri

Howard L. Taras, M.D., F.R.C.P.C.
Assistant Professor of Pediatrics
University of California, San Diego
   and District Medical Consultant
San Diego Unified School District
San Diego, California

CONSUMER HEALTH PRACTICES

Robert C. Arffa, M.D.
Adjunct Professor of
   Ophthalmology
Medical College of Pennsylvania
Allegheny General Hospital
Pittsburgh, Pennsylvania

Bertram V. Dannheisser, Jr., D.D.S.
Florida Dental Association
Pensacola, Florida

John D. Durrant, Ph.D.
Professor of Otolaryngology and
   Communication and Director
   of Audiology
University of Pittsburgh
   Medical Center
Pittsburgh, Pennsylvania

NUTRITION

Janet L. Durrwachter, M.N.S., R.D.
Nutrition Consultant
Cogan Station, Pennsylvania

Maryfrances L. Marecic, M.S., R.D.
Consultant
Montville, New Jersey
   (Former Instructor in Nutrition,
   The Pennsylvania State
   University)

Linda Fox Simmons, M.S.H.P., R.D./L.D.
Registered Dietician
Austin, Texas

EXERCISE AND FITNESS

Steven N. Blair, P.E.D.
Director, Epidemiology
Cooper Institute for Aerobics
   Research
Dallas, Texas

Deborah Waters, M.D.
Colorado Springs, Colorado
   (Former Team Physician,
   The Pennsylvania State
   University)

MEDICINE

Donna Hubbard McCree, M.P.H., R.Ph.
Assistant Professor
Pharmacy Administration
Howard University
College of Pharmacy
Washington, D.C.

Judith Ann Shinogle, R.Ph.
M.S. Candidate
Harvard School of Public Health
Boston, Massachusetts

SUBSTANCE ABUSE

Robert N. Holsaple
Supervisor of Prevention Programs
The School Board of Broward
   County
Fort Lauderdale, Florida

SAFETY AND FIRST AID

American Red Cross
Washington, D.C.

CONTRIBUTORS AND REVIEWERS

Danny J. Ballard, Ed.D., C.H.E.S.
Associate Professor of Health
Health and Kinesiology
  Department
Texas A&M University
College Station, Texas

Linda Barnes
Teacher
Wahl-Coates School
Greenville, North Carolina

Robert C. Barnes, Ed.D., M.P.H.
Associate Professor and
  Coordinator
Health Education
East Carolina University
Greenville, North Carolina

David L. Bever, Ph.D.
Coordinator of Health
  Education
Department of Human Services
George Mason University
Fairfax, Virginia

James M. Eddy, D.Ed.
Professor and Chair
Health Studies
The University of Alabama
Tuscaloosa, Alabama

Sue Ann Eddy
Teacher
Stillman Heights Elementary
Tuscaloosa, Alabama

Ruth C. Engs, Ed.D., R.N.
Professor
Applied Health Science
Indiana University
Bloomington, Indiana

Tina Fields, Ph.D.
Associate Professor
Health Education
Texas Tech University
Lubbock, Texas

Sharon Guenther
Coordinator of Health and
  Physical Education
Wilkes County Board of Education
Wilkesboro, North Carolina

Patricia Barthalow Koch, Ph.D.
Associate Professor
Health Education
College of Health and Human
  Development
The Pennsylvania State University
University Park, Pennsylvania

Patricia Langner, P.H.N., B.S.N., M.P.H.
Health Educator and Nurse
San Ramon Valley Unified
  School District
Danville, California

Samuel W. Monismith, D.Ed.
Assistant Professor
Health Education
The Pennsylvania State University
Capital College
Middletown, Pennsylvania

Marcia Newey, P.H.N., M.P.H.
Health Educator
San Ramon Valley Unified
  School District
San Ramon, California

Brenda North
Chair of Health and Physical
  Education
Lanier Middle School
Houston, Texas

Florence R. Oaks, Ph.D.
Psychologist
San Ramon Valley Unified
  School District
Danville, California

Bea Orr
Past President of the
  American Alliance for
  Health, Physical Education,
  Recreation and Dance
Health and Physical Education
  Supervisor
Logan County Schools
Logan, West Virginia

Nancy Piña
Teacher
Braeburn Elementary School
Houston, Texas

Kerry John Redican, Ph.D., M.P.H.
Associate Professor
Health Education
Virginia Polytechnic Institute
  and State University
Blacksburg, Virginia

David Sommerfeld
Instructional Supervisor
Ysleta Independent
  School District
El Paso, Texas

William J. Stone, Ed.D.
Professor
Exercise and Wellness
Arizona State University
Tempe, Arizona

Patrick Tow, Ph.D.
Associate Professor
Department of Health,
  Physical Education,
  and Recreation
Old Dominion University
Norfolk, Virginia

Donna Videto, Ph.D., C.H.E.S.
Adjunct Professor
Health Department
SUNY College at Cortland
Cortland, New York

Molly S. Wantz, M.S., Ed.S.
Associate Professor
Department of Physiology
  and Health Science
Ball State University
Muncie, Indiana

READING/LANGUAGE ADVISOR

Patricia S. Bowers, Ph.D.
Associate Director
Center for Mathematics and
  Science Education
University of North Carolina
  at Chapel Hill
Chapel Hill, North Carolina

Contents

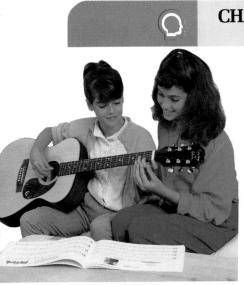

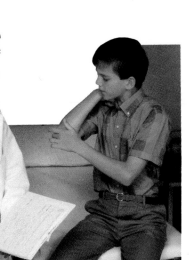

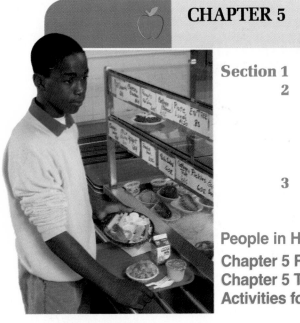

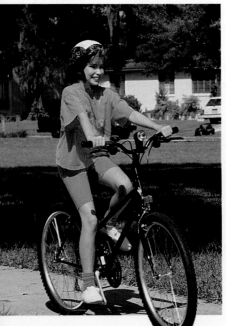

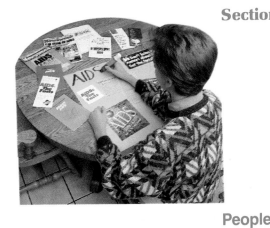
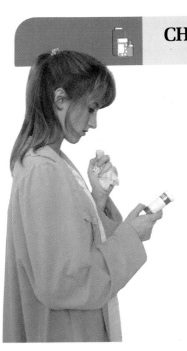

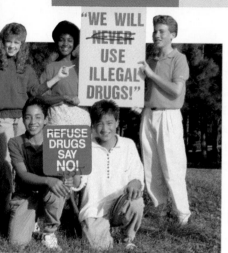

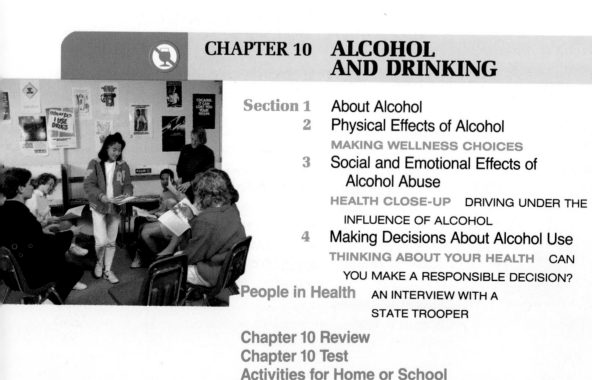

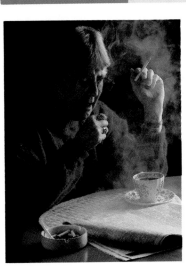
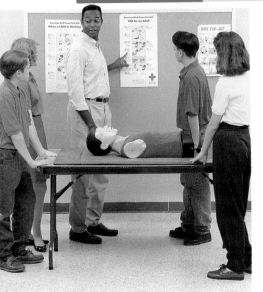

CHAPTER 13 — YOUR HEALTH AND YOUR ENVIRONMENT — 359

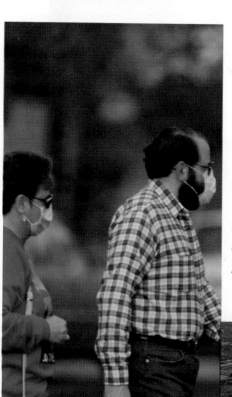

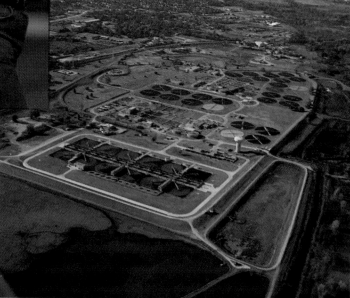

FOR YOUR REFERENCE 395

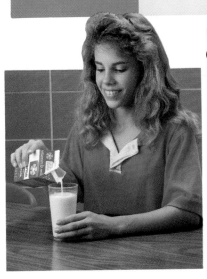

THINKING ABOUT YOUR HEALTH

xiii

REAL-LIFE SKILLS

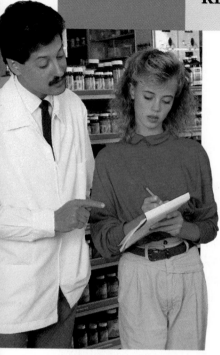

HEALTH CLOSE-UPS

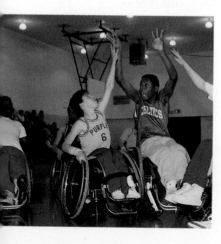

PEOPLE IN HEALTH

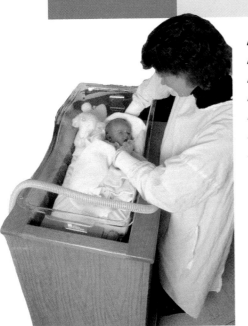

Being Healthy Is About You

You are at your best when you are healthy. When you feel good, you are able to enjoy life to its fullest. However, becoming and staying healthy can be a complex challenge. To handle this challenge, you will need knowledge—not only about health issues, but about yourself and your environment. With the right information and thoughtful preparation, you will find the challenge of being healthy both exciting and rewarding.

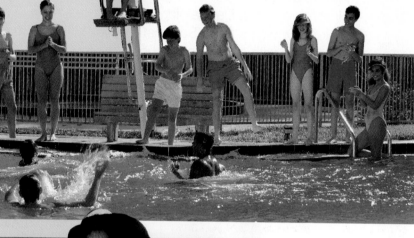

You probably think that good health requires exercise and a healthful diet. You are right; it does. However, these are not the only factors that contribute to good health. To be healthy, you must also satisfy intellectual, emotional, and social needs. In other words, your mind, feelings, family, friends, and community are also important factors in your health. Just about everything you do in the course of your day can affect your health.

As you read *Being Healthy,* you will learn about many health habits that can help keep you feeling your best. You will also learn more about the characteristics that make you a unique individual. Since everyone is different, you have the best insight into your own health. Knowing more about yourself will help you tailor your health needs to fit your personal requirements. By taking responsibility for your health now, you are preparing for a healthy future.

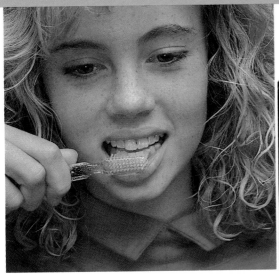

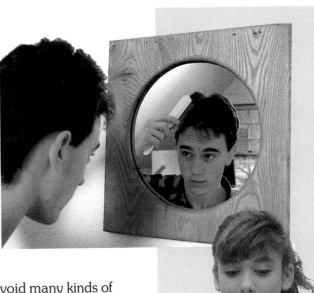

Practicing good health habits can help you avoid many kinds of diseases. Also, the healthier you become, the better you will feel about yourself. You will increase your self-esteem. When you refuse to use dangerous drugs, you will increase your self-esteem even more. By refusing harmful substances, you are saying that you have pride in yourself and value your health. Also, in refusing to be involved in substance abuse, you are protecting not only your own health, but also the health of others in your community.

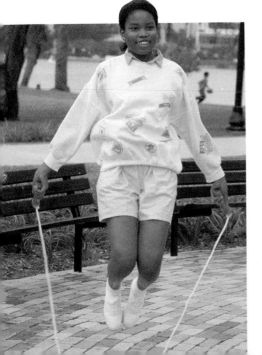

Good health habits are important factors in being healthy. Another important factor is safety. Accidents can and do happen. Fortunately, most of them can be avoided if you are careful and know what causes accidents to happen. Knowing what to do when an accident does occur can help you prevent further injury or even death.

Being healthy does not just happen. You must choose to live in a healthful way. You must take responsibility for your well-being and develop habits that will help keep you healthy. This responsibility will require you to make some important and, sometimes, difficult decisions. By reading *Being Healthy* you will help yourself prepare for these decisions. You will then be ready to make wise choices for being safe and being healthy.

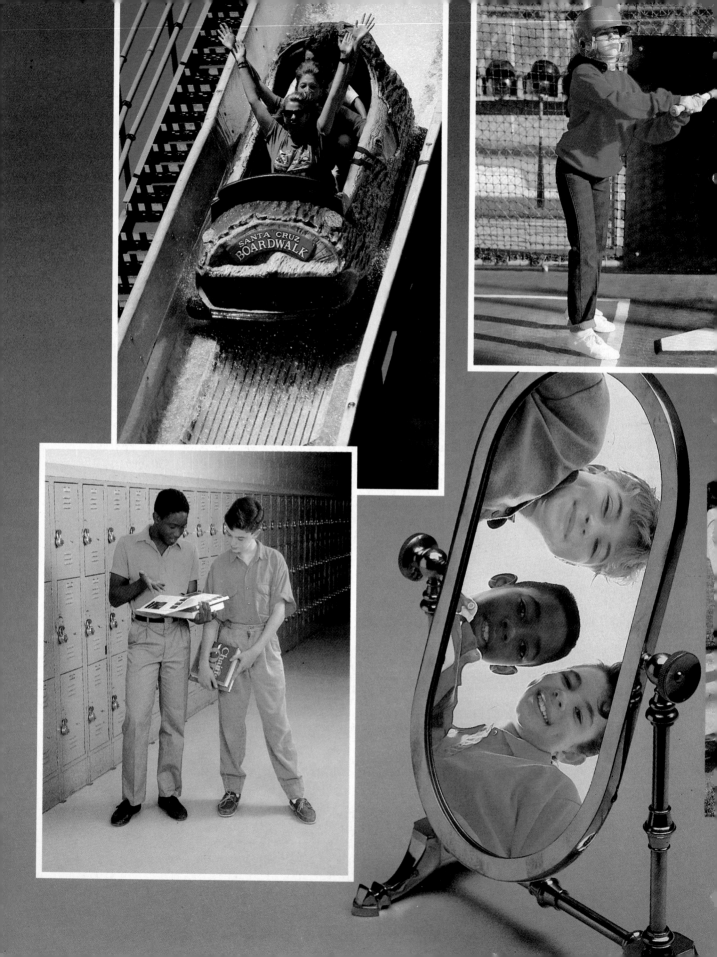

CHAPTER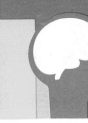

PERSONALITY, EMOTIONS, AND DECISION MAKING

Have you ever wondered why people are so different? You and your classmates are all about the same age. Yet you are all unique individuals. Even people within the same family have personalities that make them different from each other. What causes these differences in personality?

This chapter contains information that will help explain some of these differences in personality. Also described are some of the influences that your family, your friends, and your personality have on your emotions, your behavior, and your decisions.

GETTING READY TO LEARN

Key Questions

- Why is it important to learn about yourself?
- Why is it important to know how you feel about yourself?
- What can you do to feel good about yourself?
- How can you take more responsibility for the way you act and feel?
- How can you learn to make choices that help you solve problems?

Main Chapter Sections

1 Your Personality
2 Understanding and Expressing Your Emotions
3 Making Decisions

1 Your Personality

traits (TRAYTS), ways a person looks, acts, thinks, and feels.

personality (puhrs uhn AL uht ee), the sum of all of a person's traits.

How would you describe yourself? You could describe the way you look—the kind of clothes you wear or the style of your hair. You could also describe the ways you act, think, and feel. If you were to list all the words that tell how you look, act, think, and feel, you would have a list of your **traits.** All of these traits make up your **personality.** A description of your personality would give someone you have never met an idea of who you are and what you are like.

Just as no one looks exactly like you, no one has a personality just like yours. Family members and friends may have some traits that are the same as yours, but you are unique. Your personality is as unique as your fingerprints. Your personality makes you someone special.

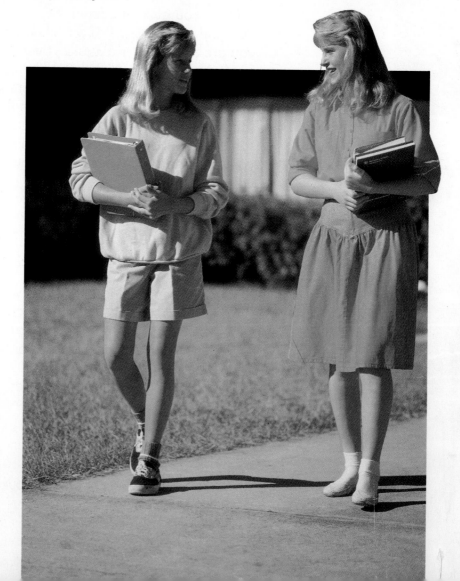

■ Your appearance and the ways in which you act, think, and feel are all traits that help make up your personality.

2

What Shapes Your Personality?

Why do you have some traits and not others? Is it possible for you to develop new traits or get rid of the ones that you do not like? Many people, especially those your age, often ask themselves questions such as these.

physical

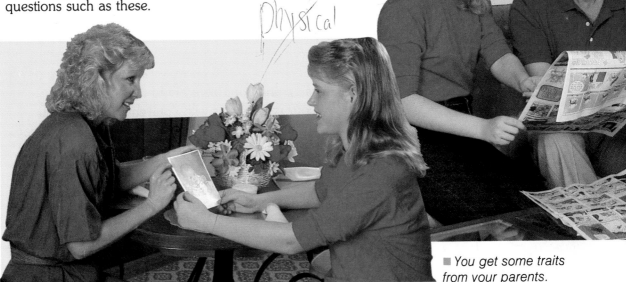

Amina
Rule
Mr.
ni x
(roob

■ *You get some traits from your parents.*

Your Heredity. You received certain traits from your parents. These traits are known as *inherited traits*. Your **heredity** is the sum of all of the traits you received from your parents. You have had these traits since birth, although some may not become obvious until later in your life. The traits easiest to recognize are those that contribute to the way you look. These are your *physical traits*. The color of your hair, your eyes, and your skin are physical traits. So are the features of your face and the general size and shape of your body. You received these traits from your parents. As a result, you probably resemble your parents in one or more ways. If you have brothers and sisters, you probably resemble them as well, because they inherited their traits from the same parents. However, your own combination of physical traits is unique to you.

Besides physical traits, you inherited traits that contribute to the development of your personality. These are *personality traits*. These traits influence the way you act and the way you are likely to think and feel. For example, one of these traits, called your **temperament,** has a lot to do with how you react to people and to situations. People who tend to be easygoing are said to have calm temperaments. People who get upset easily are said to have excitable temperaments.

heredity (huh REHD uht ee), the sum of all the traits a person received from his or her parents.

temperament (TEHM pruh muhnt), a personality trait for the general way a person reacts to people and situations.

3

environment (ihn VY ruhn muhnt), the combination of people, places, and things around a person.

attributes (A truh byoots), qualities of a person.

Your Environment. Your personality was not fully formed the day you were born. It developed and continues to develop as a result of your experiences with your environment. Your **environment** includes your family and friends, your home, your school, and your community. It includes all the people and things in your surroundings.

Different parts of the environment affect your personality in different ways. The food you eat affects your health, and your health, in turn, affects how energetic you feel. The community you live in helps determine who you meet. People influence the interests you develop and your ideas about right and wrong.

As a result of your experiences with your environment, you add **attributes,** or certain qualities, to your personality. You may also change attributes that you already have. These added or changed attributes are called *acquired attributes*. If your friends like soccer, for example, you might develop an interest in soccer, too. If you are a shy person but want to make more friends, you might try to start more conversations. In ways such as these, your environment affects how you look, think, act, and feel.

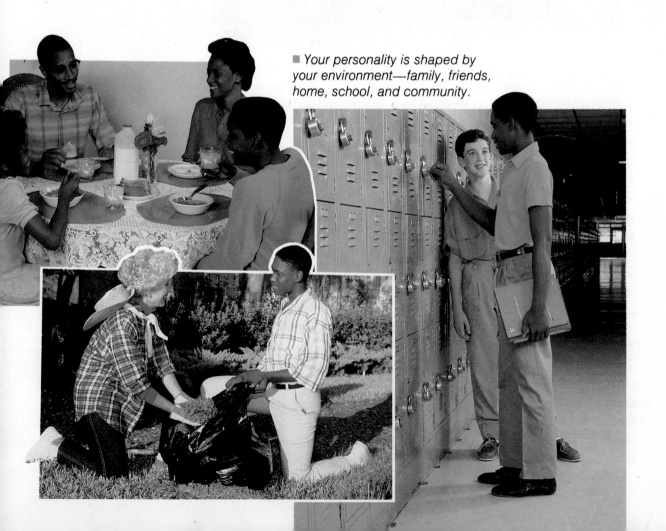

■ *Your personality is shaped by your environment—family, friends, home, school, and community.*

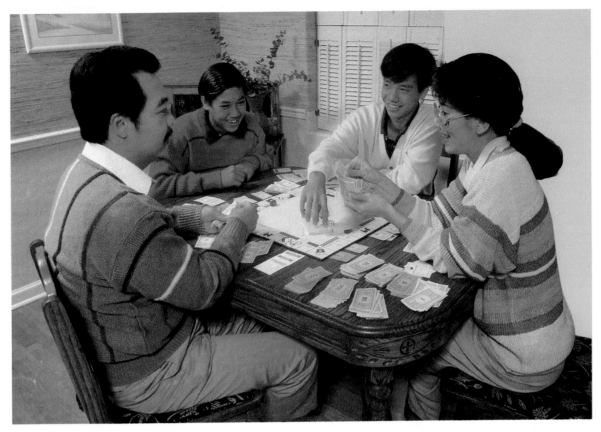

Who Shapes Your Personality?

Over a lifetime, a person may make many changes in his or her attributes. These changes, along with the influences of family and peers, affect the development of personality.

Your Family. Families are influenced by different cultural and religious traditions. Because of these influences, families differ in their structures and beliefs. The cultural background of your family helps shape your developing personality.

The first role models for most young people are their parents or guardians. **Role models** are people whose behavior is copied by others. People learn about honesty, trust, self-respect, and respect for others from their parents or guardians and other family members. The way people behave is often influenced by these role models.

Having a mature personality means behaving in a way that is proper for one's age and stage of development. Being mature also means accepting responsibility appropriate to one's age. Responsibility includes knowing that one's actions always have results, or **consequences,** and expecting to be accountable for those results.

■ *Your parents were your first role models. From them you learned behaviors that influenced your personality.*

role models, people whose behavior is copied by others.

consequences (KAHN suh kwehn suhz), results.

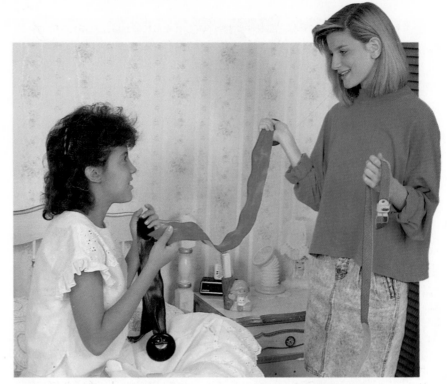

■ *During adolescence, peers become strong influences on one another's personalities.*

Your Peers.   Family influence is strongest on children. This is because children depend most on parents or guardians and other family members. Once young people start going to school, they spend more time with their peers. Peers are people of about the same age and stage of development who share many of the same interests and needs. During a person's school years, peer relationships begin to have a very strong influence on personality. This strong influence is called **peer pressure.**

peer pressure (PIHR · PREHSH uhr), the influence on someone by other people of about the same age.

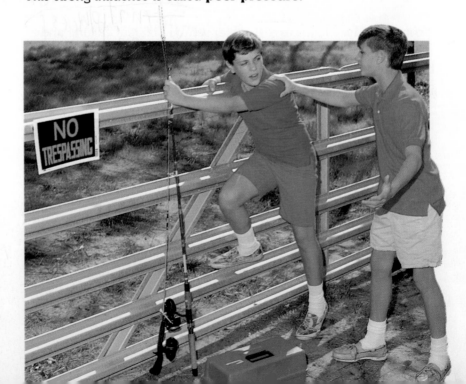

■ *Positive peer pressure may make a person choose not do something he or she knows is wrong.*

When peer pressure helps a person, the influence is known as positive peer pressure. This kind of peer pressure may have an effect in the areas of personal appearance, exercise habits, and schoolwork. Positive peer pressure is often displayed by example. By working hard in school, you may influence some of your peers to work harder. If you follow an exercise plan, you may influence some of your peers to do the same.

There is also negative peer pressure. This kind of peer pressure can influence others to behave in ways that are harmful to a person's health. For example, peers might try to get others to skip school, smoke cigarettes, or use alcohol or other drugs. A mature person usually chooses not to be influenced by negative peer pressure. He or she can confidently say, "No, thanks."

Your Self-Concept. You form a self-concept as a result of the way you feel about yourself and the way you think other people see you. Your **self-concept** is the way you see yourself, with all your strengths and weaknesses. This view you have of yourself influences your personality, as well.

If you have a negative self-concept, you probably see yourself as not able to do well at anything at home or at school. You may be comparing yourself unrealistically to a brother or sister. You may think parents or teachers have unrealistic expectations of you. If you have a positive self-concept, you probably see yourself as capable of learning new skills or forming new friendships.

MYTH AND FACT

Myth: There is someone in the world who looks exactly like you.

Fact: Unless you have an identical twin, it is nearly impossible for you to have a look-alike. The number of possible combinations of inherited physical traits is unlimited.

self-concept (sehlf KAHN sehpt), the way a person sees himself or herself.

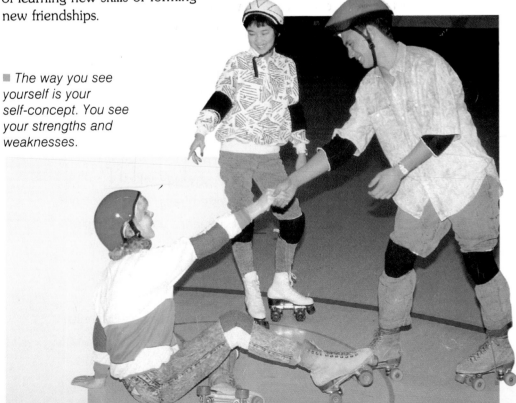

■ The way you see yourself is your self-concept. You see your strengths and weaknesses.

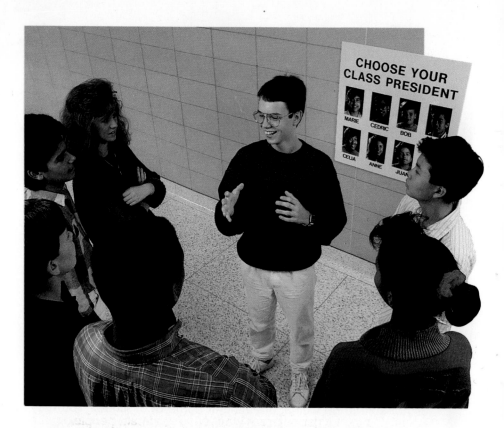

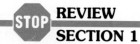

■ *A positive self-concept will help you develop new skills and form new friendships.*

wellness, a high level of health.

A positive self-concept can help you maintain wellness. **Wellness** is a high level of physical, intellectual, social, and emotional health. Wellness includes being comfortable with your personality and liking yourself as a person. By maintaining wellness, you can live your life to the fullest.

STOP **REVIEW**

SECTION 1

REMEMBER?

1. What are three examples of physical traits?
2. What are two kinds of inherited traits?
3. How do family and peers influence your personality?
4. What is wellness?

THINK!

5. How is it possible to change certain personality traits?
6. How can you tell if peer pressure is negative or positive?

8

2 Understanding and Expressing Your Emotions

Like everyone else, you experience many kinds of feelings. At different times, you might feel angry, happy, excited, or sad. Everyone, of course, has these feelings, although everyone does not feel the same way in the same situation. Certain feelings are usually stronger than others. Love, anger, fear, sorrow, and joy are strong feelings, or **emotions.** People do not always express their emotions in the same ways, either. The ways you express your emotions are a part of your personality.

Where Do Your Emotions Come From?

It may seem to you that your emotions are influenced by many events and people in your life. When you make a new friend, you may feel happy. When someone harms you, you may feel angry.

Your emotions come from the events that happen around you and the ways you understand those events. That is why the same situation may trigger different emotions in different people. Making a new friend, for example, might make some people feel worried, not happy.

■ *People, news, or situations can cause your emotions to change.*

emotions (ih MOH shuhnz), strong feelings.

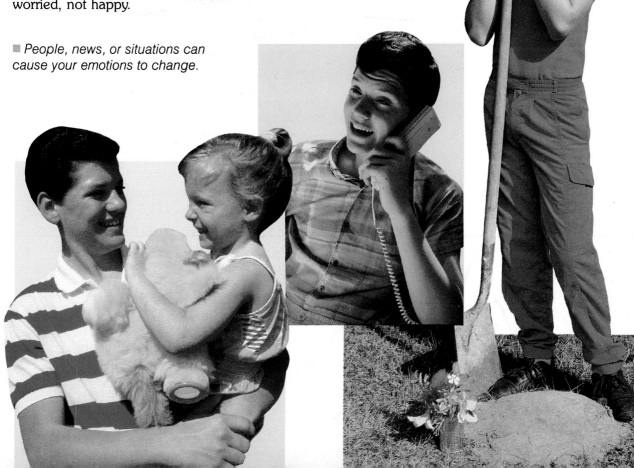

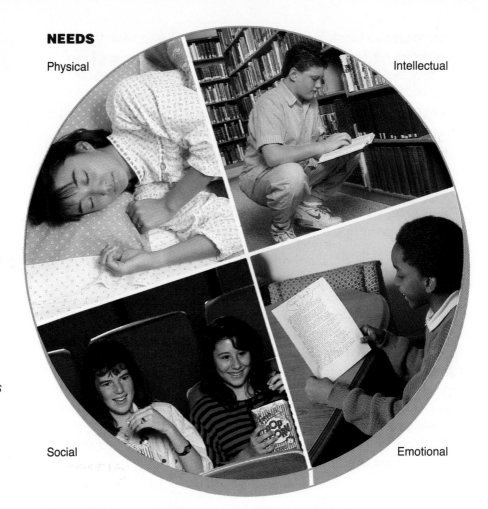

NEEDS

Physical

Intellectual

Social

Emotional

■ *A variety of activities helps you meet your physical, intellectual, emotional, and social needs.*

needs, requirements for wellness.

self-esteem (sehl fuh STEEM), the feeling a person has of being worthwhile.

Your Needs. What is going on in your body at a certain time can also affect your emotions. Many of your feelings and emotions come from your **needs,** or requirements for wellness. Needs related to your body are called *physical needs*. All people have certain physical needs. These include the needs for food and water, rest and sleep, and shelter and warmth. You also have *intellectual needs*. They have to do with your mind. You have *social needs*, which have to do with getting along with other people. You also have needs known as *emotional needs*. For example, you need to feel safe. You need to feel that you are loved and accepted. You need **self-esteem,** or a feeling that you are a worthwhile person. Mastering a new skill helps build self-esteem. Earning the approval and respect of other people helps a person build self-esteem.

Your Needs and Feelings Are Linked Together. You can think about some of your feelings as messages to your brain from your body about your needs. Feeling hungry can be a message that you need food. Feeling tired may be a message

10

that you need sleep. You can probably think of other examples that show how physical needs produce certain feelings.

Your feelings can also be linked to your social and emotional needs. When these needs are not satisfied, you may feel unhappy. For example, not having a friend to talk with can make you feel lonely. When your social and emotional needs are met, you feel good about yourself. You tend to feel confident in your ability to do well.

You probably have no trouble understanding why you have some feelings. Thirst, for example, is clearly a message that you need to drink some liquid. Other feelings can often be puzzling. This may be because there is not always a clear relationship between the feeling and the need you are experiencing. If you skip breakfast, the need for food may make you feel impatient and irritable as well as hungry. You may get into arguments with your friends. You may not be able to concentrate in order to learn new information in school.

Young people often experience times when they have very strong feelings that they are unable to explain. Sometimes these feelings may be expressed in ways that are not healthful. You may say or do things that hurt both yourself and other people.

■ *The need for food is linked to your feelings.*

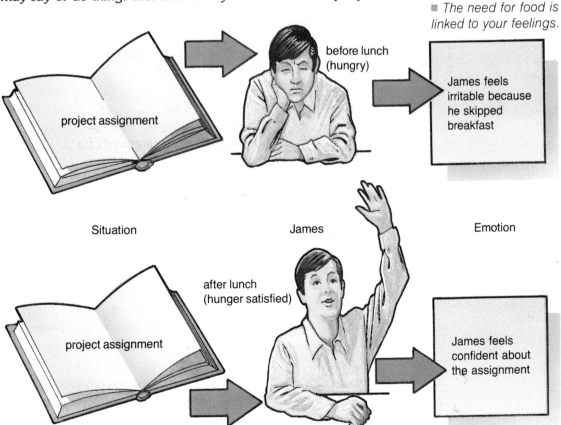

project assignment

before lunch (hungry)

James feels irritable because he skipped breakfast

Situation · James · Emotion

project assignment

after lunch (hunger satisfied)

James feels confident about the assignment

11

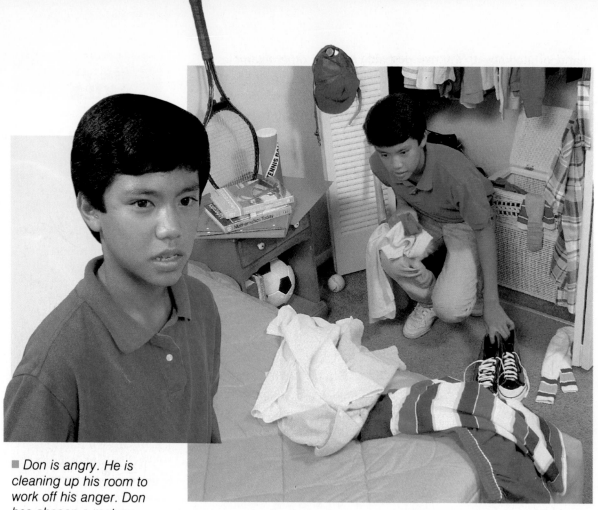

■ *Don is angry. He is cleaning up his room to work off his anger. Don has chosen a mature way of handling his anger.*

Most of these feelings are a normal part of adjusting to the rapid changes taking place in your body. As you become more comfortable with the changes taking place in your body, you can more easily cope with such feelings.

How Do Emotions Affect Your Behavior?

As a small child, you expressed your emotions in childish ways. When you were hungry, you cried until you were fed. You may have expressed your anger by hitting. When you were afraid, you may have yelled. Now that you are older, you still have feelings of hunger, anger, and fear. But you have learned new ways of expressing your feelings. There still may be times when you are so angry that you want to break something. But by now you realize that this behavior may get in the way of meeting your other needs. For example, you know that people who express anger a great deal usually do not feel good about themselves. They may not have high self-esteem. They may also have a hard time making and keeping friends.

12 Go to page 16

Part of growing up involves learning how to express your feelings and emotions in ways that will take care of your needs without hurting or offending others. Instead of hitting someone or saying something cruel when you are angry, you may decide to take a long walk. In this way, you can work through your feelings by physical activity. You might talk about how you feel with friends or family members. Or better yet, you might talk directly with the person who has angered you. Being able to handle your emotions and feelings in healthful ways is a sign of being a responsible person.

■ Feeling good about yourself can help you handle your emotions in mature ways.

How Can You Handle Emotional Problems?

Finding healthful ways of expressing your emotions contributes to your wellness. When you take care of your emotional needs, you feel good about yourself. You are more likely to eat and sleep well. You have the energy you need for the things you want to do. When you are not able to express your feelings and emotions in healthful ways, your wellness may be affected. You may worry. Because of this, you may not sleep well. If you have anger or fear that you are unable to express, you may develop some physical health problems. Headaches, ulcers, rashes, and high blood pressure often result from emotional problems.

13

Talking with Someone Who Makes You Angry

- Think about the situation before you speak.
- Be responsible for your feelings. No one can make you feel any way you do not want to feel.
- Tell the person exactly why you are angry.
- Try to resolve the situation by suggesting an outcome that will be positive for both of you.

Talking Things Over.   Sometimes people do not share their feelings with others. They may be ashamed of the way they feel, or they may think no one will understand them. They may believe they are the only ones who feel the way they do. By keeping their feelings to themselves, they believe the feelings will go away. Often, however, their feelings become stronger and they become more upset.

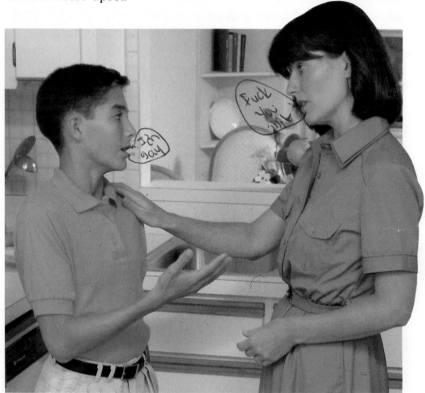

■ *Talking with a parent or a friend can help you express your emotions.*

When your feelings build up until you are troubled about them, it helps to talk things over with another person. Sometimes you may want to share your feelings with a friend. A friend may have had similar feelings and may be able to help you understand your feelings. Talking things over with a friend may help you fill your need for love, acceptance, and self-esteem.

You might want to discuss your feelings with a parent or other trusted adult. Many older people have had the same feelings as yours, and they may want to share their experiences with you. Talking often with a parent or guardian about a variety of topics can help you both have a good relationship. You will both be able to discuss feelings and problems whenever they occur. There are also people such as school counselors and religious leaders to whom you might go when problems arise. These people can suggest still others in your community who know how to help with serious problems.

Managing Stress. The response of your body to physical or emotional demands or pressures is called **stress.** Some stress, such as preparing for your first camping trip or another realistic goal, is *positive stress.* Positive stress can help make life enjoyable and challenging. Other stress can interfere with your happiness and performance. Family troubles, unrealistic goals, noise, illness, and many other factors can cause *negative stress.* Negative stress can make you feel tense, pressured, unhappy, and out of control. You may even become ill if negative stress becomes too great and lasts too long. Negative stress is not healthful.

Stress is a fact of life in today's world. The key to living with stress is learning what might cause negative stress for you and how to handle it in healthful ways. First, you must learn to recognize the signs that you are feeling negative stress. Some common signs are confusion, lack of concentration, and nervousness. Second, you must learn how to reduce negative stress by determining ways within your control to avoid situations that cause it. Third, you can try to change how you feel about situations you cannot avoid. Fourth, you can find healthful and pleasant ways to release the feelings that negative stress creates.

stress (STREHS), the response of the body to physical or emotional pressure.

■ *Getting involved in activities can help people manage stress.*

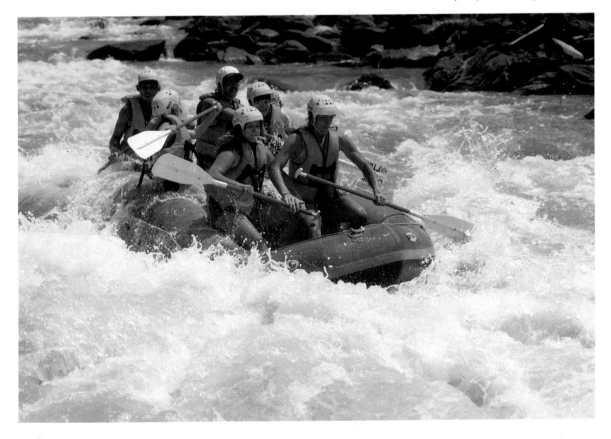

Taking a brisk walk or reading an interesting book is a healthful way to relieve negative stress. Taking part in activities you enjoy can also be healthful for reducing negative stress, especially if you cannot change what is causing it.

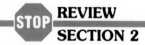

REVIEW SECTION 2

REMEMBER?

1. Where do emotions come from?
2. How do emotions affect your behavior?
3. How do emotions affect your health?
4. What is negative stress?

THINK!

5. How might a negative feeling toward a teacher keep you from being successful in class?
6. Explain how talking over a problem with a trusted adult or friend can help you better understand your feelings about that problem.

Thinking About Your Health

How Can You Be a More Effective Communicator?

Read the statements and answer the questions to explore how effective communicating can help you have better relationships with both your family and your peers.

- People often respond to others in ways that prevent further communication. They may make negative remarks or jokes at someone else's expense. How might these kinds of remarks cause communication problems between people? In what ways can people feel hurt by these kinds of comments?

- Negative communication does not meet people's needs to be liked and to feel good about themselves. Why, do you think, do people who use negative communication often find themselves with fewer friends than they would like to have?

- In what other ways do some people close the lines of communication?

Health Close-up

Preventing Youth Suicide

Depression is a condition in which a person is very sad. The sadness continues for much longer than it should. In some cases, a person who is depressed may think that a situation is hopeless. Feeling this way for a long time may cause a person to think of himself or herself as worthless. At some point, the person may think about attempting suicide. *Suicide* is taking one's own life. It is the second leading cause of death among young people ages 15 to 24. (Accidents are the leading cause.)

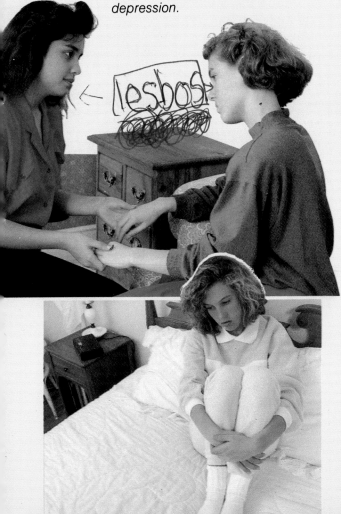

■ *Talking with a good friend may help you overcome feelings of depression.*

There are some early warning signs that might mean someone is likely to attempt suicide. They are

- sudden change in sleeping or eating patterns or in weight.
- withdrawal from family and friends.
- restlessness or lack of concentration.
- giving or throwing away of favorite possessions.
- sudden changes in mood or behavior.
- loss of interest in favorite activities or hobbies.
- feelings of loneliness, rejection, and hopelessness.
- abuse of drugs, including alcohol.

A suicide attempt or talking about suicide is a cry for help. You can call (800) 621-4000 to get help for someone who is thinking about suicide. You can also do the following:

- Take all suicide comments seriously. Let the person know that he or she needs to talk to someone about his or her feelings.
- Listen. Do not lecture or criticize.
- Encourage and support the person without judging.
- Get help. Do not try to solve the person's problem by yourself.

Thinking Beyond

1. What, do you think, makes some young people attempt suicide?
2. Why is it important to get professional help for a person who is thinking about suicide?
3. Why, do you think, are young people often angry and hurt when someone they know attempts suicide?

17

3   Making Decisions

decisions (dih SIHZH uhnz), choices made after considering various possibilities.

Decisions are choices you make after considering different possibilities. Throughout your life, your personality affects your decisions. The influence of your family and peers on your personality also has an effect. You will probably display self-confidence in making decisions if you are mature and have a positive self-concept. Mature people also take responsibility for the outcomes that result from their decisions.

What Are the Reasons for Choices?

Making a decision means choosing one thing over another. When you choose to watch a particular television show,

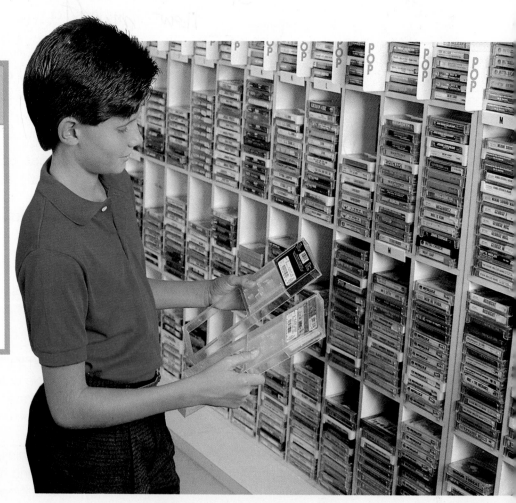

■ *You make a decision every time you choose one thing over another.*

you are also choosing not to watch other shows. You make many decisions every day. There may be a number of reasons for the choices you make.

Some choices are made because you like one thing better than another. Maybe some of your friends are going to play ball after school and other friends are going to see a movie. You like watching movies better than playing ball, so you choose to see the movie.

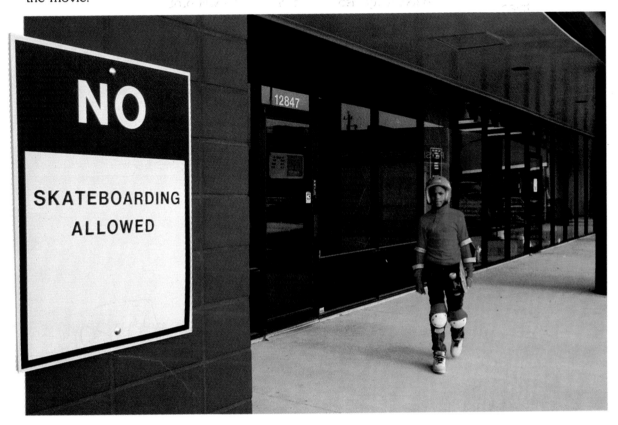

■ *Many of the decisions people make are influenced by rules or laws.*

Other choices are made because one thing is more important to you than another. Perhaps you have time after school to either practice a musical instrument or play video games. It may be more important to practice your instrument today because you have a lesson tomorrow.

The choices you make may depend on rules. Suppose your friends want to ride their skateboards in the shopping center parking lot. However, there is a rule against this. You know that you might get into trouble if you break this rule. You know that you might run into someone or get hurt by a car. You consider both the rule and safety when making your decision. You decide not to join your friends, because you would be breaking a rule and someone could get hurt.

How Can You Solve Problems?

When you first wake up in the morning, you decide what clothes to wear and what to eat for breakfast. Making most decisions is relatively easy. Solving problems, however, means making more important decisions.

Suppose that you are about to leave for school on your bicycle. You discover that your bicycle has a flat tire. Now you have a problem. The first step in solving a problem is knowing one exists.

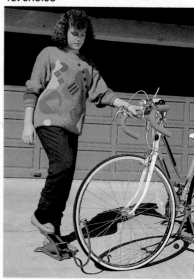

1st choice

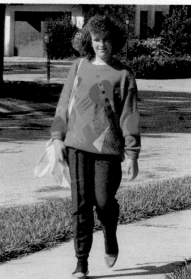

2nd choice

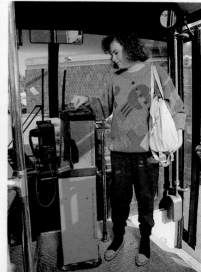

3rd choice

■ *Solving a problem may involve making a series of important decisions.*

Problem

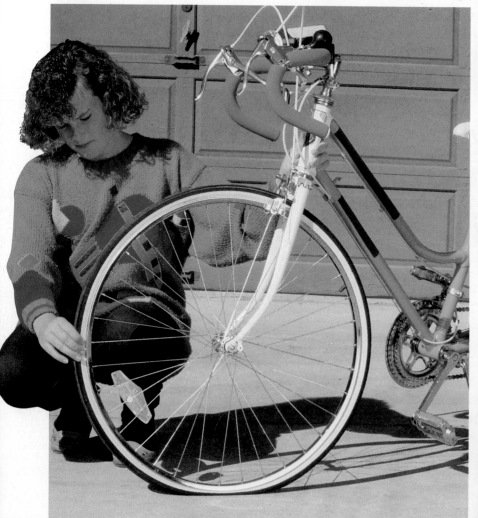

Getting to school involves realizing you have a problem, thinking of solutions to the problem, identifying possible results of each solution, and choosing a solution.

After realizing what the problem is, you must think of possible solutions. Possible solutions for getting to school include fixing the tire, walking to school, using part of your allowance for bus fare, and staying home.

Next, you must consider the results of each possible solution. If you fix the tire or walk to school, you may be late. Being late means that you will have to stay after school to make up the time. Staying home means that you will miss an important science test. Paying for bus fare means that you will have less money for yourself.

Finally, you must choose one solution. You may decide to spend your money for the bus fare because you do not like the consequences of the other solutions. Although you will have less money, you will get to school on time and will not miss the science test. Choosing a positive solution to a complex problem is difficult, but it is necessary and it lets you end the problem. Many people feel better after they have made a choice.

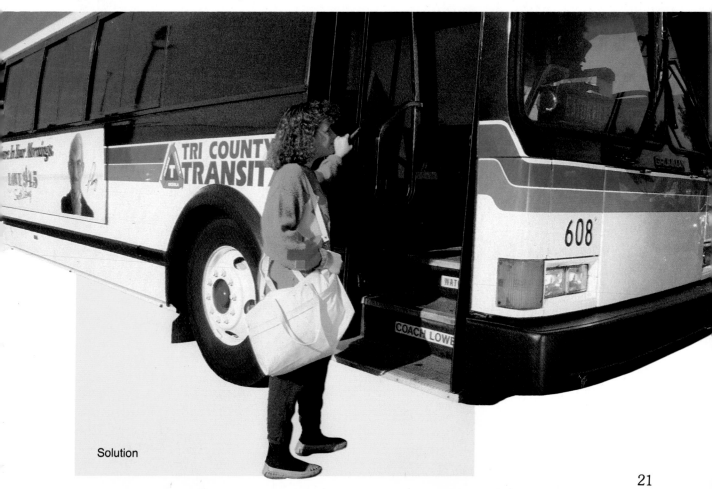

Solution

21

What Is a Responsible Decision?

There are four signs of responsible decision making. First, your decision should not conflict with your knowledge or feelings. Second, your decision should be made only after you think of all the things you could do about the problem. These are called **alternatives.** Third, you should consider what could happen because of each choice. Finally, your decision should be based on your best judgment.

Suppose you know that drinking alcohol is wrong because of family rules and because it can harm your health. You also know it is against the law for someone your age to drink. One day your friend offers you a beer. You say no, but your friend tells you that everyone is doing it and that you will be more "grown-up" if you drink. What should you do?

alternatives (awl TUR nuht ihvz), all the things a person could do about solving a problem.

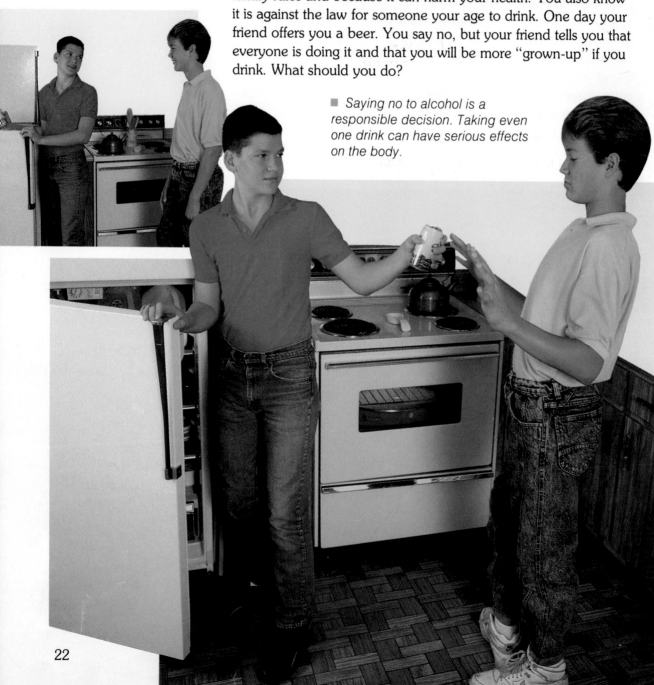

■ Saying no to alcohol is a responsible decision. Taking even one drink can have serious effects on the body.

22

If you are a responsible decision maker, you will refuse. Drinking the beer would conflict with your knowledge. If you are not confident about your knowledge, you could consider the results of choosing to drink. You might lose control of yourself, and your parents might find out. You may decide not to drink because the consequences are not what you want.

It is often hard to live with the consequences of an irresponsible decision. However, many people make irresponsible decisions. The responsible decision maker thinks before acting and evaluates each decision after it is made.

STOP · REVIEW SECTION 3

REMEMBER?

1. What are two reasons for making a choice?
2. What are the steps of problem solving?
3. What are the signs of responsible decision making?

THINK!

4. Explain how personality influences decision making.
5. Describe a situation that shows that responsible decision making does not conflict with feelings.

Making Wellness Choices

Tim has had a busy day—like most of his days recently. He can hardly keep up with all the clubs and school groups he has joined. Knowing that he is short of time, Tim has begged his brother Evan to do Tim's chore of raking the leaves in the yard. In return, Tim promised that later he would do Evan's chore of washing the dishes. Now Tim is late for his Scout meeting, and Evan has not yet raked the leaves. The boys' parents will be angry when they notice the leaves in the yard. Tim's first thought is to find Evan and shout at him for not raking the leaves.

? What would be better for Tim to do in this situation? Explain your wellness choice.

23

People in Health

An Interview with a School Guidance Counselor

Irene Flores helps students solve problems and plan for success. She is a school guidance counselor at a high school in San Antonio, Texas.

What does a school guidance counselor do?

Counselors are in the schools to help students. They help many students solve problems. They also help students make decisions about their futures. To help students solve problems or make career decisions, school guidance counselors work with school administrators, teachers, parents, and the community.

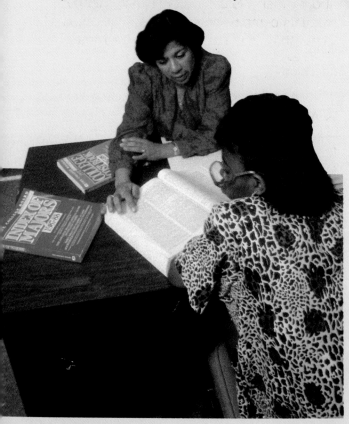

What are some of the problems that students have?

Different students will have different problems. One might worry about getting good grades. Another might worry about staying in school at all. Some students have family troubles that make them unhappy. Others are lonely. Those students may not know other adults they feel they can trust.

How do you help students who come to you with problems?

I listen. The students do most of the talking. I try to give them the confidence they need to solve many of their own problems. If students are having trouble with getting passing grades, I might tell them about the importance of learning study skills and forming good study habits. If students are having personal problems, I try to help them work on a positive self-concept. A positive self-concept, after all, can help people handle almost any problem they might face.

What do you do if a student does not want to talk to you?

Sometimes I can tell that a student would feel more comfortable discussing a problem with someone his or her age. When this happens, I refer him or her to our high school's student counseling program. We have 23 students who are trained to help their peers. A student counselor and the student looking for help talk in a private office near my own. That way, if a student needs more help than the student counselor can give, an adult counselor is nearby.

■ *Ms. Flores helps students plan their futures.*

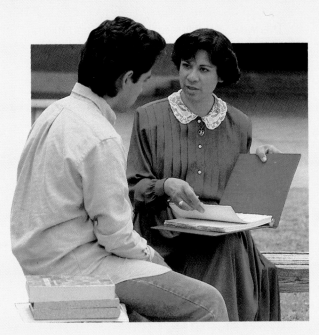

■ *Many students need help in solving their problems.*

What are some of the worst problems you have heard students talk about?

There are many serious problems. Some students talk about running away from home or dropping out of school.

Do you spend all your time talking with students who have problems?

A big part of my job every day is helping students plan their future. I often meet with students and parents to talk about career plans. I help students choose classes they need for jobs or college. I also advise students about ways to match careers with their personalities. I also give career information. Sometimes I organize career days at school, where students can learn about different kinds of work. For example, I recently distributed information about programs and schools that teach skills for specific jobs.

What training does a person need to become a school guidance counselor?

In most states, school guidance counselors need to have four years of college plus one or two years of training in counseling. Many states require that school guidance counselors have teaching experience. In addition to a college education, counselors must have an interest in helping others. Good counselors need patience and understanding with people who go to them for help.

What do you like best about being a school guidance counselor?

I like helping students make decisions about their future. Sometimes former students come back to visit me. I feel good when they tell me that I helped them succeed.

What general advice do you like to give to students?

The most important thing students should know is that help is available to them for all kinds of problems. Students can always discuss a problem with a school counselor if they need advice.

> *Learn more about people who work as school guidance counselors. Interview a counselor. Or write for information to the American School Counselor Association, 5999 Stevenson Avenue, Alexandria, VA 22304.*

25

Main Ideas

- Attributes are added to your personality as a result of your experiences with your environment.

- Your self-concept forms as a result of family and peer influences.

- Your emotions and the ways you express them make up part of your personality.

- When you take care of your emotional needs, you feel good about yourself.

- Positive stress may be good for your wellness, and unmanaged negative stress may be bad for it.

- Your personality can affect the decisions you make.

Key Words

Write the numbers 1 to 17 in your health notebook or on a separate sheet of paper. After each number, copy the sentence and fill in the missing term. Page numbers in ( ) tell you where to look in the chapter if you need help.

traits (2)	self-concept (7)
personality (2)	wellness (8)
heredity (3)	emotions (9)
temperament (3)	needs (10)
environment (4)	self-esteem (10)
attributes (4)	stress (15)
role models (5)	decisions (18)
consequences (5)	alternatives (22)
peer pressure (6)	

1. The ways that you look, act, think, and feel are your ___?___ .

2. Your ___?___ is the sum of all your traits.

3. The way you generally react to situations is determined by your ___?___ .

4. ___?___ are strong feelings.

5. A high level of health is called ___?___ .

6. Requirements for wellness are ___?___ .

7. The feeling that you are a worthwhile person is called ___?___ .

8. Traits that you develop as a result of experiences with your environment are called ___?___ .

9. Your ___?___ is the sum of the traits you received from your parents.

10. People whose behavior is copied are called ___?___ .

11. The way that you see yourself is your ___?___ .

12. The response of the body to physical or emotional pressure is ___?___ .

13. Another word for choices is ___?___ .

14. The people, places, and things around you are part of your ___?___ .

15. The strong influence a friend may have on you is called ___?___ .

16. Responsibility includes knowing that your actions have ___?___ , or results.

17. Your ___?___ are the different possible solutions to a problem.

Remembering What You Learned

Page numbers in ( ) tell you where to look in the chapter if you need help.

1. What traits might someone inherit from his or her parents? (3)

2. Why might you have some of the same physical traits as your grandparents? (3)

3. If a person is involved in many arguments and fights, what kind of temperament does he or she have? (3)

4. How might a person's environment affect the development of his or her personality? (4)

5. What physical needs are common to everyone? (10)

6. Why is self-esteem important? (10)

7. The need to have friends is an example of what kind of need? (10)

8. Why do people have similar feelings and emotions? (11)

9. What physical needs could make you feel irritable at school? (11)

10. How can you work through feelings of anger in a useful way? (13–14)

11. What health problems might occur if a person does not express anger or fear? (13)

12. What emotional needs can your family help you satisfy? (14)

13. What should you do if your feelings build up to a point where they begin troubling you? (14)

14. Describe some examples of positive stress and negative stress. (15)

15. Why is positive stress good for your wellness? (15)

16. Why do people choose some things instead of others? (19)

17. What is the process of making responsible decisions? (20–21)

Thinking About What You Learned

1. Why is it unlikely that there could be two people, except for identical twins, who have the same combination of physical traits?

2. How are physical and emotional needs related to each other?

3. Explain how influences from family and peers may lead to negative stress.

4. Describe what your day might be like if you were not allowed to make any choices for yourself.

Writing About What You Learned

1. Describe another member of your family. Try to include some physical and personality traits that you and your relative have in common.

2. Write a brief report about a famous person. Tell how you think environment and heredity interacted to influence the person's personality and behavior.

3. Describe a situation in which you were forced to make difficult choices in order to solve a problem.

Applying What You Learned

LANGUAGE ARTS

Look at a recent picture of yourself. How would you describe your physical traits to someone who has never seen you? Write a paragraph about yourself that will paint a word picture of you for someone else to "see."

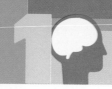

Modified True or False

Write the numbers 1 to 15 in your health notebook or on a separate sheet of paper. After each number, write *true* or *false* to describe the sentence. If the sentence is false, also write a term that replaces the underlined term and makes the sentence true.

1. Someone you admire is a <u>role model</u>.

2. <u>Peer pressure</u> is the response of the body to physical or emotional pressure.

3. Your <u>temperament</u> is the combination of people, places, and things around you.

4. <u>Self-concept</u> is the way you see yourself.

5. If your bicycle has been damaged, one of your <u>alternatives</u> is to buy a new one.

6. Your <u>personality</u> is unique.

7. <u>Personality traits</u> are the easiest to recognize.

8. Wanting to get along with people is an <u>emotional</u> need.

9. Mastering new skills will help you build <u>self-esteem</u>.

10. Having too much work to do is an example of <u>positive</u> stress.

11. The influence of your family on your personality may affect your <u>decisions</u>.

12. Your decisions should not conflict with your knowledge or <u>feelings</u>.

13. Your <u>emotion</u> is the sum of all the traits you received from your parents.

14. People who get angry easily have excitable <u>temperaments</u>.

15. Getting a ticket is one <u>alternative</u> of speeding.

Short Answer

Write the numbers 16 to 23 on your paper. Write a complete sentence to answer each question.

16. How is positive peer pressure usually demonstrated?

17. Describe how to make a mature decision.

18. How can positive stress help you reach goals?

19. How can your environment affect your personality?

20. Why are role models important?

21. Why is it important to think about the consequences of actions before making a decision?

22. How does your self-esteem affect your self-concept?

23. How does your self-concept affect your wellness?

Essay

Write the numbers 24 and 25 on your paper. Write paragraphs with complete sentences to answer each question.

24. Describe the personality difficulties you think a person might have if he or she grew up alone on a desert island.

25. Describe what decision-making steps you would take in the following situation: You tried out for a position on the softball team and a part in the school play. You got both. Now you find out that practice and rehearsal will be on the same day at the same time.

Projects to Do

1. Using photographs, drawings, and magazine and newspaper clippings, create a scrapbook of your personal environment. Show the parts of your environment that have most strongly influenced how you look, think, act, and feel.

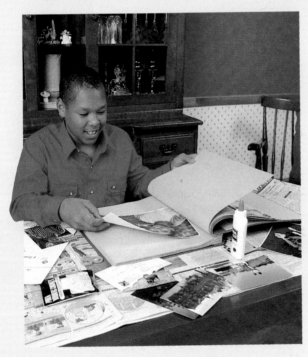

■ *You can describe your environment.*

2. Think of an experience that can bring about strong feelings—for example, speaking before a large group or visiting an unfamiliar place for the first time. Discuss with your classmates the types of feelings you might experience in each situation. On a sheet of paper, list descriptive words such as *excited,* *terrified,* or *proud* to describe the way you might feel in each situation. Then compare your lists with those of your classmates. Does everyone feel the same way about the same experiences? Why or why not?

Information to Find

1. Scientists have found that when physical needs for food and sleep go unsatisfied for long periods, an individual's personality can change in important ways. Prepare a written or oral report about the effects of lack of food or sleep on personality. Also include how these factors can affect a person's wellness. Your school or public library should have books with the information you need. Remember, your personality includes all the ways you look, think, act, and feel.

2. Some young people have family problems. Where can a young person with family problems go for help in your community? Your school counselor can help you locate the resources and get details.

Books to Read

Here are some books you can look for in your school library or the public library to find more information about personality and emotions.

Cohen, Daniel, and Susan Cohen. *Teenage Stress.* Evans and Company.

Laiken, Deidre S., and Alan J. Schneider. *Listen to Me, I'm Angry.* Lothrop, Lee & Shepard.

Shaw, Diana. *Make the Most of a Good Thing: You.* Atlantic Monthly Press.

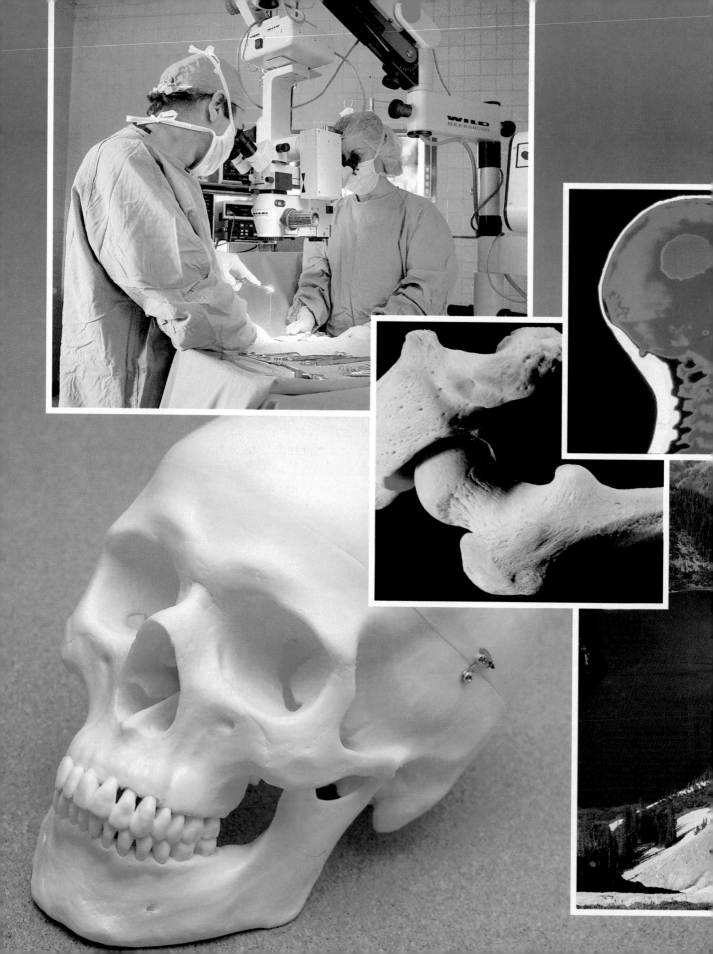

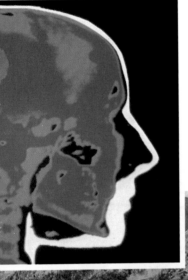

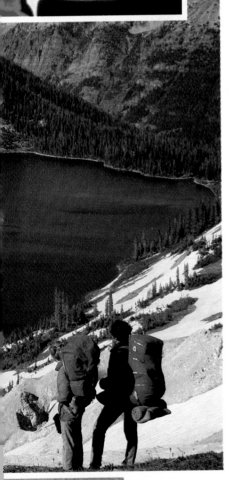

CHAPTER 2

ABOUT YOUR BODY

Your body is made up of millions of parts. Each part of your body is important to the work of every other part. When you are in good health, all the parts of your body work together in harmony. This harmony can be achieved and maintained by developing good health habits. As you get older, you are expected to take more responsibility for your own health habits. You will need to know how these habits can affect your body systems.

GETTING READY TO LEARN

Key Questions

- Why is it important for you to learn how your body works?
- Why is it important for you to know how you feel about your body?
- What can you do to feel good about your body?
- What can you do to become more responsible for maintaining the wellness of your body?

Main Chapter Sections

1 How Your Body Is Organized
2 Your Skeletal and Muscular Systems
3 Your Nervous System
4 Your Endocrine and Reproductive Systems
5 Your Circulatory and Lymphatic Systems
6 Your Respiratory System
7 Your Digestive System
8 Your Excretory System

1 How Your Body Is Organized

KEY WORDS

epithelial tissue
connective tissue
muscle tissue
nerve tissue
organ
body systems

A body can learn to do many different tasks. It can do the fine work of making a watch or the heavy work of building a dam. During your busy day, you do not even think about all the things that your body is able to do.

For you to live, grow, and stay healthy, all the parts of your body must work together. The way your body is organized allows each body part to carry out its own special function. These functions affect other parts in a body system.

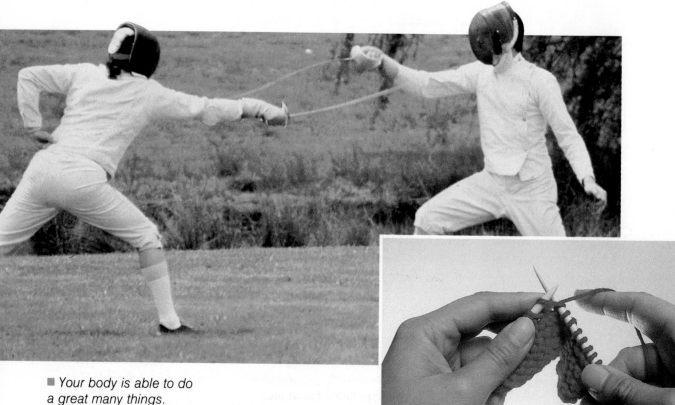

■ *Your body is able to do a great many things. Different parts of your body must work together to enable you to do these things.*

What Are Cells?

The smallest living parts of your body are cells. Your body is made up of many different kinds of cells. You know that when a fuel, such as coal, is burned, energy is released. Although your cells do not really burn food, food provides fuel for your body. To give your body energy, the food you eat must be broken down into nutrients. This fuel is then "burned" by your cells. In order to burn the fuel provided by food, cells need oxygen,

32

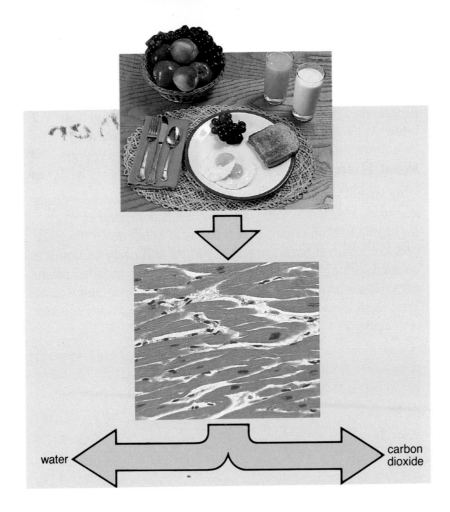

water ← → carbon dioxide

■ *Your cells use nutrients from the foods you eat to make energy for your body. This process also produces wastes, water, and carbon dioxide.*

a gas found in air. The process by which cells use nutrients and oxygen to release energy is called *oxidation*. Along with energy for your body, oxidation makes two waste products—water and carbon dioxide.

What Is Tissue?

Groups of similar cells that perform a certain function form a tissue. Your body has four major kinds of tissues. The skin that covers your body is **epithelial tissue.** Epithelial tissue also covers many of your internal body parts, such as your heart and your stomach.

The framework of your body is held together by **connective tissue.** Connective tissue holds bones and muscles together. Blood is also a kind of connective tissue.

Muscle tissue is made up of groups of muscle cells. These cells have qualities that help you move. Muscle tissue in your legs allows you to walk. Muscle tissue in your heart pumps blood to all parts of your body. Muscle tissue in your stomach helps break down food.

epithelial tissue (ehp uh THEE lee uhl • TIHSH oo), tissue that covers the outside of a structure.

connective tissue (kuh NEHK tihv • TIHSH oo), tissue that unites and supports various parts of the body.

muscle tissue (MUHS uhl • TIHSH oo), tissue that contracts to move parts of the body.

33

nerve tissue (NURV • TIHSH oo), tissue that carries information to and from parts of the body.

Groups of nerve cells working together make up **nerve tissue.** Nerve tissue receives information from around you. Nerve tissue also sends messages all through your body. By receiving and processing all this information, you see, taste, feel, and hear. Your brain, which is made of nerve tissue, allows you to think.

What Is an Organ?

organ (AWR guhn), a body part made up of tissues that work together to carry out a body function.

An **organ** is made up of two or more different kinds of tissues that work together to carry out a body function. Your stomach, for example, is an organ. Its function is to break down the food you eat. Your stomach is made of muscle and nerve tissues. It is covered with epithelial tissue. These tissues work together as an organ. Your heart is another organ. Its function is to pump blood. Your heart is also made up of muscle and nerve tissues covered with epithelial tissue.

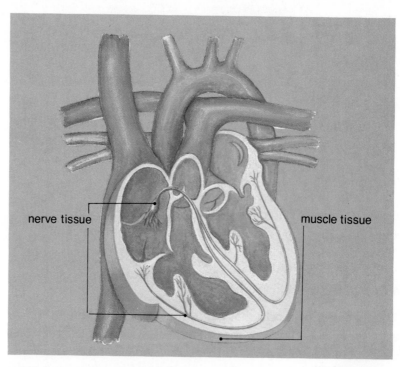

nerve tissue   muscle tissue

■ The heart is mostly muscle tissue, covered with epithelial tissue. Nerve tissue is also present in the heart.

What Are Body Systems?

body systems, groups of organs that work together.

Cells form tissues. Different kinds of tissues form organs. Groups of organs work together in **body systems.** Your digestive system, for example, has many organs, such as your mouth, your stomach, and your intestines. These organs work together to digest, or break down, the food you eat.

Your body is made up of many systems. Each system carries out one or more functions. Your skeletal and muscular systems let you move and protect your vital organs. Your nervous system

34

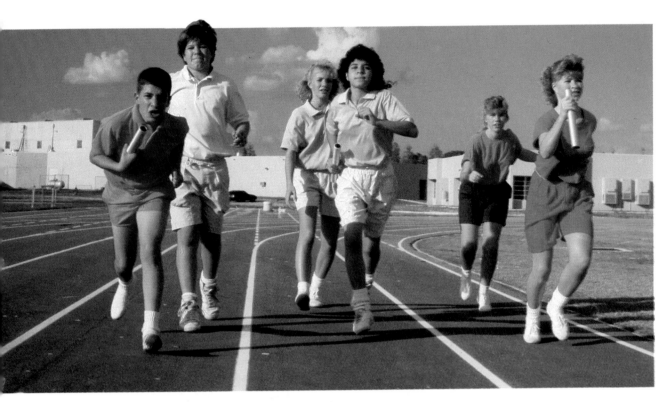

sends messages and receives information. Your circulatory system carries oxygen and nutrients to every cell in your body. All the systems of your body work together so that you can live, grow, and stay healthy.

■ *Running requires the coordination of several body systems.*

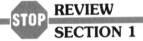 **REVIEW**
SECTION 1

REMEMBER?

1. What is the name of the process by which cells use oxygen to form energy?
2. What are four kinds of body tissues?
3. What is the name for a group of organs that work together to carry out a certain function?

THINK!

4. Explain why the stomach is considered an organ.
5. How might the breakdown of one organ affect the functioning of an entire system?

2 Your Skeletal and Muscular Systems

Of all your body's parts, you may be most aware of your bones and muscles. You may have broken a bone at one time. A physician probably put a cast around the broken bone to hold it in place until it healed. You may have exercised to develop stronger muscles. Bones and muscles support your body and let you move about. They also give your body its size and its shape. However, bones and muscles have other important functions.

What Are the Functions of Your Skeletal System?

You have 206 bones in your body. Together with other connective tissues, they form the frame that supports your body. This frame is your skeletal system. Some bones have additional functions. For example, your ribs protect your lungs and your heart. The bones of your skull protect your brain. Tiny bones in each of your ears help you hear. They vibrate when sound waves reach them. Your brain translates these vibrations into sounds.

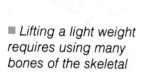

■ Lifting a light weight requires using many bones of the skeletal system.

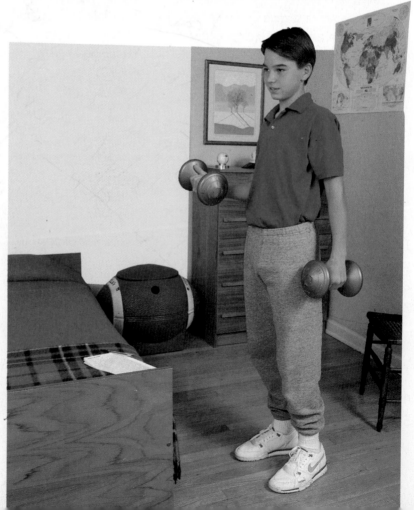

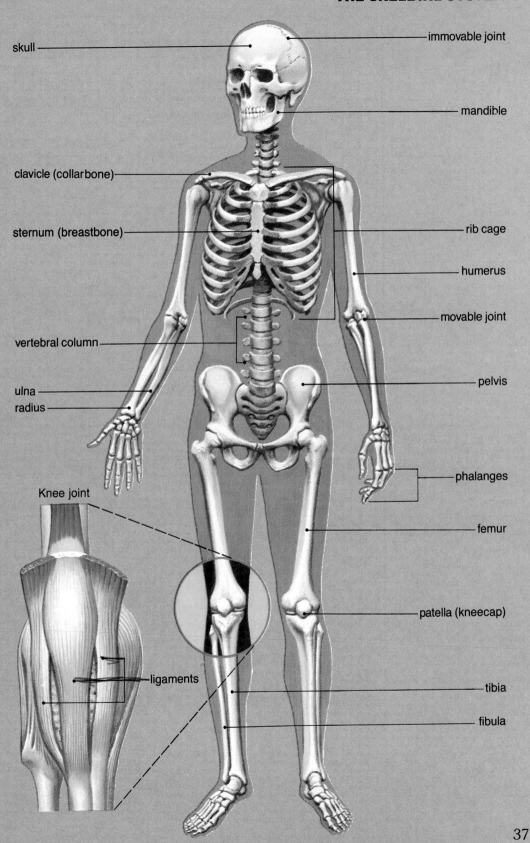

skull

immovable joint

mandible

clavicle (collarbone)

sternum (breastbone)

rib cage

humerus

movable joint

vertebral column

pelvis

ulna

radius

phalanges

Knee joint

femur

patella (kneecap)

ligaments

tibia

fibula

go to page 12

The bones in your body vary greatly in size and shape. The bone in each upper leg, for example, is long and thick. It is heavy and rigid in order to support the weight of your upper body. The bones in your hands are short and slender. They are light in weight and jointed to allow you to make fine movements with your fingers.

■ *Growth of a long bone occurs near each end of the bone, in the growth plates. Here cells divide, forming cartilage. The cartilage slowly hardens into bone.*

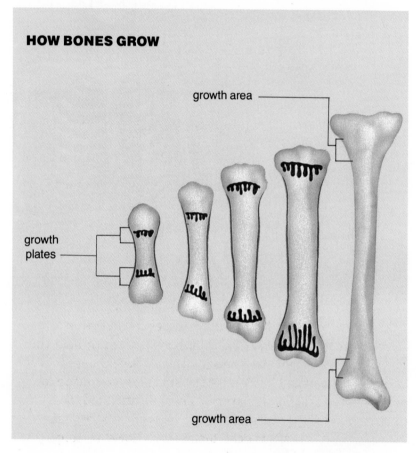

HOW BONES GROW

growth area

growth plates

growth area

As you grow, your bones grow in size. The *growth plate* in a bone is a layer of cells that divide to allow new bone tissue to form. Bone growth stops when these growth plates harden into bone. This will happen when you are in your late teens. Throughout your teenage years, you need a lot of minerals for proper bone growth. Milk and other foods with minerals are excellent for helping your bones to grow.

Your bones connect with each other at **joints.** Joints that allow bone movement are called *movable joints.* Your body has several kinds of these. For example, knees, hips, and wrists are different kinds of movable joints. *Immovable joints* do not allow the bones to move. The bones in your skull are connected by immovable joints. They fit tightly together like pieces of a jigsaw puzzle.

joints (JOYNTS), connections between bones.

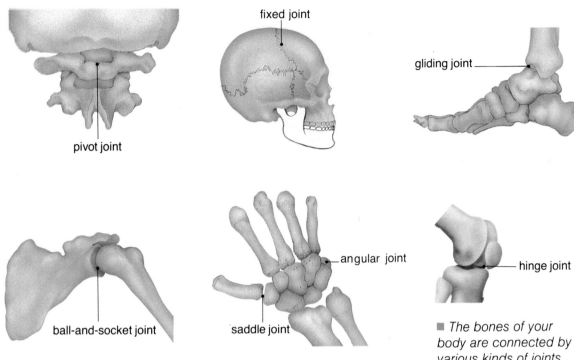

fixed joint

gliding joint

pivot joint

angular joint

hinge joint

ball-and-socket joint

saddle joint

■ *The bones of your body are connected by various kinds of joints. Some joints are fixed, while others allow a range of movement.*

Bones are held together by strong tissues called ligaments. **Ligaments** are strong bands of connective tissue that hold your bones together at movable joints. Ligaments allow bones to move only in certain directions. When a joint is twisted too far or in the wrong direction, the ligaments may be stretched, or sprained. If a joint is severely twisted, the ligaments may tear. Torn ligaments can often mend themselves. However, surgery is sometimes required to repair them.

ligaments (LIHG uh muhnts), strong bands of connective tissue that hold bones together at movable joints.

A strong, flexible material called **cartilage** covers the ends of most of your bones. Cartilage acts as a cushion between bones. It keeps the hard parts of your bones from grinding together. There is also a fluid around your joints to lubricate bone movements.

cartilage (KAHRT uhl ihj), connective tissue that acts as a cushion between bones.

How Does Your Muscular System Help You?

Your muscular system works with your skeletal system to hold you upright and allow you to move. Muscles are made of very strong tissue. Muscle tissue can contract, or get shorter, and relax, or get longer. Muscles move by first contracting and then relaxing. Muscles work in pairs. When you bend your arm, for example, one set of muscles contracts and another set relaxes.

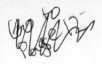

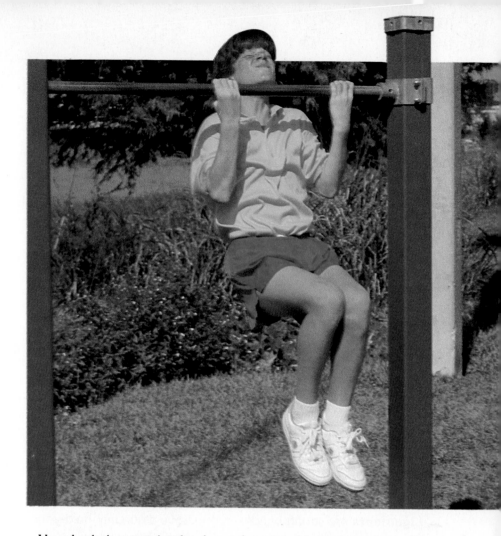

involuntary muscles
(ihn VAHL uhn tehr ee • MUHS uhlz), muscles that work without any direct thought on the part of the individual.

voluntary muscles
(VAHL uhn tehr ee • MUHS uhlz), muscles that are under the conscious control of the individual.

tendons (TEHN duhnz), connective tissue that connects muscles to bones.

Your body has two kinds of muscles—involuntary muscles and voluntary muscles. **Involuntary muscles** work without any direct thought on your part. For example, some involuntary muscles make your stomach contract so that food can be broken down. Involuntary muscles also move food through your intestines. Your heart is a kind of involuntary muscle. You do not have to think about making your heart beat.

Voluntary muscles contract or relax when you decide to make them do so. When you walk, voluntary muscles in your legs are contracting and relaxing. You decide when and where you want to walk.

Voluntary muscles are sometimes called skeletal muscles because they are connected to bones. Muscles are connected to bones by means of tough cords called **tendons.** The tendons that connect muscles to bones are also connective tissue. However, unlike your muscles, tendons cannot contract or relax. Like ligaments, tendons can be stretched, strained, or torn. Injuries to tendons, such as "tennis elbow" and "joystick hand," can also result from overuse.

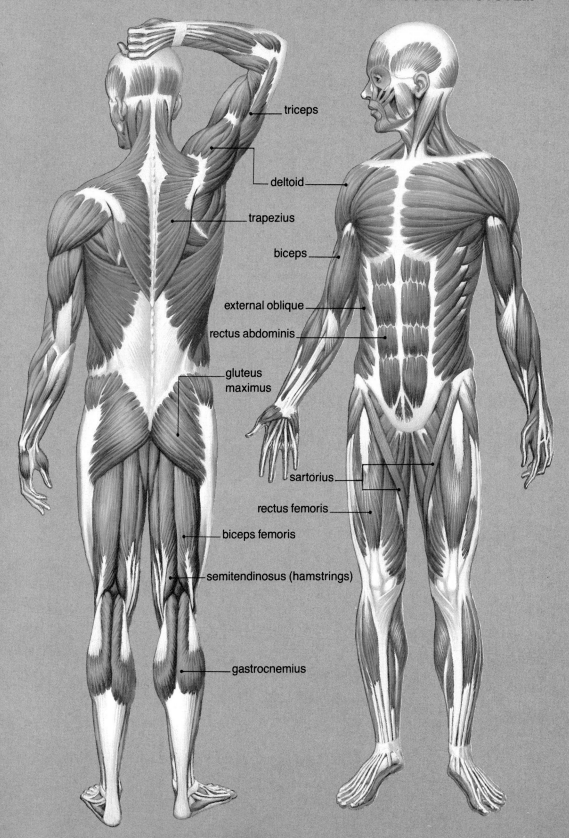

triceps

deltoid

trapezius

biceps

external oblique

rectus abdominis

gluteus
maximus

sartorius

rectus femoris

biceps femoris

semitendinosus (hamstrings)

gastrocnemius

Exercise, rest, and good nutrition help muscles grow strong. After a lot of exercise, muscles sometimes feel tired and sore. With rest, healthy muscles will recover and be stronger. Muscles should be warmed up before heavy exercise. Warming up involves slowly and gently stretching muscles that will be used later. Failure to warm up can result in muscle cramps or even injury. Muscles that are greatly stretched or torn are painful and need the care of a physician to heal properly.

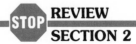

STOP REVIEW
SECTION 2

REMEMBER?

1. Where do bones connect with each other?
2. What does cartilage do?
3. How do muscles produce movement?
4. What are the two kinds of muscles?

THINK!

5. Why are healthful foods needed for bones and muscles?
6. Why are healthy skeletal and muscular systems needed for movement?

Making Wellness Choices

Kay and Maria have been playing tennis every week for the last six months. Today, they arrive at the tennis court 5 minutes late for their scheduled playing time. In the past, Maria spent about 5 to 10 minutes doing stretching and warm-up exercises to prepare her muscles for a tennis match. But the girls have the court reserved for only 30 minutes, so Kay suggests that they start playing right away.

? Should Maria take the time to warm up, or should she follow Kay's suggestion and begin playing right away? How might she avoid this problem in the future? Explain your wellness choice.

Health Close-up

Bone Diseases

You may have heard of a bone disease called *osteoporosis*. Information about this disease has been presented on television and in many newspapers and magazines. The name *osteoporosis* means "porous bones." People with osteoporosis have bones that break very easily because they are thin and brittle. The bones of the back may break without the person feeling any pain. When this happens, the bones in the back may compress, the spine may curve, and the person may lose as much as 7 inches (18 centimeters) in height.

Many older women have osteoporosis. The exact cause of the condition is not known. Scientists believe that there is not enough calcium in the bone tissue to keep the bones hard and strong. Regular exercise and a diet high in calcium are important in maintaining strong bones.

Scientists are finding out more about bones. One discovery is a way to make new bones from old ones. First, old bone tissue is ground into a powder. This powder is then treated with certain chemicals that help change the powder into new bone tissue. This new tissue is called *demineralized bone matrix*. Scientists hope that this new bone tissue can be used during surgery to replace bone tissue that is destroyed by disease or injury.

Bone diseases are not new. Scientists who study the bones of people who lived thousands of years ago have found evidence of bone diseases. This is easy to see in old skeletons. Bone diseases often caused these bones to be much thicker or thinner than normal. Sometimes the bones are bent or worn down because of bone diseases.

Although bone diseases are common, many of them can be avoided. Getting enough rest and exercise and eating foods high in calcium and other minerals can help a person to have strong, healthy bones. Not drinking carbonated soft drinks may help, also. Scientists have found that the phosphorus and caffeine in carbonated drinks reduce the calcium in bones and teeth.

■ *Osteoporosis may cause bones in the spine to break.*

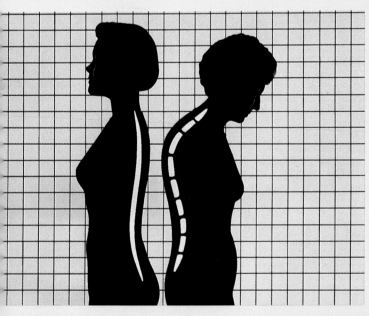

Thinking Beyond

1. Why is it wiser to prevent bone diseases than to treat them?
2. Why are milk and other foods containing calcium important for preventing bone diseases?

43

3 Your Nervous System

Your body helps you keep track of your world by means of your nervous system. Your nervous system is made up of your brain and all the nerves in your body. Nerves are special tissues that receive messages from the world around you. They also send messages to and receive them from all parts of your body.

Your brain, the control center of your nervous system, is made up of billions of nerve cells. A thick bundle of nerves, the spinal cord, connects the base of your brain to most of the nerves in your body. Protected by the bones of your spinal column, the spinal cord runs down to the lower part of your back. Your brain and spinal cord make up your central nervous system. Other nerves branch off from your spinal cord, reaching most parts of your body.

Your brain is divided into three major parts. Each part controls different activities within your body. One part is called the *cerebrum*. The cerebrum controls your emotions, your thinking, and your memory. The cerebrum also receives and interprets information from your sense organs. Your sense organs are your eyes, ears, nose, tongue, and skin. **Sensory nerves** bring information from these organs to your brain.

Another part of your brain is called the *cerebellum*. The cerebellum coordinates movements. It coordinates the messages along **motor nerves** to the body parts that are to be moved. Motor nerves are connected to skeletal muscles. They carry messages from the brain that cause skeletal muscles to contract in a coordinated manner. These messages are impulses that cause the body part to move.

sensory nerves (SEHN suhr ee • NURVZ), nerves that carry information from sense organs to the brain.
motor nerves (MOH tuhr • NURVZ), nerves that carry messages to muscles.

■ *Sensory nerves carry information from sense organs to the spinal cord and brain. The brain and spinal cord send messages along motor nerves to the parts of the body to be moved.*

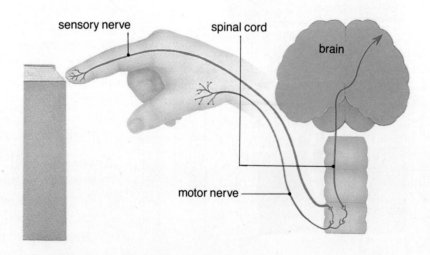

sensory nerve

spinal cord

brain

motor nerve

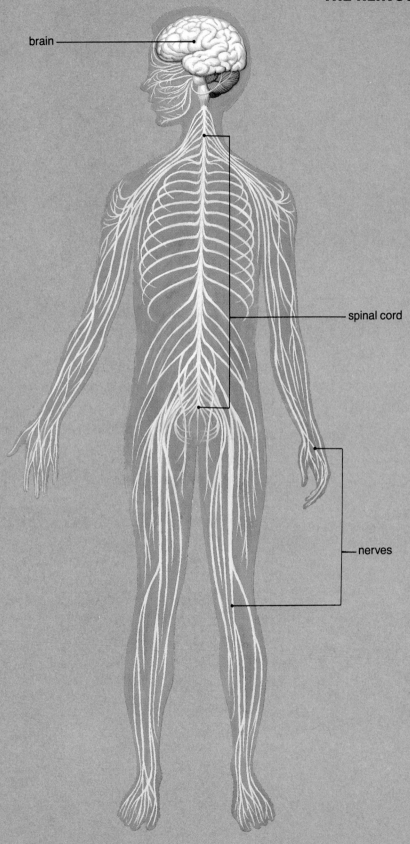

brain

spinal cord

nerves

autonomic nerves (awt uh NAHM ihk • NURVZ), nerves that send messages to vital organs without any thought by the individual.

REAL-LIFE
SKILL

Testing Reaction Time

Hold your right arm out. Keeping the back of your hand up, put a coin on the center of the back of your hand. Tilt your hand to the side so that the coin slides off. Try to catch the coin. Do this five times. Graph the results. Do you improve? Try it with your left hand.

Other nerves, called **autonomic nerves,** control involuntary activities. Autonomic nerves are connected to your spinal cord and *brain stem,* the third part of the brain. Autonomic nerves send messages without any thought on your part. Autonomic nerves control your breathing and your heartbeat, for example.

Your nervous system lets you react quickly. In an emergency, your reaction time is especially important. A fraction of a second can mean the difference between a minor injury and a major one, or even no injury at all. For example, touching a hot pan activates the sensory nerves in your finger. A message moves along the nerve to your spinal cord. Your spinal cord interprets this information as an emergency. The information about the hot pan continues up your spinal cord to your brain. But at the same time, another impulse moves out from your spinal cord to the muscles of your arm. It causes your arm muscles to contract before your brain has even processed its message of pain.

Sometimes the nerves and the spinal cord work together in this way to produce a response without involving the brain at all. When the brain is not involved, the reaction is called a *reflex.* Shivering, for example, is a reflex to being cold.

Proper body control depends on a healthy nervous system. Disease organisms, injuries, poisons, and alcohol and other drugs can all interfere with the functioning of your nervous system. Safe recreation and healthful habits, such as eating a nourishing diet and balancing rest with physical and mental activity, will help you keep your nervous system healthy.

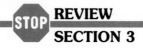

REVIEW
SECTION 3

REMEMBER?

1. What are the two parts of your central nervous system?
2. What kind of nerves carry messages from your eyes and your ears to your brain?
3. What kind of body functions are controlled by your autonomic nerves?

THINK!

4. How might substances such as alcohol, tobacco and caffeine affect your nervous system?
5. How is the nervous system related to the functioning of the skeletal and muscular systems?

4 Your Endocrine and Reproductive Systems

Your body has a system of organs that make certain chemicals. These chemicals are called **hormones.** Hormones direct body activities such as reproduction, growth, and development. They also control your reactions to certain situations. The organs of this system are called **endocrine glands.**

Hormones are made by the endocrine glands. They are chemicals that enter the blood and move through the body to other organs. Once in these other organs, they regulate how the organs work. Only very small amounts of hormones are needed to direct certain activities of your body.

The **pituitary gland** is found under your cerebrum. It is one of the most important glands in your body. The pituitary gland is only about as large as a kidney bean. It produces hormones that direct the activity of many other endocrine glands. The pituitary gland also makes hormones that direct your body's growth and development.

During the early teenage years, your pituitary gland releases hormones that cause the development of your reproductive organs. Reproductive organs make up your reproductive system.

hormones (HAWR mohnz), chemicals, produced by endocrine glands, that control the functioning of organs.

endocrine glands (EHN duh krihn • GLANDZ), glands that secrete hormones into the blood.

pituitary gland (pih TOO uh tehr ee • GLAND), the endocrine gland that controls other glands and directs body growth and development.

■ *The endocrine glands produce hormones that direct activities such as growth and reproduction.*

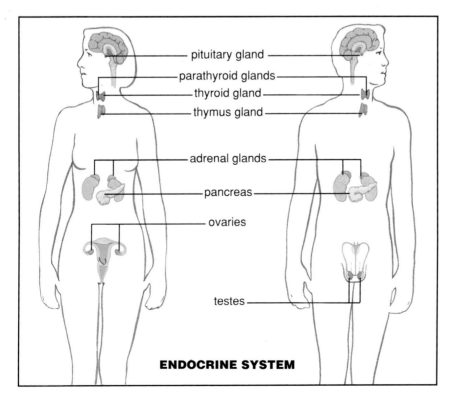

pituitary gland
parathyroid glands
thyroid gland
thymus gland

adrenal glands

pancreas

ovaries

testes

ENDOCRINE SYSTEM

47

SOME GLANDS OF THE ENDOCRINE SYSTEM

Glands	Some Functions of the Hormones Produced by the Glands
Adrenals	make the body alert and quick to respond in stressful situations
Ovaries	develop female body characteristics
Pancreas	helps cells take in certain nutrients
Parathyroids	regulate the use of calcium in the body
Pituitary	directs the activity of other endocrine glands causes the development of reproductive glands regulates the balance of water in the body stimulates involuntary muscles of organs
Testes	develop male body characteristics
Thyroid	regulates growth and the rate at which the body uses energy
Thymus	affects the body's immune system

testes (TEHS teez), male reproductive organs.

ovaries (OHV uh reez), female reproductive organs.

In males the reproductive organs are called the **testes.** The testes produce the male reproductive cells, or sperm cells. Female reproductive organs are called **ovaries.** The ovaries produce the female reproductive cells, or ova. Reproductive organs also make hormones that control other aspects of your physical development as you grow into an adult. You will learn more about the endocrine and reproductive systems in Chapter 3, "Growth and Development."

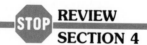

REVIEW
SECTION 4

REMEMBER?

1. What do hormones do?
2. Why is the pituitary gland so important?
3. What are the male and female reproductive organs called?

THINK!

4. Why might the pituitary gland be called the master gland?
5. Why are the reproductive organs part of both the endocrine and reproductive systems?

5 Your Circulatory and Lymphatic Systems

Your circulatory and lymphatic systems are complex body systems. These two systems carry oxygen, nutrients, water, and other materials to the cells of your body. These systems also help fight disease and remove waste materials from your body. They keep your body's cells moist and healthy.

What Are the Functions of the Circulatory System?

Your circulatory system is a great transportation system in your body. It is like an interstate highway with access roads. The circulatory system allows the fast transportation of nutrients and water to all parts of your body. The major parts of your circulatory system are your blood, your heart, and your blood vessels.

Your Blood. Blood is a tissue that is made up of both liquid and solid parts. The liquid part of blood, called **plasma,** is pale yellow and nearly clear. Plasma makes up more than 55 percent of your blood. About 90 percent of plasma is water. Blood plasma carries food nutrients, blood cells, and cell wastes.

plasma (PLAZ muh), the liquid part of the blood.

■ The solid part of blood consists of red blood cells, left, white blood cells, center, and platelets, right.

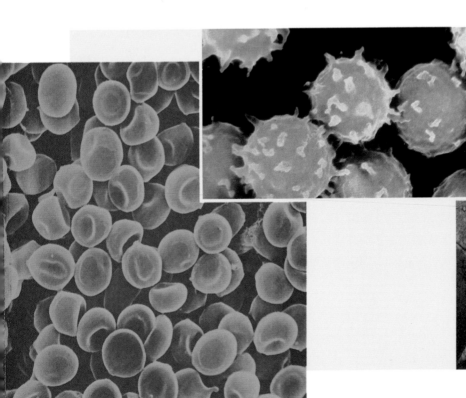
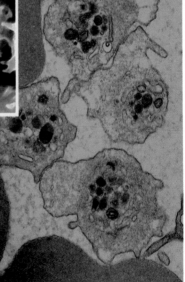

THE CIRCULATORY SYSTEM

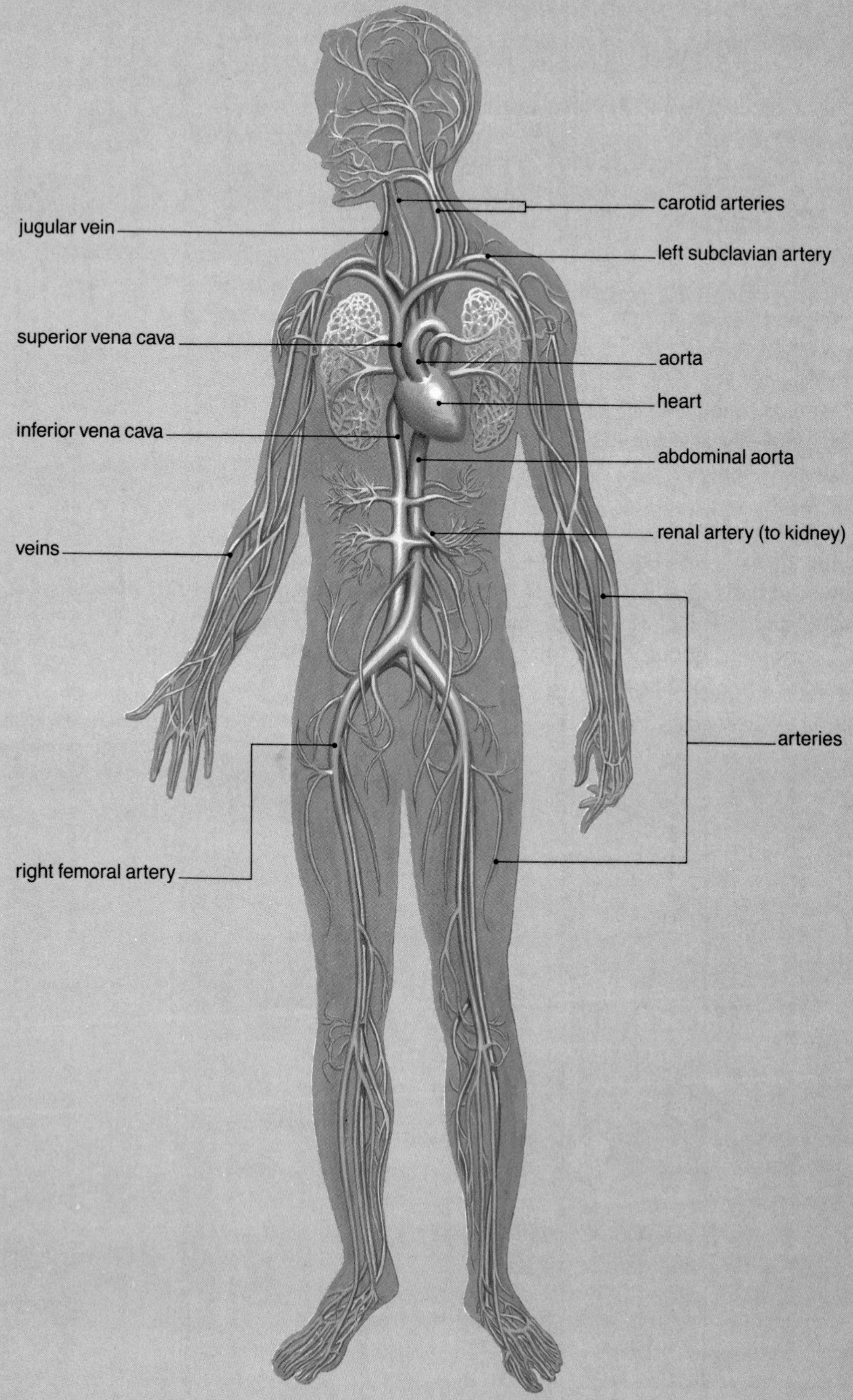

jugular vein

carotid arteries

left subclavian artery

superior vena cava

aorta

heart

inferior vena cava

abdominal aorta

renal artery (to kidney)

veins

arteries

right femoral artery

Two kinds of blood cells make up most of the solid part of your blood. These cells float in the plasma. Each kind of blood cell does a different job. One kind of cell is the red blood cell. Red blood cells are the most numerous, and they give the blood its red color. They carry oxygen to your body's other cells.

A second kind of blood cell is the white blood cell. White blood cells help defend your body against organisms that cause disease. When disease-causing organisms enter your blood, white blood cells surround and kill them.

Platelets are pieces of cells. These pieces help your blood to clot. When you cut yourself, some of your platelets break open and release a chemical. This chemical helps form a clot, or plug of thickened blood. Red and white blood cells become trapped in the clot, and the bleeding stops.

You have about a gallon (4 liters) of blood in your body. The body replaces plasma only if blood is lost. Blood cells, however, are replaced by new blood cells all the time. Red blood cells last about 120 days.

Your Heart. Your heart is a muscular organ in your chest and is about the size of your fist. Your heart keeps your blood moving through your body. It is really composed of two pumps that work side by side. Blood is sent from your lungs to the left pump. The left pump circulates the blood throughout your body. The blood is returned from your body to your heart's right pump.

platelets (PLAYT luhts), pieces of cells that help blood clot.

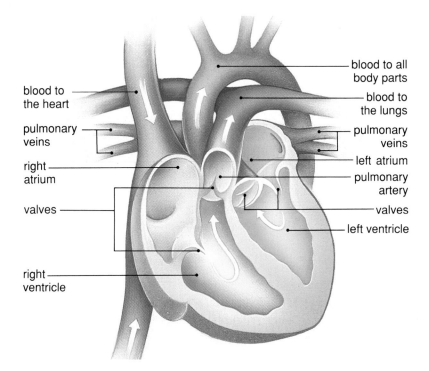

The heart is really two separate pumps. One pump sends blood to the lungs, while the other pump sends blood to the rest of the body. Both pumps work at the same time.

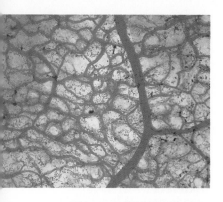

■ *Every cell of the body can receive nutrients and oxygen from a nearby capillary.*

lymph (LIHMF), tissue fluid, similar to blood plasma.

The right pump sends it back to your lungs where it picks up oxygen. Then the blood is returned to the left pump and is sent out on another trip around your body.

Your Blood Vessels.   Blood moves through your body in tubes called blood vessels. Some blood vessels near the heart are nearly an inch (2.5 centimeters) in diameter. However, most are so small that they can be seen only with a microscope. This network of blood vessels reaches all the tissues of your body.

The blood vessels that carry blood away from your heart are *arteries*. Arteries have thick, muscular walls. Arteries branch out, forming smaller and smaller vessels.

The smallest blood vessels are *capillaries*. Capillaries have very thin walls and are so narrow that blood cells must sometimes flow through them in single file. Food nutrients and oxygen carried by your blood reach your body cells by passing through the thin capillary walls. Cell wastes pass into the blood through these same walls.

The capillaries join to form larger blood vessels again. The blood vessels that carry blood back toward your heart are *veins*. Unlike arteries, veins have thin walls. The veins also have one-way valves that keep the blood from flowing backward. Activities such as walking help push the blood up the veins of the legs, toward the heart.

What Does Your Lymphatic System Do?

The lymphatic system is another transportation system in your body. This system keeps your body tissues moist and helps fight disease organisms.

As blood flows through capillaries, some plasma leaves through the capillary walls. Plasma that leaves the capillaries in this way is called *tissue fluid*. Tissue fluid bathes body cells and collects wastes from them.

Tissue fluid collects in vessels that lie next to your veins. These vessels are called *lymph vessels*, and the fluid inside is called **lymph.** Lymph later returns to the blood of your circulatory system. The lymph vessels join large veins near your neck.

Small, round lumps of tissue, called *lymph nodes*, are found at several places in the lymph vessels. Lymph nodes are filters in which white blood cells trap and destroy disease-causing microbes. When your body is fighting a disease, your lymph nodes may become sore and swollen because of the large numbers of microbes they hold. A common term for this condition is "swollen glands." In fact, they are swollen lymph nodes.

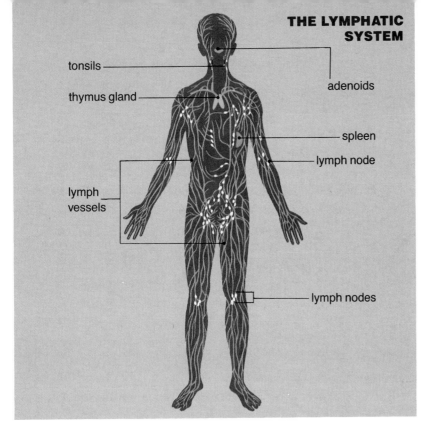

THE LYMPHATIC SYSTEM

tonsils

adenoids

thymus gland

spleen

lymph node

lymph vessels

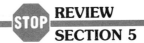

lymph nodes

■ *Tissue fluid collects in lymph vessels that empty into veins.*

The health of your circulatory and lymphatic systems is important to your general wellness. Maintaining a healthy circulatory system requires that you eat properly, exercise regularly, and not smoke or take drugs that will harm your heart and blood vessels.

STOP REVIEW SECTION 5

REMEMBER?

1. What are the three major parts of your circulatory system?
2. What is the liquid part of blood called?
3. Name the two kinds of blood cells.
4. Name three kinds of blood vessels.
5. What are the two major functions of your lymphatic system?

THINK!

6. Why is a healthy circulatory system necessary for general body wellness?
7. How are good nutrition and regular exercise helpful to your circulatory system?

6 Your Respiratory System

KEY WORDS

mucus
cilia
trachea
bronchial tubes
alveoli

mucus (MYOO kuhs), a thick, sticky secretion that traps dust and dirt.

cilia (SIHL ee uh), tiny hairs lining the respiratory passages.

trachea (TRAY kee uh), the windpipe.

Every time you breathe, you are using your respiratory system. The organs of this system allow your body to take in the oxygen your cells need. These organs also allow your body to get rid of the carbon dioxide formed by your cells.

When you inhale through your nose, the air goes through your nasal passages. These passages are lined with tiny hairs and a sticky substance called **mucus.** Mucus traps dust and dirt from the air. The nasal passages also warm the inhaled air before it enters your lungs.

The tiny hairs lining your nasal passages are called **cilia.** Cilia are always sweeping outward in a wavelike motion. This action helps carry the mucus containing dirt and dust particles out of your respiratory system.

From your nasal passages, air passes into your windpipe, or **trachea.** Like your nasal passages, your trachea is also lined with mucus and cilia that trap any remaining dirt. In your chest,

■ Air enters the respiratory system through the nasal passages. Air travels through the trachea and bronchial tubes to the lungs. In the alveoli of the lungs, oxygen is absorbed by the blood as carbon dioxide is released.

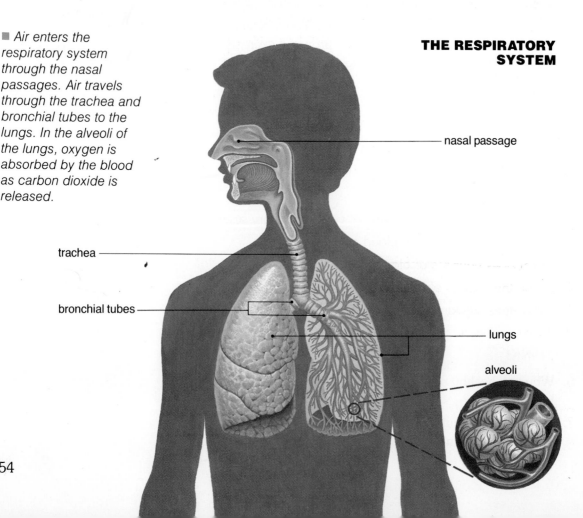

THE RESPIRATORY SYSTEM

nasal passage

trachea

bronchial tubes

lungs

alveoli

54

your trachea divides into two **bronchial tubes.** One tube leads to your right lung and the other to your left lung. Inside your lungs, the bronchial tubes branch many times, becoming smaller and smaller. Air passes through these small tubes until it reaches clusters of tiny air sacs called **alveoli.** Alveoli are like small balloons. Every time you inhale, the alveoli fill with air and get larger. Every time you exhale, they empty and get smaller.

The walls of the alveoli are very thin and have many capillaries. Oxygen passes into your blood through the walls of these capillaries. Oxygen is then carried by your red blood cells through your arteries to all the other cells in your body.

When food is used by your cells, carbon dioxide, a waste gas, is made. The carbon dioxide is carried back to your lungs through your veins by your red blood cells. There the carbon dioxide passes through the walls of the capillaries into the alveoli and then into your bronchial tubes. When you exhale, carbon dioxide goes up your bronchial tubes, trachea, and nasal passages and leaves your body through your mouth or your nose. Along with carbon dioxide, the air you breathe out also contains water vapor.

Eating healthful foods, exercising regularly, and breathing clean air will help you keep your respiratory system healthy. The alveoli and the cilia of the trachea can be damaged by air pollution and cigarette smoke. It is not easy for damaged alveoli to exchange oxygen and carbon dioxide with the blood. A loss of cilia may allow disease organisms to enter the trachea and lungs. You can prevent these kinds of damage by avoiding smoky or polluted areas.

bronchial tubes
(BRAHNG kee uhl • TOOBZ), tubes through which air passes from the trachea to the lungs.

alveoli (al VEE uh ly), tiny air sacs within the lungs.

FOR THE
CURIOUS

If all of the surfaces of your lungs were laid out flat, they would cover an area as large as a tennis court.

STOP REVIEW
SECTION 6

REMEMBER?

1. What does your respiratory system allow your body to do?
2. How does mucus help clean the air you breathe?
3. How does oxygen reach your cells?
4. What two waste materials leave your body when you exhale?

THINK!

5. Why is a healthy respiratory system necessary for general wellness?
6. How could heavy smoking make a person feel tired?

SECTION

7 Your Digestive System

Your digestive system is made up of organs that break down, or digest, food so that it can be used by your cells. This process is known as **digestion.** Digestion takes place in many small steps. For example, if you eat an apple, many things must take place before your cells can use the food nutrients of the apple.

The first step in digestion takes place in your mouth. Your teeth chew the food into pieces small enough to be swallowed. These pieces mix with saliva formed in your mouth. The saliva begins to soften the food. Saliva also has chemicals in it that begin to digest the starches in foods such as bread and pasta.

How Does Food Get from Your Mouth to Your Stomach?

When you swallow, the food in your mouth passes into a tube called the *esophagus*. Muscles in your esophagus squeeze the food along to your stomach. More digestion takes place in your stomach. Strong stomach muscles churn the food into smaller and smaller pieces. The wall of your stomach also makes fluids that break down certain kinds of foods even further. These fluids are called *digestive juices*.

After a few hours in your stomach, the food has been turned into a thick liquid called **chyme.** At this point, some of the food has been digested. However, very little of the food has been absorbed by your body.

What Is the Function of Your Small Intestine?

Muscles in your stomach push the chyme into your small intestine. Your small intestine is a narrow tube that is about 20 feet (6 meters) long. The small intestine is coiled and folded to fit in your abdomen below your stomach. Muscles in your small intestine keep pushing the chyme along. More digestive juices, made by the wall of your small intestine, mix with the chyme and digest it even more.

Chyme in your small intestine also receives digestive juices from two other organs. One of these organs is your pancreas. Your pancreas makes juices that enter your small intestine and help the small intestine finish digestion. The other organ that makes juices is your liver. One of the largest organs in the body, the liver makes a fluid called *bile*. Bile helps break down fats.

KEY WORDS

digestion
chyme

digestion (dy JEHS chuhn), the process of breaking down food.

chyme (KYM), partly digested food in the form of a thick liquid.

56

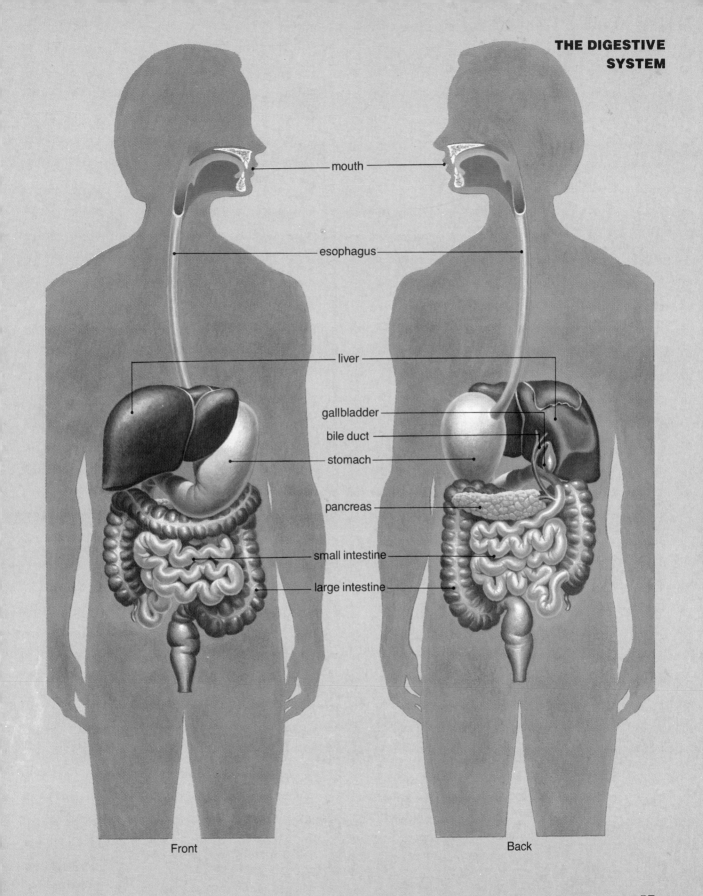

mouth

esophagus

liver

gallbladder

bile duct

stomach

pancreas

small intestine

large intestine

Front

Back

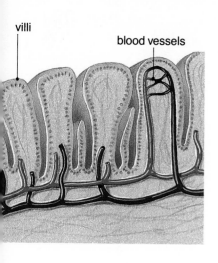

villi

blood vessels

■ *When food is digested, nutrients pass through the wall of the small intestine into the blood.*

It is stored in the gallbladder. When fats enter the small intestine, bile is squirted into the small intestine and mixes with the fats.

Most digestion takes place as the food moves through the small intestine. When the food is completely digested, nutrients are able to pass into capillaries and lymph vessels in the thin wall of the intestine. As blood passes through your liver, excess nutrients are removed and stored. The rest of the nutrients are then carried by your blood to all the cells of your body.

What Is the Function of Your Large Intestine?

Your body cannot digest everything you eat. For example, fiber cannot be digested. Fiber is the stringy part of some vegetables. Some seeds and fruit skins are not digested, either. These parts of your food pass from your small intestine into your large intestine. Your large intestine is about 4 feet (1.2 meters) long. It is wider and shorter than your small intestine.

Water is also carried into your large intestine with the undigested food. Most of this water passes through the wall of your large intestine and into your blood. The remaining water and the undigested food form solid wastes. These wastes stay in your large intestine until they are eliminated from your body in a bowel movement.

Along with maintaining overall wellness, eating a variety of healthful foods is necessary for the proper working of your digestive system. Drinking plenty of water and eating foods high in fiber will keep food from staying too long in the large intestine.

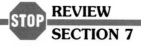

REVIEW

SECTION 7

REMEMBER?

1. What is digestion?
2. How does the liver help in digestion?
3. What happens to food while it is in your stomach?
4. What happens to the parts of food that cannot be digested?

THINK!

5. How is the work of the digestive system important to all the other systems?
6. How does fiber help food move through the digestive system?

8 Your Excretory System

Besides the solid wastes in your large intestine, your body must get rid of other wastes. Some of these wastes come from cell activities. If these wastes stay in your body, they may build up and harm your cells. Your body's excretory system removes these wastes and carries them out of your body. The excretory system works closely with the digestive and circulatory systems to help you stay healthy.

What Are the Excretory Functions of Your Lungs and Your Skin?

Perhaps you have never thought of your lungs and your skin as part of your body's excretory system. Your lungs rid your body of carbon dioxide. Your lungs also remove water from your body. You can see this moisture by breathing on a mirror.

Your skin helps your body get rid of excess water and some cell wastes. There are tiny sacs in your skin called *sweat glands*.

KEY WORDS

urine
ureter

FOR THE CURIOUS

An English coal miner holds the record as having sweated 1.8 British gallons (8 liters) in 5.5 hours. He lost 18 pounds (8 kilograms) as a result.

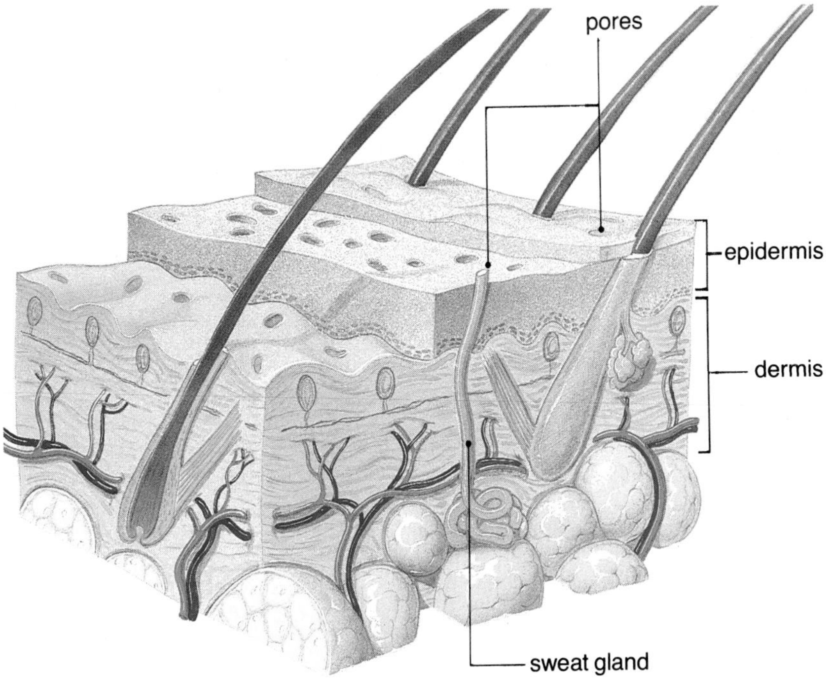

pores

epidermis

dermis

sweat gland

■ *The skin acts as an excretory organ to get rid of wastes. Excess water and cell wastes are released from the body as sweat.*

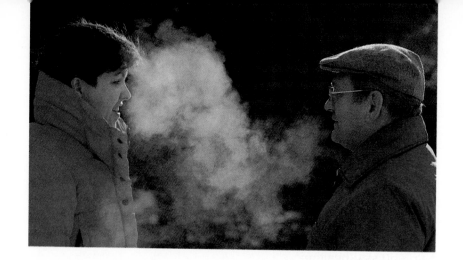

■ *The lungs help rid the body of excess water. On a cold day, you can see water vapor as you exhale.*

Water and some cell wastes pass from your body through your sweat glands. Sweat made by these glands leaves your skin through small openings called *pores*.

What Are the Functions of Your Kidneys and Bladder?

As your blood moves through your body, the blood passes through your kidneys. Your kidneys are two bean-shaped organs located in the middle of your back. They remove cell wastes and extra water from your blood. The liquid waste that results is called **urine**. If you are ill, urine may also contain viruses or bacteria.

urine (YUR uhn), a liquid containing cell wastes; filtered from the blood by the kidneys.

■ *Most of the cell wastes and excess water are removed from the blood by the kidneys. Urine is stored in the bladder until it is eliminated.*

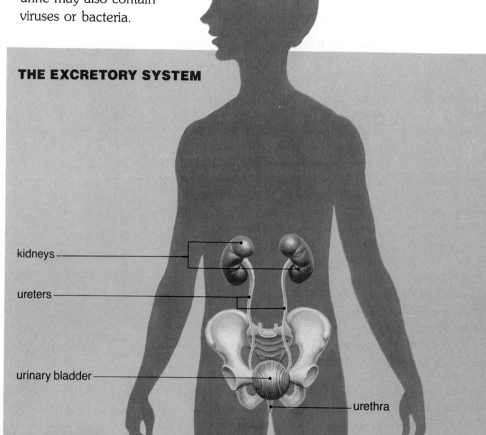

THE EXCRETORY SYSTEM

kidneys

ureters

urinary bladder

urethra

Urine leaves each kidney through a narrow tube called a **ureter.** The ureters carry urine to the urinary bladder. The urinary bladder is an expandable sac in which urine is stored. A set of voluntary muscles keeps an opening from your bladder closed. By relaxing these muscles, you let urine pass out of your body through a single tube called the *urethra.* This process is called *urination.*

ureter (YUR uht uhr), the tube that connects each kidney to the urinary bladder.

Drinking about eight glasses of water a day helps your skin and your kidneys remove wastes from your body and gives your body the water it needs. You need a healthy excretory system to maintain your wellness.

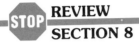

REVIEW
SECTION 8

REMEMBER?

1. What wastes are removed by your lungs?
2. What function do the kidneys perform?
3. Where is urine stored until it leaves your body?

THINK!

4. How does drinking a lot of water help rid the body of wastes?
5. Why is kidney failure a very serious problem?

Thinking About Your Health

Caring for Body Systems

Answer the following questions to learn how proper health habits are related to your wellness:

- What body systems are most directly affected by breathing clean air and exercising regularly? How might smoking cigarettes and sitting most of the day affect these systems?

- What might happen to your body systems if you did not eat healthful foods?

- Why are healthful patterns of exercise, rest, and sleep necessary for maintaining your body systems?

People in Health

An Interview with a Respiratory Therapist

Anna E. Read knows about the respiratory system. She helps people overcome breathing problems. She is a respiratory therapist in Lewiston, Maine.

What does a respiratory therapist do?

A respiratory therapist helps people who have breathing problems by using medicines and physical treatment. A respiratory therapist provides community education for the prevention of respiratory diseases.

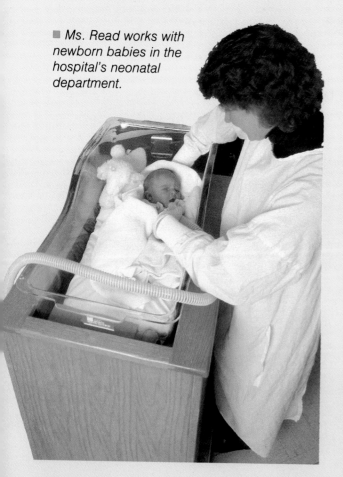

■ *Ms. Read works with newborn babies in the hospital's neonatal department.*

What breathing problems does a respiratory therapist treat?

Some patients a respiratory therapist treats have lifelong breathing problems caused by conditions such as asthma. Others have emergency breathing problems due to a sudden illness or accident. Respiratory therapists help treat these problems.

Where do most respiratory therapists work?

Most work in hospitals. Hospitals started using respiratory therapists because of the large number of patients who develop breathing problems when recovering from surgery. Sometimes the medicines taken to ease pain make people's breathing shallower than normal. It is easy for a patient to get a lung infection when breathing is shallow.

Where do you work?

I work everywhere in the hospital. Three areas are the emergency room, the intensive-care unit, and the neonatal department. *Neonatal* refers to newborn babies.

How do respiratory therapists help newborn babies?

Many premature babies are not able to breathe as they should. Their lungs are not fully developed. Respiratory therapists give these babies a little extra air pressure to help open their lungs. Some of the babies respond quickly. They need the treatment for only a few days. Other babies may need treatment for weeks or months.

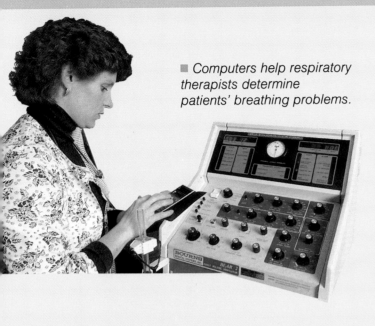
■ *Computers help respiratory therapists determine patients' breathing problems.*

Do you help older children?

The hospital where I work has a large cystic fibrosis clinic. Cystic fibrosis is a hereditary disorder of the endocrine system. Many children with cystic fibrosis have trouble breathing. I help these children by doing chest-percussion treatments and aerosol or mist treatments with medicine that helps open airways. I cup my hand and tap on the patient's chest to loosen mucus trapped inside. This technique helps them breathe more easily. Some children with allergies and asthma need help, too.

How do respiratory therapists tell what kind of breathing problem a person may have?

One way is to test the person's blood. Using a certain machine, the respiratory therapist can determine the amounts of oxygen and carbon dioxide in the blood. Oxygen is the gas in the air that people need to stay alive and healthy. Each cell in the body needs oxygen. Carbon dioxide is a waste gas produced by the cells. Too much of this waste and not enough oxygen can cause certain serious health problems.

Do you use other machines and computers?

Computers help provide the respiratory therapist with quick information about a patient. Computers can measure the volume, or amount, of a breath and a patient's breathing rate much faster than a person can. Computers help me determine the kind and extent of a breathing problem. The sooner I know the problem, the sooner I can determine the ways in which the problem might be solved.

How can a person keep the respiratory system healthy?

Breathing clean air and avoiding places where the air is unclean will help. Cigarette smoke and other forms of air pollution can cause damage to the lungs and other parts of the respiratory system. Even if you do not smoke, being around dust and other people's cigarette smoke can affect your breathing. It also helps to eat healthful foods and to get enough exercise. Vigorous exercise can help you keep your whole cardiorespiratory system healthy.

Learn more about people who work in respiratory care. Interview a respiratory therapist from a local hospital. Or write for information to the American Association for Respiratory Care, 11030 Ables Lane, Dallas, TX 75229.

Main Ideas

- Your body is made of similar cells grouped as tissues, organs, and systems.
- Your skeletal and muscular systems allow you to move and give you size and shape.
- Your nervous system controls most of your body activities.
- Your endocrine system controls growth, reproduction, and development.
- Your circulatory system moves oxygen and nutrients to your cells.
- Your respiratory system exchanges oxygen and carbon dioxide.
- Your digestive system breaks down food into nutrients your cells need.
- The kidneys, lungs, and skin are all organs of your excretory system.

Key Words

Write the numbers 1 to 10 in your health notebook or on a separate sheet of paper. After each number, copy the sentence and fill in the missing term. Page numbers in ( ) tell you where to look in the chapter if you need help

cartilage (39)	ovaries (48)
tendons (40)	plasma (49)
sensory (44)	trachea (54)
motor (44)	alveoli (55)
testes (48)	urine (60)

1. ___?___ produce sperm cells.

2. ___?___ is the liquid part of blood.

3. ___?___ join some muscles to bones.

4. ___?___ covers the ends of most bones.

5. ___?___ are tiny air sacs in your lungs.

6. ___?___ nerves carry messages from the brain to skeletal muscles.

7. The ___?___ produce egg cells.

8. The windpipe is also the ___?___ .

9. Liquid waste is called ___?___ .

10. ___?___ nerves bring information from sense organs to your brain.

Write the numbers 11 to 32 in your health notebook or on a separate sheet of paper. After each number, write a sentence that defines the term. Page numbers in ( ) tell you where to look in the chapter if you need help.

11. epithelial tissue (33)

12. connective tissue (33)

13. muscle tissue (33)

14. nerve tissue (34)

15. organ (34)

16. body systems (34)

17. joints (38)

18. ligaments (39)

19. voluntary muscles (40)

20. involuntary muscles (40)

21. autonomic nerves (46)

22. endocrine glands (47)

23. hormones (47)

24. pituitary glands (47)

25. platelets (51)

26. lymph (52)

27. mucus (54)

28. cilia (54)

29. bronchial tubes (55)

30. digestion (56)

31. chyme (56)

32. ureter (61)

Remembering What You Learned

Page numbers in ( ) tell you where to look in the chapter if you need help.

1. What is oxidation? (33)

2. What is one function of each of these tissues: epithelial, connective, muscle, nerve? (33–34)

3. What are two functions of the skeletal system? (36)

4. What are two functions of the muscular system? (39–40)

5. What do each of the three areas of the brain control? (44–46)

6. What is the difference between sensory nerves and motor nerves? (44)

7. What is the function of the endocrine glands? (47)

8. What is the function of the circulatory system? (49–51)

9. What are the functions of red blood cells, white blood cells, and platelets? (51)

10. What are two differences between veins and arteries? (52)

11. What are "swollen glands"? To what body system do these "glands" belong? (52)

12. What are cilia? (54)

13. How does carbon dioxide leave the body? (55)

14. What are three functions of your excretory system? (59–60)

15. What is the function of your kidneys? (60–61)

Thinking About What You Learned

1. Why must you keep all of your body systems healthy?

2. How is your circulatory system related to your respiratory and muscular systems?

3. How might cigarette smoke affect your circulatory system?

4. Why do the organs of the digestive system have muscles?

5. How does the excretory system use other body systems?

Writing About What You Learned

1. Select two body systems whose functions are directly related to each other. Explain how they depend on each other for performing a specific function. For example, the respiratory and circulatory systems are responsible for supplying oxygen to body cells.

2. Write several paragraphs explaining how one good health habit, such as eating a balanced diet, helps maintain several body systems.

Applying What You Learned

ART AND SCIENCE

Draw and label a diagram of the circulatory system. Be sure to show arteries and veins going to and from each major body part. Make a separate drawing of capillaries connecting an artery to a vein. Also make a separate drawing showing the flow of blood through both sides of the heart.

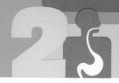

Modified True or False

Write the numbers 1 to 15 in your health notebook or on a separate sheet of paper. After each number, write *true* or *false* to describe the sentence. If the sentence is false, also write a term that replaces the underlined term and makes the sentence true.

1. Your heart, stomach, and other internal organs are covered with <u>connective</u> tissue.

2. Muscles are connected to bones by <u>tendons</u>.

3. The spinal cord is a thick bundle of <u>nerves</u>.

4. The <u>autonomic nerves</u> direct the movement of involuntary muscles.

5. <u>Platelets</u> allow bones to move only in certain directions.

6. The liquid part of blood is <u>plasma</u>.

7. Tiny hairs lining your nasal passages are <u>alveoli</u>.

8. Your stomach turns food into a thick liquid called <u>chyme</u>.

9. <u>White blood cells</u> carry oxygen to your body's other cells.

10. <u>Sensory</u> nerves send messages throughout the body without any thought on your part.

11. <u>Arteries</u> have thick, muscular walls.

12. Your <u>pituitary</u> gland releases hormones that cause the development of reproductive organs.

13. Your large intestine is <u>wider and shorter</u> than your small intestine.

14. The <u>lungs</u> removes cell wastes and extra water from your blood.

15. The liver makes a fluid called <u>bile</u>.

Short Answer

Write the numbers 16 to 23 on your paper. Write a complete sentence to answer each question.

16. What are three functions of nerve tissue?

17. What are two functions of bone, other than to frame the body?

18. What is the purpose of hormones?

19. What would happen to a person who did not have lymph nodes?

20. When does bone growth stop?

21. Why do capillaries have thin walls?

22. What would happen to a person whose liver did not produce bile?

23. How are sensory nerves different from autonomic nerves?

Essay

Write the numbers 24 and 25 on your paper. Write paragraphs with complete sentences to answer each question.

24. Describe how the circulatory and respiratory systems work together.

25. What problems might a person have if the body did not have autonomic nerves?

ACTIVITIES FOR HOME OR SCHOOL

Projects to Do

1. If a microscope is available to you, use it to observe cells and tissues. Use prepared slides if possible, rather than trying to prepare your own. Under a microscope, observe cells in the skin of an onion. You may also want to look at muscle fibers in a thin piece of uncooked meat.

2. Cut open an uncooked chicken leg. Try to identify the various kinds of connective tissues of the skeletal and muscular systems. Some parts that you may be able to identify are skin, muscle, bone, and cartilage. You may also be able to see blood vessels, tendons, ligaments, and fat tissue.

3. You may enjoy reading the science fiction book *Fantastic Voyage* by Isaac Asimov. In the story, scientists shrink to microscopic size and travel inside a human body. After you have read the book, try to illustrate some of the scientists' adventures. Or write a story about what else someone might see if he or she could make such a journey through the human body.

Information to Find

1. Some young people get a sore, swollen lump just below one or both kneecaps. This condition is called *Osgood-Schlatter's disease*. It is due to a pulled ligament between the thigh bone and the large bone in the lower leg. Ask a physician or your school nurse for information about this condition. Find out about treatment and prevention for this disease.

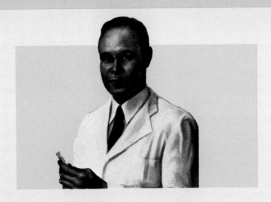
■ *Dr. Drew created the model for modern blood banks.*

2. Charles Richard Drew first discovered ways to store blood and plasma in blood banks. His work has helped save many lives. Find out more about Dr. Drew and prepare a report for your class about his discoveries. One book you might read is *Charles Richard Drew, Pioneer in Blood Research* by Richard Hardwick.

3. In recent years, surgeons have successfully transplanted eyes, kidneys, livers, hearts, and other body parts. Find out about the process of transplanting organs and why organ transplants do not always succeed. A medical society in your area can help you contact groups that help people who need transplants.

Books to Read

Here are some books you can look for in your school library or the public library to find more information about how your body systems work.

Limburg, Peter. *The Story of Your Heart.* Coward, McCann & Geoghegan.

Nourse, Alan E. *Hormones.* Franklin Watts.

Ward, Brian R. *Body Maintenance.* Franklin Watts.

67

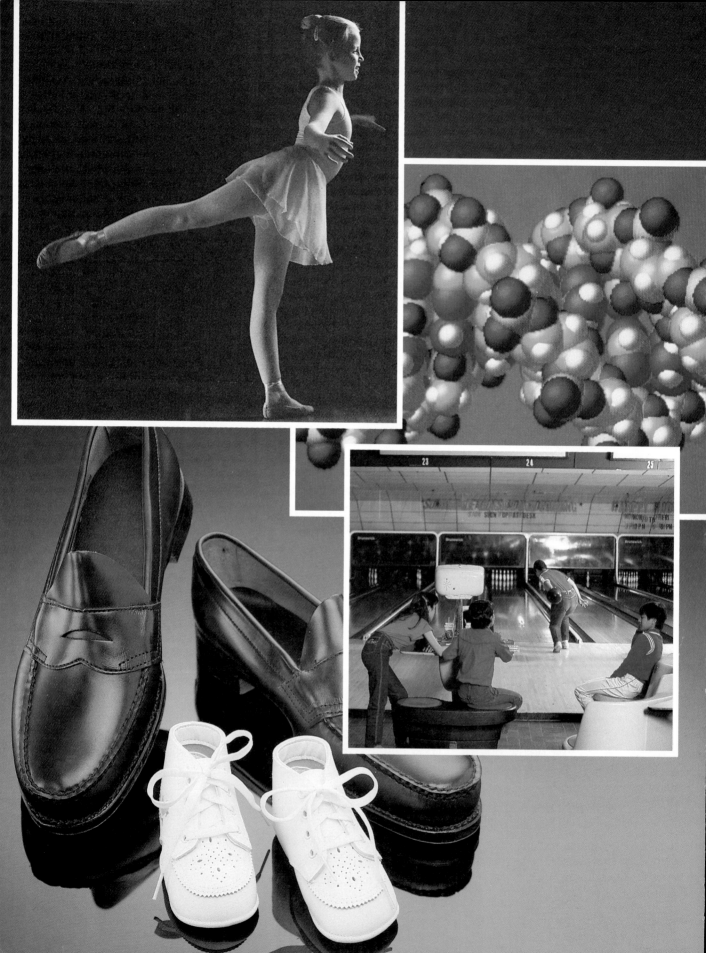

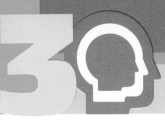

GROWTH AND DEVELOPMENT

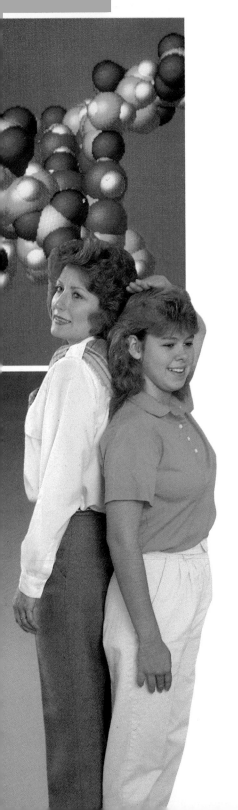

Physical changes happen to all people as they grow from children into adults. For those who do not understand what is happening to their bodies, there can be confusing or embarrassing times. But for those who are prepared with knowledge about their bodies, adolescence can be an exciting and a challenging time.

By making healthful and responsible choices about your body, you can help yourself gain greater physical, emotional, and social maturity. When you strive to maintain wellness during times of change, you feel good about yourself and you feel good about being with others.

GETTING READY TO LEARN

Key Questions

- Why is it important to learn how you grow and develop?
- Why is it important to know how you feel about the ways in which you are growing and changing?
- What can you do to help yourself feel good about your body's changes?
- What can you do to make responsible choices that will help you grow and develop as you should?

Main Chapter Sections

1 Growth and the Body's Cells
2 Physical Growth and Change
3 Emotional and Social Growth

1 Growth and the Body's Cells

KEY WORDS

mitosis
nucleus
chromosomes
meiosis
genes
dominant
recessive

mitosis (my TOH suhs), cell division in which two cells identical to the original are formed.

nucleus (NOO klee uhs), the part of the cell that controls the cell's activities.

chromosomes (KROH muh sohmz), threadlike structures made of DNA inside the cell nucleus.

Look at your hand. Each square inch of the skin of your hand contains millions of cells. The skin you are looking at is made up of dead cells. Most of them will be worn away by tomorrow. However, below the surface are live cells that are dividing to make new skin. Like skin cells, most body cells reproduce by dividing. An original cell is called a *parent cell*. The two new cells that result when a parent cell divides are called *daughter cells*.

How Do Cells Grow?

The kind of cell division by which two daughter cells are formed is called **mitosis.** During mitosis, the **nucleus,** or control center of the cell, duplicates and the cell divides into two daughter cells. Each daughter cell is exactly like the parent cell.

Before mitosis can begin, the hereditary material in the cell's nucleus must be copied. This hereditary material, or DNA, makes up threadlike structures called **chromosomes.** Chromosomes are grouped in pairs within the cell nucleus. Human cells contain 23 pairs of chromosomes, or 46 chromosomes in all.

Just as a copying machine makes exact copies of a letter, a cell can make exact copies of its chromosomes. This copying is necessary so that each daughter cell will have exactly the same number and kinds of chromosomes as the parent cell has. As a result, every cell in your body contains exactly the same DNA as was in the single fertilized cell from which you developed.

■ *During mitosis, chromosomes duplicate, line up in the center of the cell, and separate. Then the rest of the cell divides.*

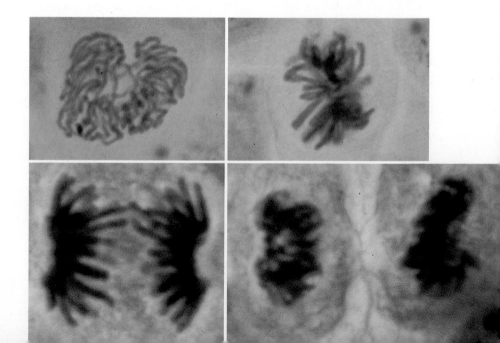

Where Did the Chromosomes in Your Body Cells Come From?

The answer to this question involves certain cells called *reproductive cells.* There are two kinds of reproductive cells. One kind, produced by females, is called the *ovum,* or egg cell. The ovum is one of the largest of all human cells. The other kind, produced by males, is called the *sperm cell.* Compared to the ovum, the sperm cell is very small.

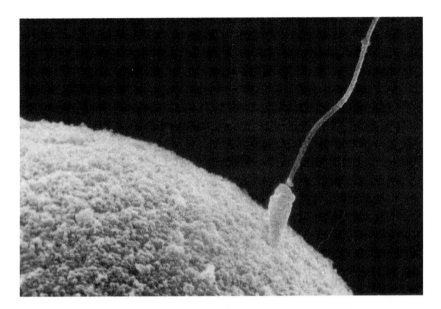

FOR THE
CURIOUS

The ovum is about 1/25 of an inch (1 millimeter) in diameter. It is about the size of the period at the end of this sentence, just visible to the human eye.

■ *During the process of fertilization, a sperm cell attaches to an ovum. The chromosomes of the sperm and the ovum then join.*

Reproductive cells are formed by a different kind of cell division, called **meiosis.** Unlike mitosis, which produces two daughter cells, meiosis results in four daughter cells. The two daughter cells produced in mitosis each have exactly the same number of chromosomes as the parent cell. However, the four daughter cells produced in meiosis each contain one-half of each pair of chromosomes found in the parent cell. Human reproductive cells, therefore, have 23 chromosomes instead of the 46 found in their parent cells.

meiosis (my OH suhs), cell division that forms reproductive cells.

When a sperm cell joins with an ovum, the process of fertilization occurs. The 23 chromosomes from the sperm pair up with the 23 chromosomes from the ovum. The new cell that results has 46 chromosomes in 23 pairs. When this new cell divides, it undergoes mitosis and produces identical daughter cells. Eventually, many cell divisions produce a new human being. Each cell in the new person's body has 46 chromosomes. Twenty-three chromosomes are identical to those that came from the sperm, and 23 are identical to those that came from the ovum.

What Do Chromosomes Do?

The DNA in each chromosome makes up small bits of hereditary information called **genes.** Genes usually occur in pairs. One gene of each pair is located on a chromosome that came from the sperm. The other gene of a pair is on a chromosome that came from the ovum. Genes determine the traits that are passed from parents to children. In humans, traits such as head shape, body build, and hair and eye color come from information that is supplied by gene pairs.

genes (JEENZ), the small bits of hereditary information on chromosomes.

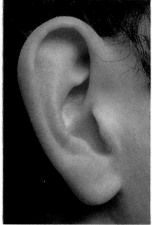

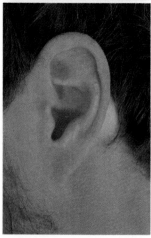

■ *A certain pair of genes determines whether your ear lobes are attached or hang free.*

SOME INHERITED HUMAN TRAITS	
Dominant	**Recessive**
curly hair	straight hair
much body hair	little body hair
long eyelashes	short eyelashes
short fingers	long fingers
cleft	no chin cleft
dimples	no dimples
ability to roll tongue	inability to roll tongue
free ear lobes	attached ear lobes
freckles	no freckles
short stature	tall stature

dominant (DAHM uh nuhnt), describes the stronger gene of a pair of genes.

recessive (rih SEHS ihv), describes the weaker gene of a pair of genes.

Some gene pairs are made up of a strong gene and a weak gene. The strong gene is called **dominant.** The weak gene is called **recessive.** A dominant gene in a pair prevents a recessive gene from being expressed as a trait in the individual. A trait determined by a recessive gene is expressed only when that gene is paired with another recessive gene.

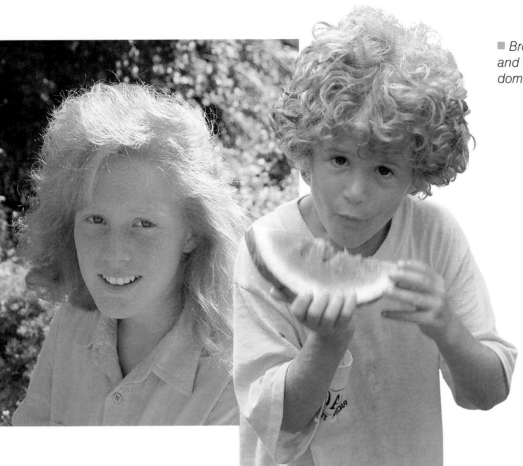

■ Brown eyes, curly hair, and dimples are all dominant traits.

In humans the gene for curly hair is dominant. The gene for straight hair is recessive. A person with straight hair must have two recessive genes for this trait, since only a pair of recessive genes results in the expression of the trait. A person with curly hair, however, may have either one gene for curly hair and one gene for straight hair, or two genes for curly hair. If the gene for curly hair is paired with the gene for straight hair, the dominant gene prevents the expression of the recessive gene.

If a parent with curly hair has only the dominant genes, any child of that parent will have curly hair. But some curly-haired parents can have straight-haired children. This can happen only if curly-haired parents each have a recessive gene for straight hair. Then these genes can form a recessive pair and the child will have straight hair.

Thousands of human traits are inherited. Some of these are determined by one pair of genes. Others are determined by two or more gene pairs. For example, hair color and eye color in people are determined by more than one pair of genes. That is why there is such a variety of shades in both hair and eye color. Some of the inherited traits are listed on page 72.

MYTH AND FACT

Myth: Some people's hair turns gray overnight.

Fact: This is not possible. However, some diseases affect cells so that they stop producing pigments. This causes the hair to turn gray as it grows out.

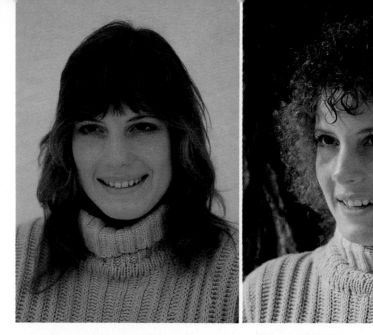

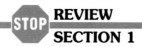
Adding curl to your hair has no effect on the genes that determined your hair traits originally.

Some other traits, although present at birth, are not inherited. Certain birth defects, for example, are caused by alcohol, other drugs, or illnesses during pregnancy. Babies whose mothers had German measles during the first three months of pregnancy may be born blind, deaf, or with heart defects. When these conditions occur, it is important to know that they were not inherited and will not be passed on to future generations.

Traits that people create for themselves, such as curly hair from having a permanent, or blond hair from bleaching, do not change the genes carried by those people. Artificially changed traits will not be passed on to children.

STOP REVIEW
SECTION 1

REMEMBER?

1. What is DNA?

2. How are genes involved in heredity?

3. What is the difference between dominant and recessive genes?

THINK!

4. What, do you think, would happen if reproductive cells divided like other body cells?

5. Compare and contrast mitosis and meiosis.

74

2 Physical Growth and Change

When an ovum is fertilized by a sperm cell, the fertilized cell divides many times. The developing new organism, which is called an **embryo,** slowly forms various tissues, organs, and body systems. The time between fertilization and birth, in humans, is usually about 266 days, or almost nine months.

What Development Occurs Before Birth?

The embryo is called a **fetus** after the second month of development. By the end of the third month of development, the fetus is about 3 inches (7 centimeters) long and all of the body systems have formed. During the second three-month period, the fetus begins to move. During the fifth month, the mother can usually feel this movement. By the seventh month, all the body systems of the fetus are functioning. During the final two months before birth, the fetus continues to grow. Lung tissue matures, and fat tissue is added to help the fetus maintain its body temperature. This growth prepares the fetus for survival after birth.

During pregnancy a woman must be very careful about what she takes into her body. The first three months are the most important, even though many women may not yet realize that they are pregnant. At this time, the developing organs of the embryo can be damaged easily by alcohol, other drugs, and tobacco. Such damage can lead to the birth of babies with mental or physical defects. Even commonly used medicines can be harmful. Aspirin, for example, can cause bleeding from the tissues of the embryo.

KEY WORDS

embryo
fetus
maturity
adolescence
puberty

embryo (EHM bree oh), the new organism developing from a fertilized cell.

fetus (FEE tuhs), an unborn baby after the second month of development.

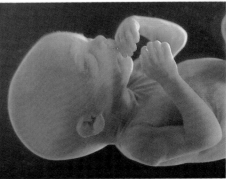

■ *Compare the features of an embryo, left, and a fetus, right.*

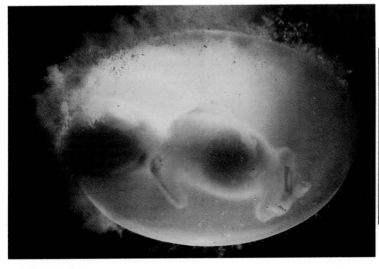

75

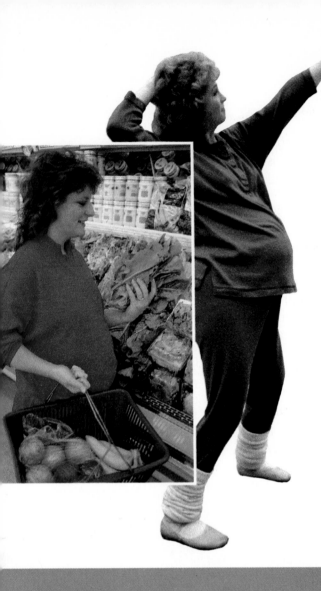

The mother's diet is important during the whole pregnancy. A balanced diet, rich in nutrients such as protein, calcium, and iron, is needed by the mother as well as the fetus. The fetus needs calcium for bone growth, and iron for blood cell development. Muscle and brain cells require large amounts of protein in order to form properly. These nutrients must be supplied through what the mother eats.

Throughout pregnancy the mother's health habits affect the development of the fetus. Tobacco smoking decreases blood circulation in the fetus. Smoking may cause a baby to be born underweight, threatening its survival. Alcohol, even in very small amounts, can harm the fetus. Regular examinations by a physician can detect and solve some problems before they become serious. Exercise helps a woman feel good about herself. It also helps her handle the job of being a mother after the baby is born.

■ *Pregnant women need to exercise and eat foods that will supply the fetus with the nutrients it needs for development.*

Thinking About Your Health

Understanding Your Attitude Toward Wellness

Taking increasing responsibility for yourself is a sign of maturity. Answer the following questions to explore your attitude toward your own wellness:

■ Why is it important to evaluate your personal health habits?

■ Do you need to be reminded to practice certain health habits, such as washing your face?

■ Why do good health habits benefit your intellectual, physical, emotional, and social health?

■ Why is it important for you to make plans to maintain and improve your wellness?

■ Which one of your health habits would you like to improve? How could you improve this habit?

What Development Occurs After Birth?

During the nine months of development before birth, the fertilized ovum grows from a single cell to a baby weighing about 6.5 pounds (3 kilograms). The changes that occur in the first two years after birth are nearly as dramatic. At no time during the rest of a person's life will growth be as rapid.

Newborn infants spend most of their time eating, sleeping, and growing. Their vision and hearing develop quickly, and they begin to take in information about their surroundings.

During the first year, babies begin to master the movement of their bodies. As their muscles develop, they learn to control their heads first. By the age of five months, most babies can roll over and hold objects. By nine months, most babies can sit upright by themselves. Some can crawl. Babies are curious and need people to talk to them and give them new objects to hold so that they can learn.

By one year of age, the baby may weigh three times as much as at birth. At one year, babies are called *toddlers*. Toddlers begin to move around on their own to explore their worlds. As they do, others need to make sure that they stay safe while they move and explore.

■ *During its first year of life, a baby develops the ability to handle objects, crawl, sit, and stand.*

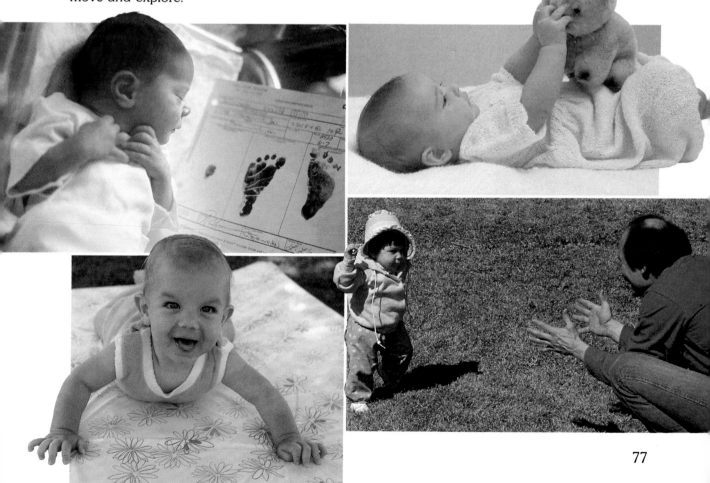

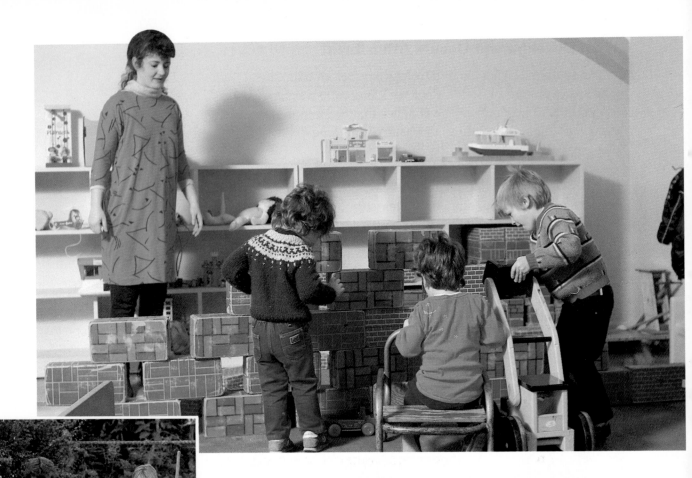

In addition to increasing in body size and strength, toddlers grow and develop in other ways. As their brains develop, they learn to speak and to understand speech. Toddlers quickly recognize new people, places, and things in their environment. As they develop more control over their physical movements, they become ready to master new tasks and activities. However, they still need caring people who will praise their efforts to learn.

Toddlers quickly develop into preschoolers and then school-age children. As their development continues, their physical and mental abilities increase. Young children like to imitate the actions and words of members of their families. When they are about five years old, they begin to form real friendships with other children. Later they develop other skills and begin to discover their physical, intellectual, and creative abilities.

■ Children continue to grow mentally by exploring their environment and by copying the actions of others.

Children's growth and development are influenced by both heredity and environment. A person's heredity only partly determines what he or she may become. As children move from the family into larger environments, their growth and development are influenced by other things as well. The people they know, their experiences at home and in school, their nutrition, and their physical activity all affect their growth and development.

78

What Development Occurs During Adolescence?

In a period of about 15 years, a person develops from a young child into a young adult. What is an adult? How does a child become an adult? Adults have reached a level of **maturity,** or full development. Children are continually growing toward maturity. Complete maturity, however, requires many changes in the body, in emotions, and in relationships. **Adolescence** is the stage of development between childhood and adulthood. Many changes occur during adolescence. These include physical changes in the body, changes in emotions, changes in relationships, and changes in responsibilities and privileges.

maturity (muh TUR uht ee), full development.

adolescence (ad uh LEHS uhns), the stage of development between childhood and adulthood.

■ *Between childhood and adulthood is adolescence. In most people, adolescence is characterized by a period of rapid physical development known as puberty.*

Physical Maturity. The time when many physical changes take place is called **puberty.** Puberty is controlled by the endocrine system. The pituitary gland makes a growth hormone, which affects the growth of bones. When the pituitary gland begins secreting growth hormone, puberty begins, and there is a period of very quick growth.

puberty (PYOO buhrt ee), the time during adolescence when rapid changes in maturity start.

Girls most often reach puberty before boys. Puberty often begins for a girl between the ages of 11 and 14, although it may start earlier or later. For boys, puberty often starts between the ages of 13 and 16. At about age 16 for girls and 18 for boys, the pituitary gland stops making growth hormone. By then the person will have reached full adult height. The person will be about 3 to 3.5 times taller than at birth.

79

All parts of the body do not grow at the same rate during adolescence. Hands and feet will probably grow first. At times, they may seem too big for the rest of the body. Next, arms and legs will begin their rapid growth. Some young people may feel clumsy because they always seem to be dropping things or tripping over their own feet. Finally, the trunk of the body will grow and catch up in size to the rest of the body.

Sexual Maturity. The physical development of puberty is accompanied by sexual development. The pituitary gland sends hormones to the reproductive organs that signal them to begin developing. As the reproductive organs develop, they secrete their own hormones, which cause other parts of the body to form the physical characteristics of an adult.

The testes in a male's body secrete a hormone called *testosterone*. Testosterone causes secondary sex characteristics such as facial hair and voice changes to develop.

A female's ovaries secrete a hormone called *estrogen*. Estrogen affects her body in many ways, causing secondary sex characteristics such as breasts to develop. These secondary sex characteristics change her body from that of a girl to that of a woman. Estrogen also causes the maturing and releasing of an ovum on a regular cycle. When this begins to occur, a female is capable of becoming pregnant. Avoiding sexual contact—or practicing abstinence—will ensure that pregnancy does not occur.

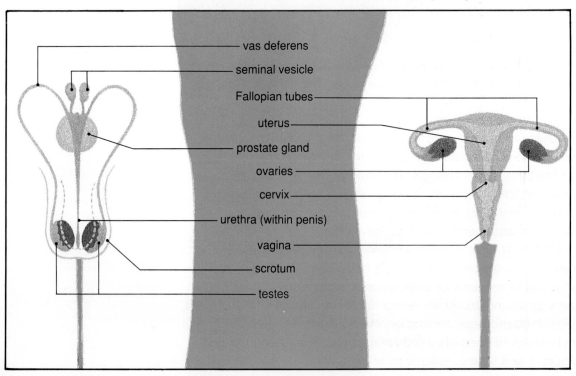

vas deferens

seminal vesicle

Fallopian tubes

uterus

prostate gland

ovaries

cervix

urethra (within penis)

vagina

scrotum

testes

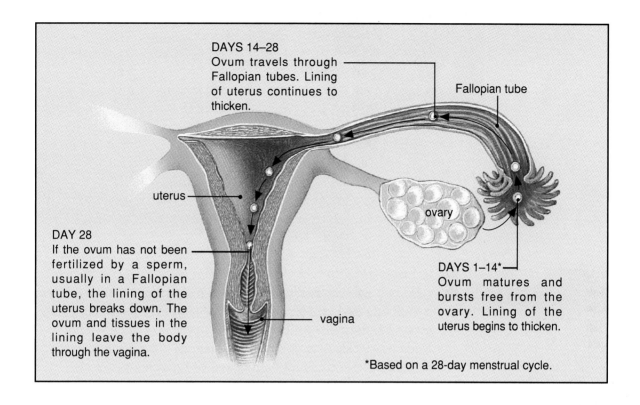

DAYS 14–28
Ovum travels through Fallopian tubes. Lining of uterus continues to thicken.

Fallopian tube

uterus

DAY 28
If the ovum has not been fertilized by a sperm, usually in a Fallopian tube, the lining of the uterus breaks down. The ovum and tissues in the lining leave the body through the vagina.

ovary

vagina

DAYS 1–14*
Ovum matures and bursts free from the ovary. Lining of the uterus begins to thicken.

*Based on a 28-day menstrual cycle.

■ The menstrual cycle prepares a female body for the possibility of an ovum being fertilized.

What Is Aging?

You have been growing older, or aging, since the day you were born. Aging does not suddenly begin when a person is 50 or 60 years old. The term *aging* is used at the time when many signs of aging appear. Aging is a natural process that happens to everyone. How it happens depends partly on heredity and partly on health habits formed as a young person.

Most people think of old age in terms of physical change. Wrinkles may appear in the skin, especially if the person has spent a lot of time in the sun. The hair becomes gray, coarse, and less full. Muscle tone and bone strength are not as easy to maintain. The older person must exercise to keep these tissues healthy.

Some characteristics considered to be a part of the aging process may actually be caused by disease that began at an early age. A heart attack, for example, is not a characteristic of old age. It is a sign of heart disease that may have been developing for many years.

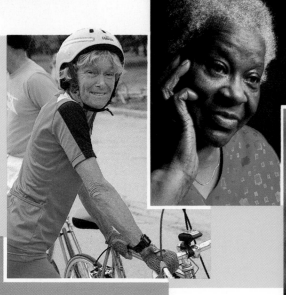
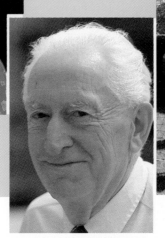
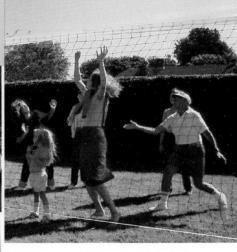
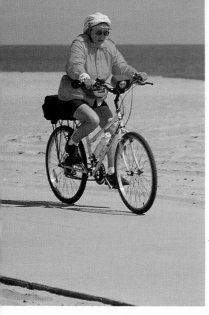

No one knows exactly what causes the changes that take place in the body as a person grows older. Aging may have something to do with the cells. An older person's cells do not grow and divide as quickly as a younger person's do. As a result, damaged or worn-out parts cannot be repaired or replaced as quickly. However, even as people age, they can still maintain wellness.

The habits you form now will contribute to your wellness and may influence how long and how well you live. For example, if you do not smoke, chew tobacco, or drink alcohol, you might live longer than people who do. If you eat healthful foods, keep your weight in a normal range, and get regular exercise and sleep, you will add to your chances of enjoying wellness throughout a long life.

■ *No one knows exactly what causes a person to age. However, good habits formed now can help you maintain wellness as you age.*

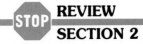 **REVIEW**
SECTION 2

REMEMBER?

1. What is an embryo?
2. What development takes place during the first year of life?
3. What happens to your body as you age?

THINK!

4. How are physical and sexual maturity related?
5. In what ways could your health habits as a young person affect your wellness in old age?

Health Close-up

Aging

Infants born in 1900 could expect to live an average of about 45 years. In contrast, infants born now can expect to live an average of about 75 years. A few people will even live beyond 100 years. But why do our bodies not last forever? Scientists who study aging have always wondered why people age. Many agree that heredity is involved in aging, but they are not sure exactly how.

Studies have shown that the chemicals produced by old cells are exactly the same as the chemicals produced by young cells. However, research shows that older cells reproduce more slowly. Older cells also take longer to repair themselves when damaged.

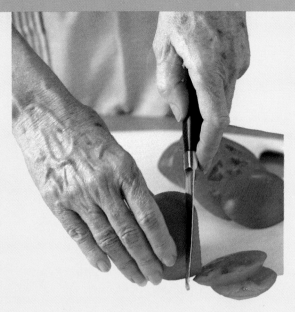

■ *Spots on the skin are one sign of aging.*

■ *The average life expectancy of a person born today is about 75 years. However, some people live beyond 100 years.*

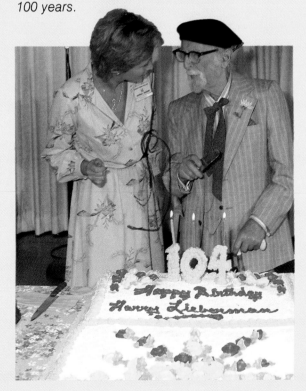

There is a law of nature that says systems become more disorganized as time passes. Some scientists think that body cells are victims of this law. Disorder in cells appears in the form of mistakes in the makeup of the cells' chemicals. The chemicals no longer do the job that they are supposed to do. Perhaps these mistakes damage cells and cause the changes we see as people age.

Today scientists are searching for the causes of these mistakes. They do not have a complete explanation for aging yet, but progress is being made. In the future, people can expect to live longer, healthier lives if they practice good health habits.

Thinking Beyond

1. Why has life expectancy increased so much since 1900 even though the aging process is still not fully understood?
2. How might good health habits add to the length of people's lives?

3 Emotional and Social Growth

Your teenage years are a time of tremendous growth. Even when physical growth has stopped, many changes will continue to occur in your personality and in your relationships with other people. You will be expected to take on new responsibilities. Most of these changes will take place because of your increasing emotional and social maturity.

■ *As children grow, they mature physically, intellectually, socially, and emotionally.*

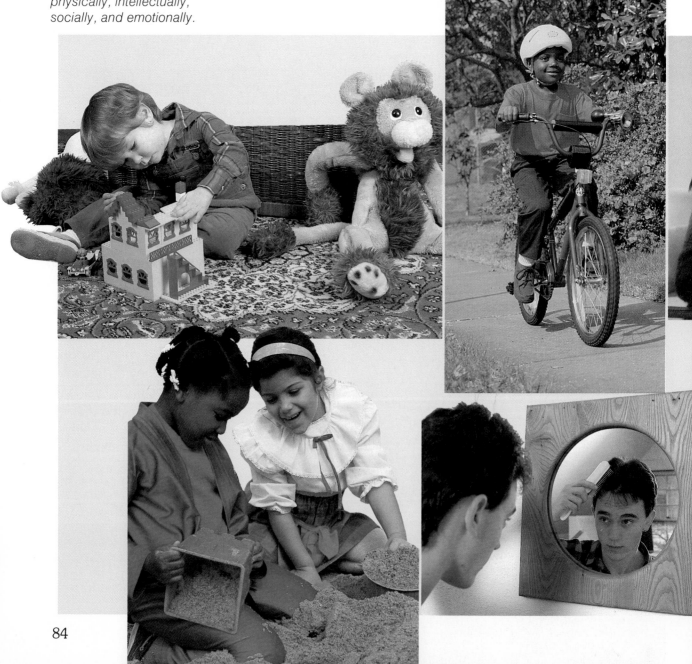

In their teenage years, many people start to think about a job or career. During their twenties and thirties, some people marry and start a family. All of these experiences contribute to growth and development. When you think of adults that you know, it may seem to you that they are no longer growing and changing. Yet many adults continue to learn new things and discover new abilities throughout their lives. They continue to try new activities and to learn from their experiences, just as you do.

■ *Growth and development continue throughout life.*

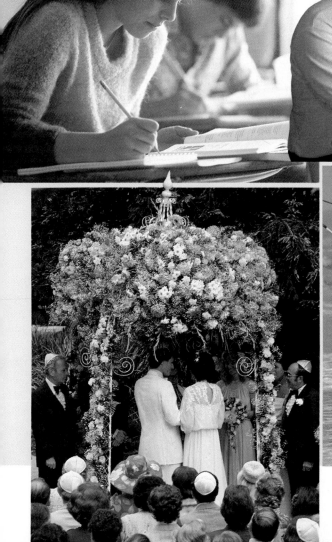

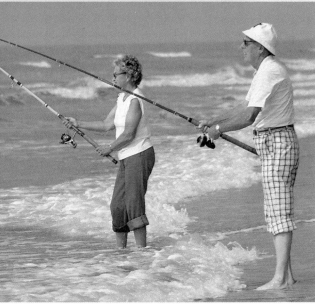

How Do Changes Affect Self-Concept and Self-Esteem?

Changes in your body affect more than just your body's appearance or functioning. They also affect how you think about yourself—your self-concept. When you are used to yourself being a certain way, it may be difficult to see yourself in a new way and to change your self-concept.

In order to feel good about yourself, or have high self-esteem, you need to deal with any negative feelings you may have about your body. It might help to realize that puberty happens to everyone. Your parents, your teachers, and your favorite movie and sports stars experienced puberty. At some time in life, all people are faced with major changes in the size, shape, and functioning of their bodies. Having information about what causes these changes can help you accept them. Talking about your feelings with people that you trust, such as your parents, helps you deal with your changing self-concept. You will find out that you are not the only person who has ever had such feelings. Knowing that all these changes and feelings are natural can help you feel better about yourself.

Another way to improve your self-esteem is to work on changing those things about your body that you do not like and that can be improved. By improving your diet, exercise program, and relaxation and sleep patterns, you can help your body look and perform better.

■ *Talking with parents about physical changes can help you develop a positive self-concept.*

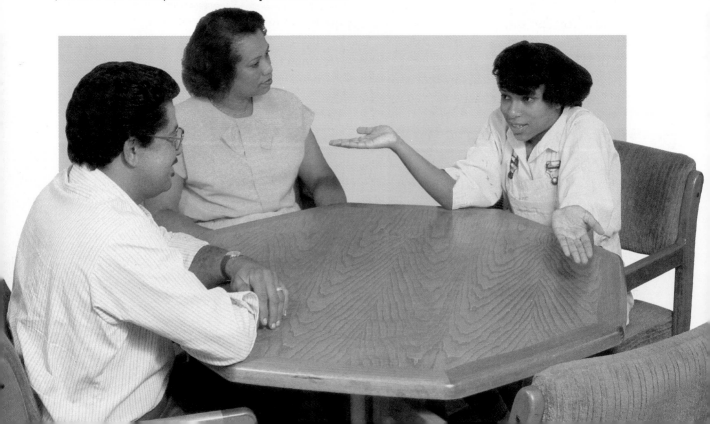

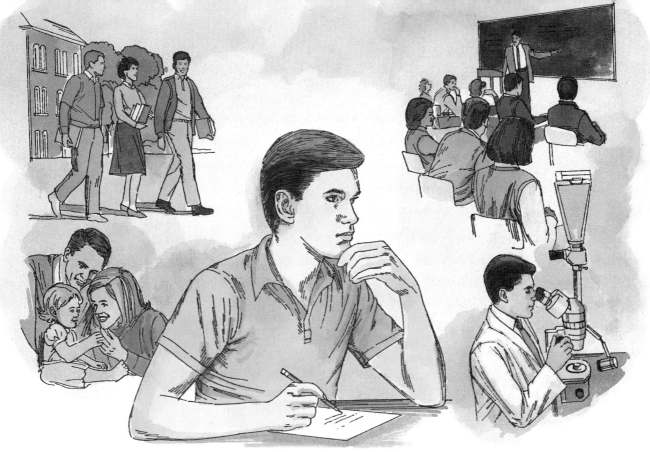

■ As changes occur in life, a person needs to maintain a positive self-concept.

An emotionally mature person has high self-esteem. Emotional maturity does not just happen. You need to develop it within yourself. You can start this by having a self-concept based on accurate information about your body. You need to accept the things about your body that you cannot change. You need to change unhealthful feelings or actions into healthful ones to improve your body's appearance and functioning.

What Is Responsibility?

Every person has a variety of needs. These include physical, intellectual, social, and emotional needs. It is impossible for a person to meet all of these needs alone. As people grow and become more mature, they learn to meet more of their own needs without having to rely on other people. They also learn how to help others meet needs. Helping others is part of becoming a more responsible person.

Maturity involves understanding what your needs are and identifying responsible ways to fulfill needs.

■ A responsible person helps others meet their needs.

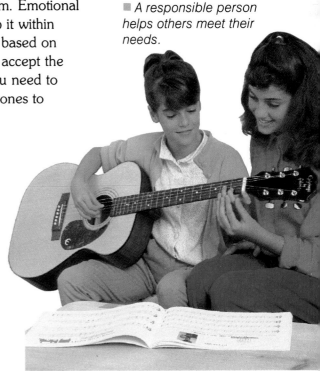

87

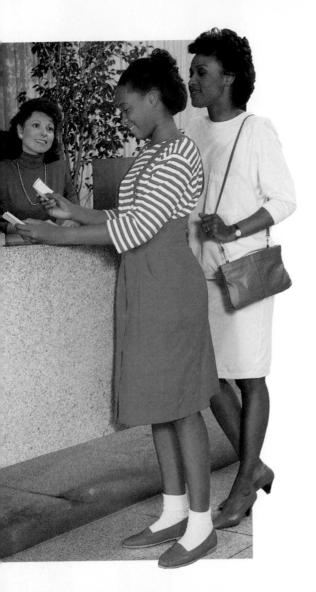

All this always takes some planning, some waiting, and some working toward goals. Maturity also means learning what other people think and feel. A mature person is concerned that other people meet their needs, too.

What Does It Mean to Be Grown-up?

As people become adults, they are expected to take care of, or be responsible for, their own physical needs. To be able to afford food, water, shelter, clothing, and health care, most people need to develop skills for which they will be paid. Besides providing money, jobs may also give people a sense of accomplishment.

In order to fulfill some of their emotional needs, many adults choose marriage and some choose to have children. By becoming parents, they are no longer responsible only for themselves, but for other lives as well. More money is needed in order to provide children with food, clothes, shelter, and other necessities. Parents need to be educated in order to get jobs and to understand their children's development.

■ *Saving money that you earn can give you a sense of accomplishment.*

Making Wellness Choices

José was excited about meeting his new co-worker at the flower shop. He took extra care while getting ready for work that day. José made sure that his uniform was clean and pressed and that his hair was combed and his nails were clean. When Jack arrived for work, he was dressed in a badly wrinkled shirt and worn jeans. His hair was messy, his nails were dirty, he was unshaven, and he needed a bath.

? What could José say to Jack about appearance and working at the flower shop? How could both of them act in responsible ways? Explain your wellness choices.

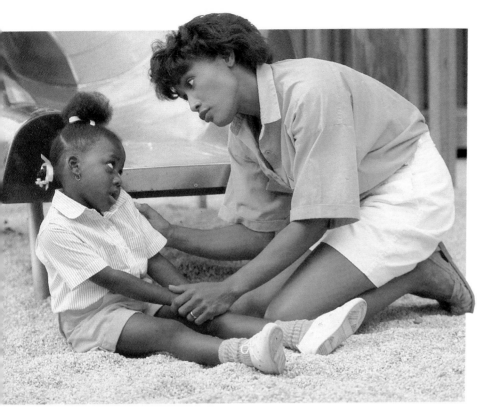

Parents need to be emotionally prepared to devote time and attention to their children. It takes many different resources to support children. Even though people may be physically able to produce babies, they may not be emotionally or socially mature enough to cope with children. Helping others fulfill their needs instead of just fulfilling your own needs is part of becoming mature, responsible, and grown-up.

STOP ═══════════════ **REVIEW
SECTION 3**

REMEMBER?

1. What is a person's self-concept?
2. During the teenage years, what conditions are likely to change a person's self-concept?
3. What are two ways a person can improve self-esteem?

THINK!

4. How would you describe an emotionally mature person?
5. How would you describe a socially mature person?

People in Health

An Interview with a Geneticist

> *Lester Weiss knows about genes and heredity. He is a geneticist at a major hospital in Detroit, Michigan.*

What do geneticists do?

Geneticists are concerned with the study of genes, particularly the ways in which genes relate to health disorders. Some geneticists are physicians and work directly with patients. Other geneticists work in laboratories, researching ways to cure or prevent genetic disorders. Geneticists also explore nongenetic causes of birth defects, such as the use of drugs, alcohol, and other chemicals during pregnancy.

How might a person's environment affect genes and cause some kinds of disorders?

Overexposure to X rays or the sun's rays can produce environmental damage that may cause a disorder such as cancer. However, not everybody exposed to the sun will get skin cancer. This is because not everybody has the *genetic predisposition,* or genetic makeup, to get cancer in this way.

How can knowing about genetic makeup help a person stay healthy?

By studying people's genes, a geneticist can identify those who are at risk for certain conditions such as heart disease. With that information, a person can modify diet and life-style to reduce the risk. The person can eat foods low in cholesterol and get more exercise.

How does a geneticist learn about people's genes?

To gather information about genes, a geneticist takes a complete medical and family history. Then the geneticist examines the patient for clues as to what might have caused a genetic disorder. A geneticist might order certain chromosome tests. If a genetic disorder is suspected in an unborn child, a geneticist may also do a prenatal diagnosis, which is a genetic study done before a child is born. About 1 in every 200 babies have some kind of chromosome problem.

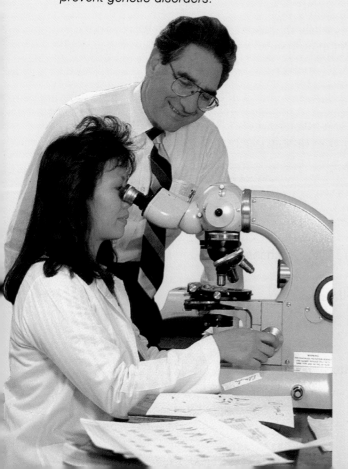

■ *Some geneticists search for ways to prevent genetic disorders.*

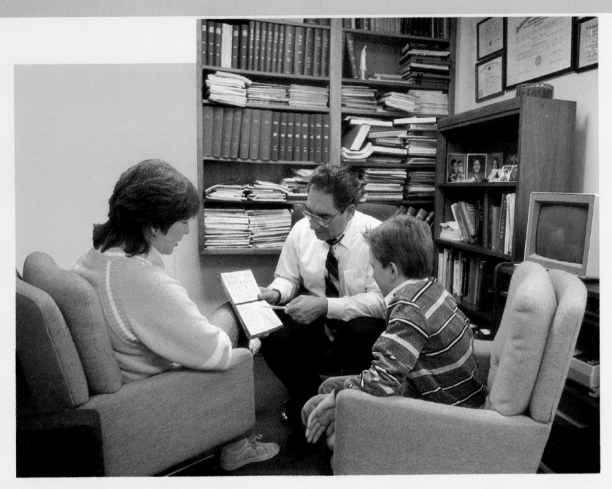

■ *Dr. Weiss discusses the details of a genetic disorder with family members.*

What can be done if you find a genetic problem?

It depends on the nature of the problem. It might mean simply modifying the diet. In the future, there may be many more options available. Genetic researchers are now working to find ways to change a person's genetic predisposition for disorders. If a person had a predisposition for a fatal disease, the ability to change the genes in that person could save his or her life.

What education does a person need to become a geneticist?

There are various kinds of geneticists. Most researchers and physicians need a medical degree or other advanced degree. Genetic counselors or genetic associates, who work with other geneticists, need a college degree.

Learn more about the work of geneticists. Interview a geneticist. Or write for information to the American Society of Human Genetics, 9650 Rockville Pike, Bethesda, MD 20814.

91

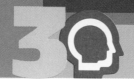

Main Ideas

- Body cells divide to make new cells by mitosis. Reproductive cells are made by meiosis.
- Heredity is controlled by factors in each reproductive cell.
- Organ development occurs during the time the developing baby is an embryo.
- Heredity and environment work together as a person develops physical and personality traits.
- During puberty, your pituitary gland produces a chemical that causes your reproductive organs to develop and mature.
- Aging is the continuous process of growing older.
- An accurate self-concept and high self-esteem are necessary if a person is to become an emotionally mature person.

Key Words

Write the numbers 1 to 12 in your health notebook or on a separate sheet of paper. After each number, copy the sentence and fill in the missing term. Page numbers in ( ) tell you where to look in the chapter if you need help.

mitosis (70)	recessive (72)
nucleus (70)	embryo (75)
chromosomes (70)	fetus (75)
meiosis (71)	maturity (79)
genes (72)	adolescence (79)
dominant (72)	puberty (79)

1. Threadlike structures called ___?___ are duplicated right before a cell divides.

2. ___?___ contain the DNA that determines inherited traits.

3. The stage of emotional and social growth called ___?___ occurs between childhood and adulthood.

4. When a person is fully developed, he or she has reached physical ___?___ .

5. The stronger gene of a pair is the ___?___ gene.

6. The weaker gene of a pair is the ___?___ gene.

7. The process of ___?___ produces two cells identical to the original.

8. The process of ___?___ forms reproductive cells.

9. The organism produced from a fertilized cell is an ___?___ .

10. The ___?___ is the part of the cell that controls the cell's activities.

11. An embryo is called a ___?___ once all of the body systems have formed.

12. The time of rapid change as a person begins adolescence is ___?___ .

Remembering What You Learned

Page numbers in ( ) tell you where to look in the chapter if you need help.

1. What are two different ways in which cells divide? (70–71)

2. What do chromosomes do before a cell divides? (70)

3. What is the function of DNA? (70)

4. What happens right after a sperm cell fertilizes an ovum? (71)

5. What determines inherited traits? (72)

6. Why are nonhereditary birth defects not passed on to future generations? (74)

7. What happens to a fertilized human cell during the nine months after fertilization? (75)

8. What are some substances that can harm the development of a fetus? (75–76)

9. What are two ways in which a baby grows and develops during the first year of its life? (77–78)

10. What is the adolescent growth spurt? When is it likely to occur? (79)

11. What causes the adolescent growth spurt? (79)

12. Why do some teenagers look more grown-up than their friends of the same age? (79)

13. What are two examples of body changes during adolescence? (80–81)

14. What are two factors that may be responsible for signs of aging? (81–82)

15. What physical changes may become noticeable as people approach old age? (81–82)

16. What kinds of experiences contribute to social and emotional growth after the teenage years? (84–85)

Thinking About What You Learned

1. Why do all 15-year-old males not grow at the same rate?

2. In what ways could a person be physically mature enough, but not emotionally or socially ready, to have a baby?

3. Will a person's self-concept be exactly the same all through his or her life? Why or why not?

4. Why does adolescence involve a change in self-concept?

5. Describe one way in which your family has influenced your wellness habits.

6. Why should women who are pregnant have medical care?

Writing About What You Learned

1. Whether you are aware of it or not, you are constantly making decisions about your health. Think about a recent health decision you have made. Write a one-page description of what that health decision was and what influenced your decision. How do you feel now about the decision you made? Would you make the same decision again? Why or why not?

2. Describe two ways in which a person who is unhappy about his or her appearance can increase his or her self-esteem.

Applying What You Learned

SOCIAL STUDIES

Every ten years, a government agency called the Census Bureau gathers information about the country's growth and development. This information includes facts about the numbers of people of different ages that make up the population of the United States. From reference books in the library or from an almanac, find out how the age distribution of the United States has changed since the year 1900.

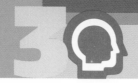

Modified True or False

Write the numbers 1 to 15 in your health notebook or on a separate sheet of paper. After each number, write *true* or *false* to describe the sentence. If the sentence is false, also write a term that replaces the underlined term and makes the sentence true.

1. The new cells that result from cell division are called <u>parent</u> cells.

2. Babies who are one year old are called <u>embryos</u>.

3. Puberty is controlled by your <u>reproductive</u> system.

4. After its third month of development, the embryo is called a <u>fetus</u>.

5. If you are <u>mature</u>, you understand what your needs are and how you can responsibly achieve them.

6. An older person's cells do not <u>grow and divide</u> as quickly as a younger person's.

7. The <u>nucleus</u> is the control center of the cell.

8. <u>Maturity</u> is the stage of development between childhood and adulthood.

9. Cell division in which two daughter cells are formed is called <u>meiosis</u>.

10. An emotionally mature person has <u>low</u> self-esteem.

11. A person's growth and development are influenced by his or her heredity and <u>environment</u>.

12. A female's ovaries secrete a hormone called <u>estrogen</u>.

13. <u>Puberty</u> is the time a mother carries the embryo and fetus.

14. The hereditary material that genes are made of is <u>DNA</u>.

15. <u>Genes</u> determine the traits that are passed from parents to children.

Short Answer

Write the numbers 16 to 23 on your paper. Write a complete sentence to answer each question.

16. What is the difference between an embryo and a fetus?

17. What is the difference between mitosis and meiosis?

18. Why do all the cells in your body have exactly the same DNA?

19. How could two parents with dimples, a dominant trait, have a child with no dimples?

20. What birth defects are not inherited?

21. Why does a fetus born at seven months have a good chance of survival?

22. What development does a toddler experience?

23. What are some factors that affect a child's development?

Essay

Write the numbers 24 and 25 on your paper. Write paragraphs with complete sentences to answer each question.

24. What steps can you take to slow down the aging process?

25. Summarize the entire human life span from fertilized egg to old age. Describe the development that can be expected at each stage.

Projects to Do

1. Interview members of your family about their family responsibilities. Make a chart listing all of the responsibilities that each person has, including yourself. Discuss with the family members how they feel about their family roles. How does each person's role indicate a stage of development?

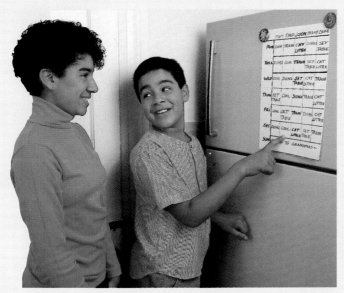

■ *All members of a family have certain responsibilities.*

2. Collect news reports about products or habits that can harm an embryo or fetus. Consider chemical pollutants, tobacco smoke, alcohol, medicines, and other drugs. Create a bulletin board display describing harmful products or habits.

Information to Find

1. Over 100 years ago, much information about heredity was discovered by Gregor Mendel. At your school library or public library, find out more about Mendel's experiments and what they revealed about heredity.

2. An organization called the March of Dimes collects money and provides funds for research into birth defects. Call or write your local March of Dimes chapter for information about the organization's work. Or write to the national headquarters at this address: March of Dimes Birth Defects Foundation, 1275 Mamaronech Avenue, White Plains, NY 10605. Prepare a report based on the information you receive from the organization.

3. Physicians believe that people's health habits contribute to their wellness. Physicians believe that these habits greatly influence life expectancy. Make a list of health habits that may increase life expectancy and a list of health habits that may decrease life expectancy. Decide which of these health habits you can develop now to maintain wellness and to increase your life expectancy.

Books to Read

Here are some books you can look for in your school library or the public library to find more information about human growth and development.

Bornstein, Jerry, and Sandy Bornstein. *New Frontiers in Genetics.* Messner.

Brister, C. W. *Becoming You.* Broadman.

Simon, Nissa. *Don't Worry, You're Normal.* T. Y. Crowell.

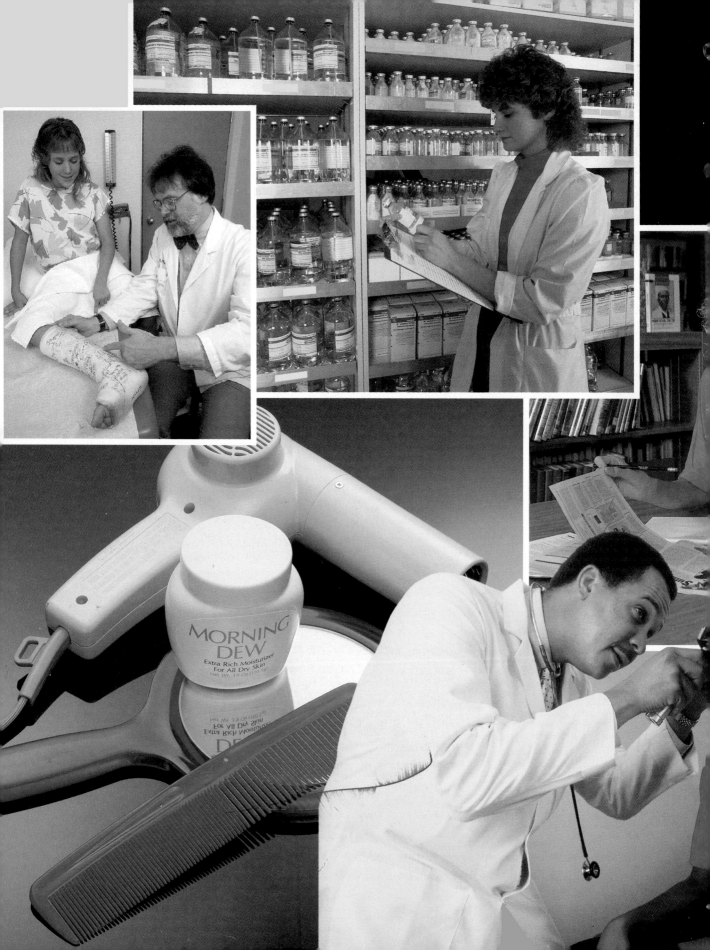

4

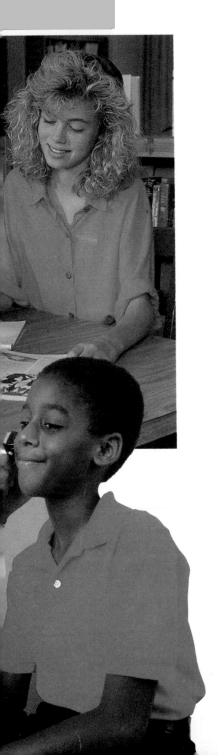

HEALTH CARE CONSUMER CHOICES

You have choices to make about products and services. The products and services you choose to buy as a consumer are important for your health. Your local, state, and federal governments work to protect you from worthless and unsafe health products. But you are still responsible for your consumer decisions.

As an adult, you will select the health professionals from whom you will receive health services. You can learn skills now that will help you inform health workers about your health needs. You can also learn questioning skills that will help you better understand the advice of health workers. You and the health workers need to communicate and work as a team.

GETTING READY TO LEARN

Key Questions

- Why is it important to learn how to care for your body?
- How can you learn to make wise health care choices?
- How are you protected from poor health services?
- How can advertising help you make wise consumer choices?
- What can you do to become more responsible for taking care of your health?

Main Chapter Sections

1 Making Wise Health Care Choices
2 Choosing Health Products
3 You and Your Health Care Team

97

1 Making Wise Health Care Choices

consumer (kuhn SOO muhr), anyone who buys or uses a product or service.

■ *Being a consumer can be confusing. There are so many of products and services from which to choose.*

What is the best treatment for dandruff? Is there a miracle cure for cancer? Is it safe to take a medicine your physician did not prescribe for you? Is it possible to buy a cheaper medicine that will work as well as the one your physician orders? These are just a few of the many health-related questions you might ask as a consumer. A **consumer** is anyone who buys or uses a product or a service. As a consumer, you may have many questions. You need to know how to make wise choices about the health services and products you use.

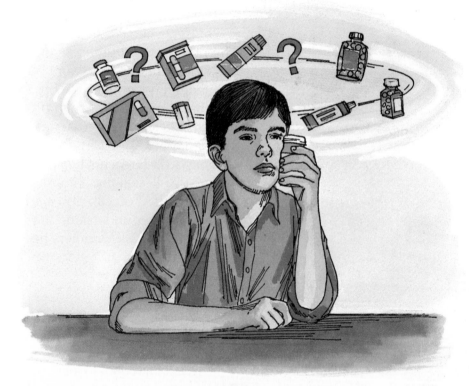

How Can You Make Wise Health Care Choices?

Anita was preparing for her summer vacation. The family was planning to spend a week at the beach, and Anita was looking forward to swimming. She had checked the weather report and found that there would be clear skies.

Anita enjoyed the beach, but she also knew about the dangers of too much sun. She knew she needed a sunscreen, but she was not sure about which product to buy. When Anita went to the pharmacy, she was surprised at the number and variety of sunscreens.

SPF (SUN PROTECTION FACTOR)	
SPF Levels	**Amount of Protection**
SPF 0 to 3	no protection
SPF 4 to 6	mild protection for skin that tans easily and rarely burns
SPF 7 to 8	extra protection that still permits tanning
SPF 9 to 10	excellent protection for skin that burns easily
SPF 11 to 15 and up	total protection that blocks the sun's rays

Anita decided to go to the library to find out more about sunscreens. The librarian recommended a magazine that evaluated consumer products. An article on sunscreens gave Anita a lot of information. Results of tests done with many brands of sunscreens were explained in the article. The best kind of sun protection for people of each skin type was recommended. Using this information, Anita was able to narrow her choice to two effective sunscreens.

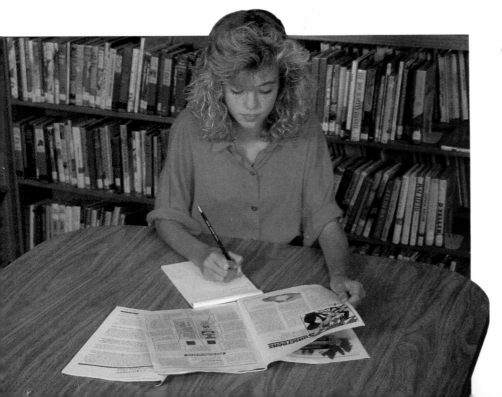

■ Reading about health products and services in a consumer magazine can help you make decisions about which ones to use.

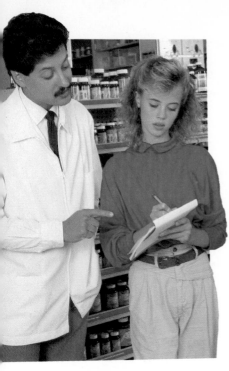

Anita went back to the pharmacy to check the price of the two brands of sunscreen. She asked the pharmacist which sun protection factor (SPF) she should use. The pharmacist told her that SPF 15 or higher of either brand would be safe for her. Anita selected SPF 15 of the less expensive brand. She saved money, yet she still got the sunscreen protection she needed.

Anita had a great time at the beach, and she did not get sunburned. She felt good about the effort she had put into her consumer decision. Working through the decision-making steps helped her make a wise choice. The following decision-making steps can be useful when making any consumer choice:

1. Realize a choice is needed.
2. Find out about all the choices that could be made.
3. Think about the consequences of each possible choice.
4. Make what seems to be the best choice.
5. Think about what happened as a result of the choice.

When making health care decisions, you should always find out about all the possibilities. There are many sources of information about health care products. You can use these sources to your advantage.

■ Your pharmacist is a good source of information about health care products.

■ Having made an informed decision about which sunscreen product to use, Anita can now have fun at the beach without worrying about sunburn.

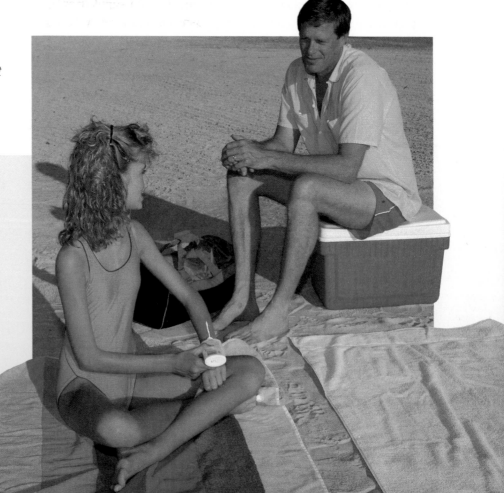

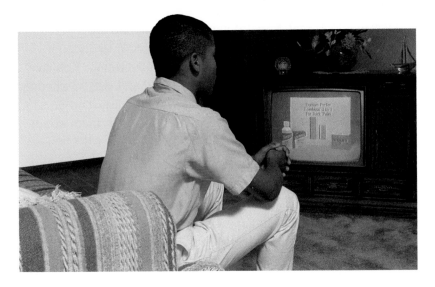

■ *Accurate, honest advertising can help you make a decision about a health product or service.*

How Does Advertising Affect Your Decisions?

There are many advertised products that you can buy to help your appearance and protect your health. **Advertising** is anything done to make consumers aware of products and services and to encourage them to buy. Advertising lets consumers know about new products and services. It describes supposed benefits. Shampoos, toothpastes, vitamin supplements, antiseptics, cold remedies, and mouthwashes are just a few of the health products that use advertising to encourage consumers to buy.

Accurate advertising can help consumers shop for safe and useful products. For example, if you need to buy an over-the-counter medicine for allergy relief, you can read advertisements to find out what symptoms the medicines are supposed to relieve. Advertising may also tell you how to use the medicines.

Advertising may give the cost of a product or service. It may tell consumers where to buy it. Competition in advertising can help lower the prices of some products. If you know what product you want to buy, you can check advertments to find the best price or the closest store.

Advertising tries to sell a product; it is not always completely accurate. But many people believe everything they hear or read in advertising messages. Most consumers say that advertising is the chief source of information they use when choosing over-the-counter medicines, for example. Misleading and inaccurate advertising can keep consumers from making wise choices.

Judging a product from advertisements is not always easy. The product may not always give you what you expected from reading the advertisement. You may have picked the lowest-priced product or service and discovered that it was of poor quality.

advertising (AD vuhr tyz ihng), anything done to make consumers aware of products and services and to encourage them to buy.

Keeping a Health Directory

You can create a directory of health services that are available to you. Begin by using a notebook to list the telephone numbers and addresses of your physician, dentist, pharmacist, hospital, and any specialists you visit. You can add community and government organizations as you learn about them.

license (LYS uhns), a permit given to an individual who meets the qualifications for a profession.

■ *Some government regulations provide protection against the spread of disease.*

For example, you may have bought something that an advertisement said would help skin problems, only to discover that it had no real effect. You cannot ignore advertising. You can, however, think about what is being advertised and decide whether or not you need the product. Your physician, dentist, school nurse, and pharmacist are experts. You can talk with them about the value of over-the-counter health products.

How Does the Government Protect Your Health?

To protect the consumer, governments have set up consumer laws and regulations. A regulation is a rule that deals with details or procedures. Local, state, and federal governments have formed agencies or departments to enforce health laws. These groups are responsible for protecting the consumer. They make sure that health products are safe.

Health products are controlled by consumer health laws. Aspirin, sunscreen, eyeglasses, shampoo, and toothpaste are just a few of the products controlled by those laws.

Besides monitoring health products for consumer protection, governments have laws and regulations to protect you from poor health services. Each state is responsible for issuing a permit called a **license** to every pharmacist, physician, dentist, nurse, and other health professional. If a health professional has a license, you know that he or she has the basic qualifications needed to give health services. People who do not pass licensing tests do not get licenses to practice health services. Under the law, people who try to practice health care without a license can be fined and sent to prison.

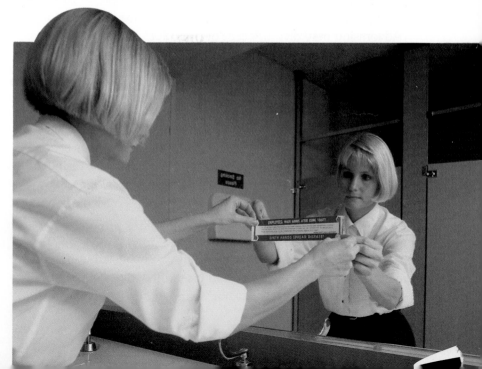

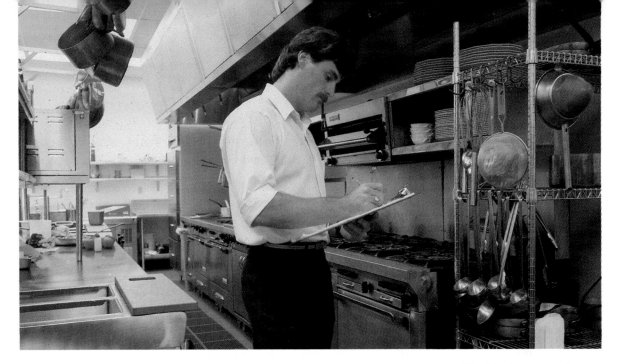

Every state and many communities have health departments. A health department is responsible for protecting the health of local citizens. One way the health department reaches this goal is by giving screening tests to find certain health problems. The health department gives other health services, such as immunization programs. Health departments check restaurants, health clubs, hospitals, and other places to be sure they are clean and to prevent the spread of diseases. Health departments keep records on health problems for the citizens they serve. Health departments also develop programs to help solve and prevent health problems.

■ *Health department inspectors check public places that prepare and serve food. The inspectors ensure that sanitary conditions are maintained.*

STOP REVIEW SECTION 1

REMEMBER?

1. What is a consumer?
2. What is the purpose of having consumer health laws?
3. List five steps for making a good health decision.

THINK!

4. How does advertising affect your own health care choices?
5. What might happen if the government did not make laws and regulations for consumers of health products and services?

2 Choosing Health Products

Health and grooming aids can help you stay healthy, feel good, and look attractive. Some examples are toothpaste, shampoo, soap, aspirin, and allergy medicine.

When you choose health and grooming aids, you may want to ask yourself these questions:

- Do I really need this kind of product?
- Which product best fills my needs?
- Which brand should I buy?
- What size is the best buy for my needs?
- Can this product harm me?

What Do Product Labels Tell You?

One way to answer your questions about health products is to read labels. Like food labels, health-product labels give several kinds of information. Information such as the kind of product, the brand name, the ingredients, and the name and address of the manufacturer may be found on the label.

Product Description and List of Ingredients.   Many labels describe what the product does. They may use phrases like "for relief of headaches," "stops wetness and odor," or "helps control dandruff." They may also have a few words of advertising.

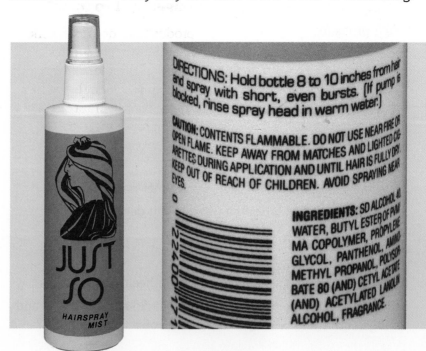

■ The labels of health products should give directions for use, a list of ingredients, and any special precautions that must be followed.

KEY WORDS

sebaceous gland
sebum
acne
deodorant
antiperspirant
fluoride

104

"Leaves hair soft and shiny" and "makes teeth whiter" are two examples of advertising phrases.

Most labels also list ingredients. By reading these lists, you can compare the ingredients of one product with those of another. You can also tell if a certain brand has an ingredient you do not want to use. For example, you might want to avoid using a cough medicine that contains alcohol. If alcohol is an ingredient, it must be listed.

Directions for Use.   Since many health and grooming aids can threaten your wellness if not used properly, most labels have directions for use. The label on a liquid medicine might say, "Take one teaspoonful every four to six hours."

Labels often have a warning of possible dangers, such as "Harmful if swallowed" or "Keep out of the reach of young children." Hair sprays and other sprays warn against storing the cans near heat. Under high temperatures, the cans might explode. Many hair care products and deodorants are also flammable and will burn if used near a flame or cigarette. This information is included on the label.

Labels often give instructions to follow in case of an accident. For example, if a skin care product, such as foot powder, is accidentally eaten, the local Poison Control Center, a pharmacist, or a physician can tell you what first aid is needed. The label will give instructions on what to do until a health worker can be contacted.

What Is an Unwise Use of Consumer Products?

It may be costly to buy a health product that does not work. But it can actually be harmful to buy and use a product for something for which it was not intended. In some cases, misusing a product may make a condition worse. It may hide discomfort that should warn of danger. If used regularly, the product may keep you from seeing your physician for proper medical treatment. For these reasons, it is important to use over-the-counter health products as recommended. Using a product in other ways can seriously threaten your health.

What Should You Know Before Buying Products for Your Skin?

Many grooming aids are made to be used on your skin. Some say they will help "teenage skin problems." Others promise to make you more attractive. It is not always easy to know which products will help and which will irritate your skin.

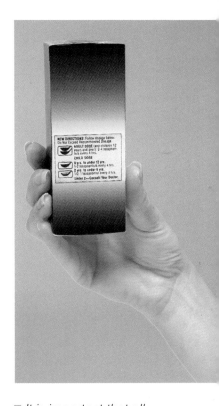

■ *It is important that all directions for use of a health product be followed. Some products may threaten your wellness if used incorrectly.*

About Your Skin. The more you know about your skin, the better you are able to choose products to help you care for it. The skin has three distinct layers. The outer layer, called the *epidermis,* is about as thick as a sheet of paper. Beneath the epidermis lies the *dermis,* where most of the life of the skin goes on. The third layer of skin, beneath the dermis, is called *subcutaneous tissue.*

In the dermis are hair follicles. A single hair grows out of each hair follicle. An oil gland, called the **sebaceous gland,** is connected to each hair follicle. The sebaceous gland makes an oily substance that passes out of tiny ducts to the surface of the skin. The oil, or **sebum,** helps keep your skin soft and moist.

The dermis also contains sweat glands, which carry liquid waste to the surface of the skin. This liquid waste is perspiration. Perspiring, or sweating, is one way in which your body keeps its temperature constant.

Some Skin Problems. Some of the hormone changes that take place in your body during puberty affect your skin. The hormone testosterone causes your sebaceous glands to make much more sebum. Sometimes, the lining of a hair follicle blocks the sebum. Bacteria in the sebum multiply in the plugged follicle. The follicle wall then becomes irritated and bursts. This infection causes the bumps you see as pimples.

Having many pimples on your skin is a sign of **acne.** The skin on your face, neck, chest, and back is most often affected because the sebaceous glands in these areas are large and numerous. Acne is common in adolescence. It usually clears up later in life.

sebaceous gland (sih BAY shuhs • GLAND), an oil gland attached to a hair follicle.

sebum (SEE buhm), oil produced by the sebaceous glands to help keep skin soft and moist.

acne (AK nee), a skin condition in which the person has many pimples.

■ *If a hair follicle becomes blocked by excess sebum, the follicle may become irritated and infected.*

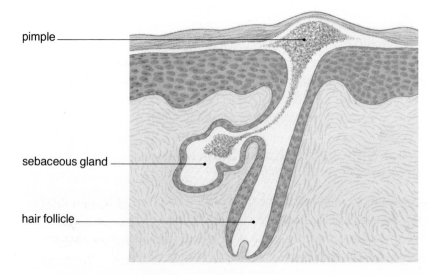

pimple

sebaceous gland

hair follicle

Acne is caused by a hormone that stimulates production of sebum in the hair follicles. This action does not seem to be caused by eating certain foods. Acne does not start because of emotional upsets, although they can make acne worse.

Caring for Your Skin. Eating a balanced diet and getting enough sleep and exercise can help keep your skin healthy. Wash your face with soap and warm water twice a day. Do not squeeze blackheads and pimples, because this can cause scarring. Do not use oily creams and lotions on your skin. They can plug up the openings of the hair follicles.

A physician can help you with acne. If you have a serious case, your physician may suggest that you visit a dermatologist. A *dermatologist* is a physician who treats skin problems.

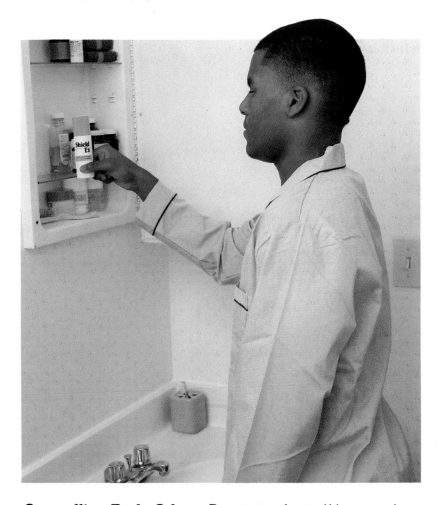

■ *An antiperspirant and deodorant will reduce the amount of sweat your glands produce and will stop the growth of bacteria that cause odor.*

Controlling Body Odor. Perspiration by itself has no odor. Odor comes when perspiration acts with bacteria on the skin. Perspiration comes from sweat glands all over the body. Most perspiration odor seems to come from the area under the arms.

107

deodorant (dee OHD uh ruhnt), a product that helps stop perspiration odor by blocking the growth of bacteria on the skin.

antiperspirant (ant ih PUR spuh ruhnt), a product that reduces the amount of perspiration given off by the sweat glands.

Washing with soap and warm water removes some bacteria. Bathing often, wearing clean clothes, and using a deodorant or an antiperspirant can also help take care of body odors. A **deodorant** has chemicals that stop odor by keeping bacteria from growing. An **antiperspirant** cuts down the amount of perspiration given off by the sweat glands.

If you perspire a lot, you may want to use a product that is both a deodorant and an antiperspirant. The label will give you this information. Most deodorant and antiperspirant labels warn against using the products on broken skin, because the products were not meant to get inside the body. They also advise you to stop using the products if your skin becomes irritated or breaks out in a rash. These reactions may mean you are allergic to an ingredient in the product.

What Should You Know Before Buying Products for Your Hair?

Most people want clean, healthy hair. Many products promise to make your hair look shiny. The more you know about your hair, the better you will be able to decide which products are best for you.

Dandruff forms when oil from sebaceous glands in your scalp dries and mixes with dead skin cells. This causes flakes of dandruff and often an itchy scalp.

Making Wellness Choices

Bob and Todd have been friends since grade school. They have both recently begun to have skin problems. Bob has only a few pimples. But Todd has severe acne, and it has hurt his self-esteem. He has been taking good care of his skin, but he still has trouble. His dermatologist has told him that his skin is very oily right now. His acne will heal when his skin becomes less oily.

Todd does not want to wait. He wants his skin to look better now. He has shown Bob an advertisement in the back of a magazine. The advertisement says a product is able to cure acne "overnight." With this product, which is based on a "scientific breakthrough," acne goes away "like magic." The product, which sells for $30.00, is not found in stores. Todd asks Bob to lend him some money so that he can buy the product.

 What should Bob tell Todd? Explain your wellness choice.

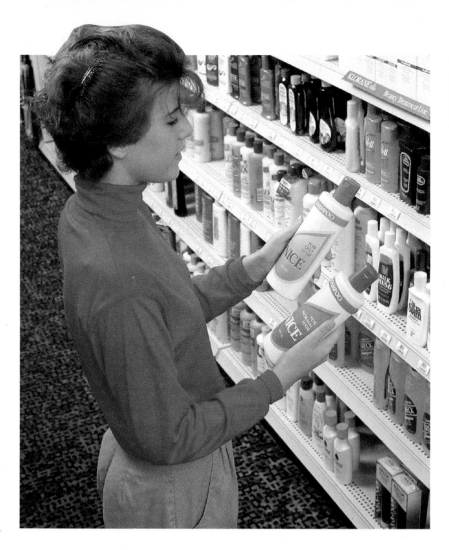

Daily brushing and frequent shampooing can help get rid of dandruff. Certain shampoos have special ingredients to control dandruff. You can buy these shampoos without a prescription. Their labels have phrases like "antidandruff shampoo" or "helps fight dandruff."

In some cases of dandruff, the scalp becomes red and sore. This condition should be treated by a dermatologist. He or she may order a prescription for a shampoo with medicine in it.

What Should You Know Before Buying Dental Health Products?

Healthy teeth and gums are important for eating and speaking properly, looking your best, and maintaining wellness. Proper nutrition is one part of dental care. Regular examinations with thorough cleanings are also important. Keeping your teeth and gums healthy can prevent problems such as tooth decay and gingivitis, a gum disease.

■ Regular brushing with a fluoride toothpaste and daily flossing can help prevent tooth decay and gum disease.

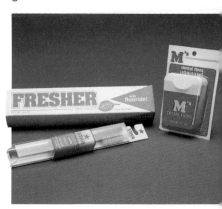

109

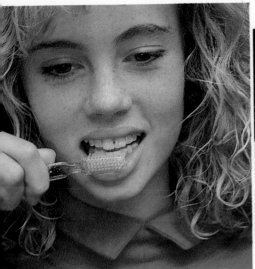

Brush gently at the gumline.

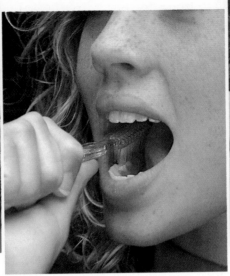

Brush the chewing surfaces.

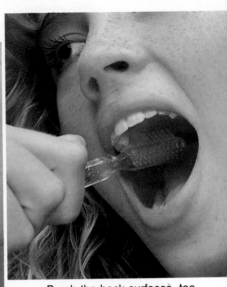

Brush the back surfaces, too.

fluoride (FLUR yd), a substance that strengthens tooth enamel.

One kind of preventive care is the use of a fluoride rinse or toothpaste. **Fluoride** is a substance that helps make tooth enamel strong. Enamel covers each tooth. It is the hardest part of the tooth, yet it can be damaged. Every day, a sticky substance called plaque builds up on your teeth. Plaque acts quickly on certain foods in your mouth, such as white sugar and white flour, and forms a strong acid. This acid can slowly dissolve tooth enamel, leaving cavities. Plaque also causes bad breath.

Brushing the teeth removes plaque from the outer, inner, and chewing surfaces of the teeth. Many dentists tell their patients to brush their teeth with fluoride toothpaste and a toothbrush that has soft bristles and rounded tips.

Use unwaxed dental floss.

Gently work the floss between the teeth.

Floss up and down.

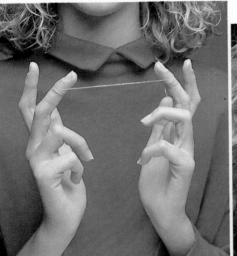

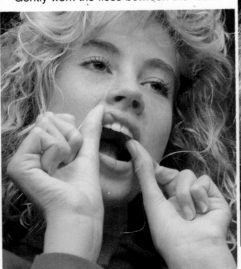

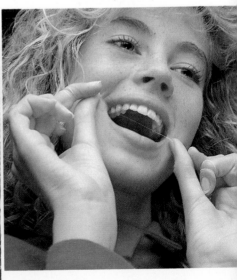

Flossing the teeth removes plaque that builds up between teeth and at the edge of the gums. These are areas where a toothbrush cannot reach. Most dentists recommend the use of unwaxed dental floss. The fibers that make up unwaxed dental floss scrape the teeth cleaner than waxed dental floss can. Also, waxed dental floss may leave wax deposits on the teeth, and more plaque can build up on waxy teeth.

STOP REVIEW SECTION 2

REMEMBER?

1. Why is it important to read directions on health aids?
2. What are two ways to take care of your skin?
3. What are two ways to take care of your teeth and gums?
4. How are deodorants and antiperspirants different?

THINK!

5. What could you do if you discovered you had accidentally used a health product in the wrong way?
6. How could you apply the steps of decision making to selecting a toothpaste?

MYTH AND FACT

Myth: If you wear braces, you can chew gum that is not supposed to stick to braces.

Fact: Any chewing gum can stick to braces. Chewing gum can stick or pull on the wires attached to the braces, preventing the wires from working as they should.

Thinking About Your Health

Are You a Wise Consumer?

How do you know if you are making wise consumer choices for your own good health? Ask yourself whether all of the following statements describe your health habits. You need to talk about your consumer choices with a parent, guardian, school nurse, or teacher.

- You follow the directions on medicines and over-the-counter products.
- You always ask your physician questions about any medicine prescribed for you, to be sure you know its name and expected action.
- You never let advertising be the only reason for your choice of products.
- You have seen your physician's license to practice medicine and your dentist's license to practice dentistry.
- You ask a pharmacist to explain any directions you do not understand on labels of health care products that you have bought.

111

Health Close-up

Health Care in the Future

Because of the rising costs of care for disease and injury, people must be more responsible for their own health care. Computers will become more and more important to consumers in watching their health status. One example of this self-monitoring is known as the Sleep Sentry®. The Sleep Sentry is a device worn on the wrist. It gives off an alarm when skin temperature drops. A drop in skin temperature in a person who has diabetes is a symptom of an insulin reaction. The Sleep Sentry can awaken a person who has diabetes and let him or her know there is a problem.

Computers in the home may also help people monitor their health. The advice of physicians could be given on home computers. The computers would be linked to many programs for watching diet, exercise, stress and other parts of wellness. By answering certain questions from the computers, consumers could check on their health and receive qualified medical advice.

Computers may some day become part of an in-home early warning system. This system would warn consumers of health crises about to occur, such as heart attacks and strokes, based upon preprogrammed health histories. With this information, consumers may be able to avoid the crises through the use of medicines or through changes in life-style.

Computers are playing larger roles in hospitals, where they help cut costs. In one hospital, for example, computers monitor the patient's blood pressure, heart rate, and temperature. This information is shown on a screen by the person's bed. At another hospital, computers measure stomach acid and then graph the information.

Physicians also use computers as medical references. The computer is a source of medical information. The physician can type in the person's symptoms, and the computer will list disorders that have those symptoms. It may also recommend further tests. The physician, however, must still make the medical diagnosis and recommend treatment.

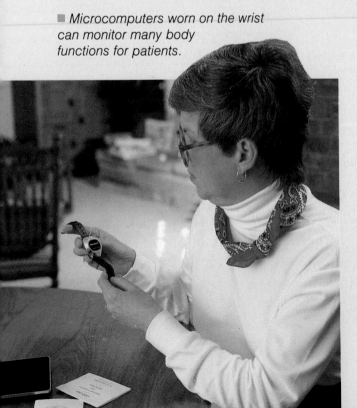

■ *Microcomputers worn on the wrist can monitor many body functions for patients.*

Thinking Beyond

1. What are some other ways in which computers might help people make good health decisions?
2. What might be some disadvantages of using computers in health care?

3 You and Your Health Care Team

The government licenses health care providers. However, each person must still learn how to protect his or her own health. What steps can you follow to select good health care providers?

How Should You Choose a Physician?

Suppose your family moves to a new community and needs to find a new physician. To decide whether a certain physician will meet your needs, you should try to talk with him or her when you are not ill. During that visit, you and your parents should ask questions about fees, services, office hours, and emergency procedures. Your parents might also ask about the physician's medical training. The physician's license to practice medicine should be displayed somewhere in his or her office. If it is not, you should ask to see it.

Choosing a physician when you are healthy and able to make sound judgments is being a wise consumer. It is also important that you find a physician with whom you can talk openly. Your physician depends on you for information about the

KEY WORDS

quacks
medical insurance

■ *It is important to choose health professionals who are qualified and who make you feel comfortable.*

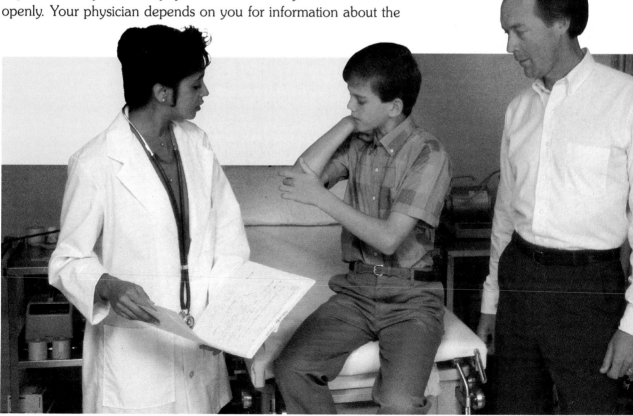

signs or symptoms of any illness or injury. The history of your problem includes a description of what you have done already to help yourself feel better. This information is important to the physician who is deciding how to treat your health problem.

You and your physician need to work as a team. The physician is an expert in diagnosing and curing illness. You are the expert about your body and habits. You may be given a prescription for medicine, an exercise plan, or a diet plan. Your responsibility is to use the medicine, do the exercise plan, or follow the diet as directed. You may need help from other members of a health care team, such as a nurse or therapist, in order to restore and maintain your health.

BEING A MEMBER OF YOUR HEALTH CARE TEAM

You need to ...

- ask what treatment the health worker plans for you.
- ask what technical words mean.
- ask what your test results mean; do not just accept that they are "normal."
- tell what you have done to help yourself feel better.
- answer truthfully when asked about your daily habits.
- say what worries you about your illness, feelings, symptoms, or injuries.
- ask for a picture or sketch to explain what is happening inside your body.
- ask what to expect from treatment and how long it will take.
- ask what symptoms you need to report to the health worker before the next visit.

How Can You Protect Yourself from Quacks and Quackery?

quacks (KWAKS), people who pretend to be health professionals.

Sometimes people pretend to be health professionals. These people are called **quacks.** These people cannot admit someone to a hospital or write a prescription to be taken to a pharmacist. They may say they have a "miracle drug," "secret formula," or "scientific machine" that regular physicians will not use. They may promise that you will be cured of a disease physicians say is incurable. They might offer a quick and easy way to do something that is hard, such as losing weight or quitting cigarette smoking.

114

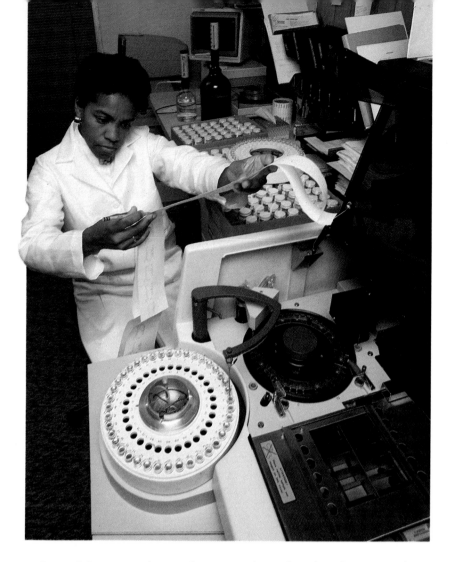

■ *The FDA conducts research to ensure the safety and effectiveness of health products before they can be sold.*

One of the worst things about quacks is that they keep people from getting the proper treatment. Quacks do what they do to make money. Selling a product or service that cannot work as promised is called a *deceptive trade practice*.

Many government and business groups have been formed to protect consumers from quacks. These groups test drugs and other products to make sure that they are safe and effective. The U.S. Food and Drug Administration (FDA) reviews research on food and medical products before they can be sold. The FDA makes sure the products meet certain standards.

How Do People Pay for Health Care?

The amount of money people are spending each year on health products and services is rising. The expense of a major illness can wipe out a family's life savings. Even regular health care for minor problems can use up much of a family's monthly budget. Cost is an important issue for health consumers.

medical insurance,
a plan that can be purchased to help pay a person's medical expenses.

■ *Medical insurance provides the money for expensive medical care that some people could not otherwise afford.*

Parents cannot tell when they or their children will become ill. Many families try to protect their budgets from sudden large medical bills by buying medical insurance. **Medical insurance** is a plan by which people pay a company a certain amount of money regularly. The company guarantees to pay certain amounts to help cover the costs of a serious illness. Insurance is a way people pool money. Each person pays a little knowing that if large health expenses should come up, they can get help. These payments from many people add up to a large amount. Since many people will never need help, there will be enough money for those who do.

1. Mrs. Hall sends a certain amount of money —called a premium—to her insurance company every month.

2. One day, Mrs. Hall's son Lewis breaks his arm and needs medical care.

3. Mrs. Hall takes Lewis to have his arm treated by a physician.

World Care Insurance

4. The insurance company pays the physician for treating Lewis's arm. It costs much more than Mrs. Hall pays the insurance company each month. But the Halls were able to pay for medical treatment through insurance instead of having to come up with the money all at once.

A person usually buys a medical insurance policy from an insurance company by making monthly payments called premiums. If an insured person needs medical care, the company then pays all or part of the medical costs from the money they hold from premiums. The exact amount is set by the original agreement between the buyer and the insurance company.

Many people buy insurance through group plans offered to them as employees of large companies. About 85 percent of all workers in the United States are protected by some kind of health insurance. However, some people who need medical

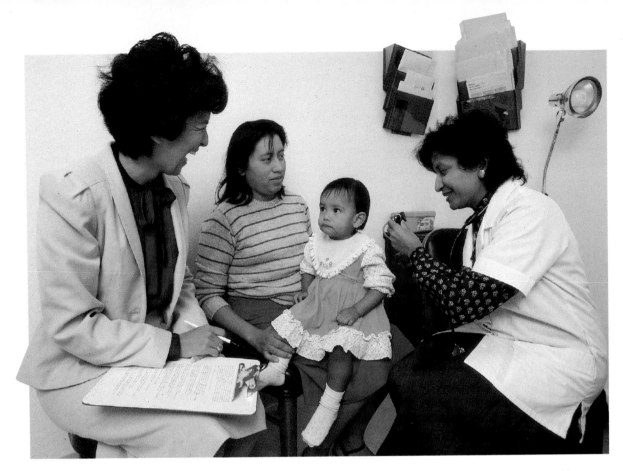

Some communities provide free or low-cost medical care through health department clinics.

care and medical insurance do not have it. Although the government pays for insurance and clinics to help with medical costs for some who cannot afford it, the coverage is different from state to state. Nearly 35 million people in the United States have no insurance at all. About one-third of this number are young people.

STOP **REVIEW SECTION 3**

REMEMBER?

1. What steps should you take in choosing a physician?
2. What steps can you take to participate actively with health workers to help them give you good health care?
3. How does a medical insurance plan work?

THINK!

4. What makes some people go to quacks for health care?
5. How might your physician use information from you to decide on a treatment?

117

People in Health

An Interview with a Dermatologist

Henry W. Lim understands the importance of good skin care. He is a dermatologist in New York City.

What does a dermatologist do?

A dermatologist is a medical doctor who treats skin diseases and other skin problems. A dermatologist uses many treatments, such as creams, lotions, oral medicines, and injections. Sometimes a dermatologist even does surgery to correct a skin problem.

What is the most common skin problem you treat for young people?

By far the most common problem is acne. Acne is a skin condition marked by many pimples on the skin.

■ *A dermatologist is a physician who specializes in the treatment of skin diseases.*

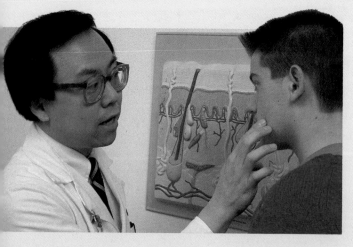

Why is acne so common among young people?

Around the start of puberty, the sebaceous glands begin to work more. This increased activity is brought on by a hormone that is beginning to be made. Young children do not often have acne because their hormone level is so low. But some adults will continue to have acne well after puberty because their hormone level remains high.

Do all young people get acne?

Some individuals are more likely to get acne than others. Heredity can be a reason for this.

What can people do to care for acne?

Keeping the skin clean will lower the number of bacteria that make acne worse. Washing the face at least twice a day with soap and warm water is a healthful practice in caring for acne. For some people, certain foods can make acne worse. It all depends on the person.

Is there another skin problem that is common among young people?

Another common skin problem is eczema. Eczema is a condition in which the skin becomes very dry and itchy. To relieve the itching, a person might scratch the skin. Unfortunately, when they scratch the skin, they cause it to become thick and irritated. Bacteria can get into the irritated areas and cause an infection.

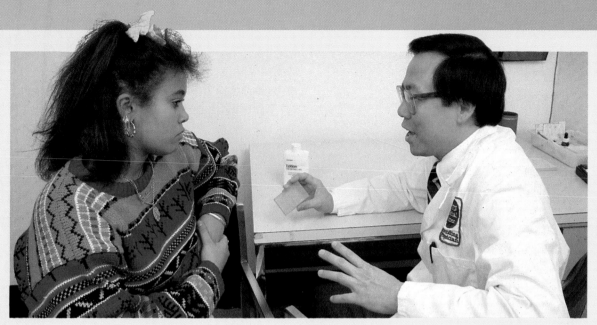

■ *Dr. Lim often treats young people with acne problems.*

How can eczema be treated?

There are several ways. One way to relieve the dryness is to use a moisturizer on the skin. A moisturizer helps trap water on the skin. I often also suggest that people who have eczema use an oil-based soap. This kind of soap will also help keep the skin soft and moist. Severe cases of eczema might need certain medicines, such as cortisone cream. Cortisone keeps the skin from becoming inflamed. It is easy for inflamed skin to become infected.

Can stress cause skin problems?

Emotional stress can make certain skin conditions, such as acne and eczema, much worse. However, stress will not cause these skin problems to develop in people who do not have the tendency to develop them.

What have been the latest advances in skin care?

Dermatologists are adding to their understanding of the skin as an organ. It has been found that the skin is not only an organ that covers the body, but it is also an important organ in protecting the body from disease. For example, it has been found that too much sunlight can change the ability of the skin to fight off disease. The fact that the sun can change the skin's immunity explains why some people get skin cancer.

How can people protect themselves from getting too much sun?

I simply tell people not to stay in the sun for a long time. If they must be in the sun, they should always use a sunscreen.

Learn more about skin care and about the work of dermatologists. Interview a dermatologist. Or write for information to the American Academy of Dermatology, P.O. Box 4014, Schaumburg, IL 60168.

119

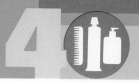
Main Ideas

- You can make wise health choices by following a decision-making process.

- Local, state, and federal governments help protect the consumer.

- Advertising is a major source of health information for many consumers.

- You can use the information on product labels to help you choose products and use them correctly.

- Understanding how your body works will help you make informed decisions about health products.

- You should choose a health professional who seems to understand your needs and with whom you can talk openly.

- It is important to be able to distinguish between good health workers and quacks.

- A person can plan for health care expenses by buying medical insurance.

Key Words

Write the numbers 1 to 11 in your health notebook or on a separate sheet of paper. After each number, copy the sentence and fill in the missing term. Page numbers in ( ) tell you where to look in the chapter if you need help.

consumer (98)
advertising (101)
license (102)
sebaceous gland (106)
sebum (106)
acne (106)

deodorant (108)
antiperspirant (108)
fluoride (110)
quacks (114)
medical insurance (116)

1. People who try to make money by selling unsafe or ineffective health products or services are ___?___.

2. A ___?___ is anyone who buys or uses a product or service.

3. A skin condition that involves having many pimples is called ___?___.

4. ___?___ is a plan that can be purchased to help pay a person's medical bills.

5. A ___?___ produces oil that keeps the skin soft and moist.

6. A ___?___ is a permit that shows that a person meets certain qualifications for a profession.

7. Manufacturers use ___?___ to help sell products or services.

8. ___?___ is the oil produced by the sebaceous glands.

9. Using ___?___ helps stop perspiration odor by blocking the growth of bacteria on the skin.

10. Using ___?___ cuts down the amount of perspiration given off by the sweat glands.

11. A chemical called ___?___ helps strengthen tooth enamel.

Remembering What You Learned

Page numbers in ( ) tell you where to look in the chapter if you need help.

1. What steps should you take when selecting a health product? (100)

2. How can advertisements for health products be helpful to consumers? (101)

3. How can advertising be harmful to consumers? (101–102)

4. What is the purpose of consumer health laws and regulations? (102)

5. What does a license tell you about a health care professional? Why are licenses important? (102)

6. Name four services your local health department provides. (103)

7. What information do product labels give you? (104)

8. What are some ways in which health products are sometimes misused by people? (105)

9. What could be some benefits for the consumer if health professionals advertised? (113)

10. What are four things a quack might promise in order to get you to use his or her product? (114–115)

Thinking About What You Learned

1. Describe what you think would happen if the government did not help protect the consumer.

2. What are some benefits of talking with your physician about any medicine prescribed for you?

3. What are some things you and your family can do to control your health care expenses?

4. Compare and contrast accurate and inaccurate advertising for personal health products.

5. Describe what you can do to work effectively with a physician to treat an illness or injury.

Writing About What You Learned

1. Imagine that you are an advice columnist. What advice would you give to a person who is misusing a health product? Write to him or her explaining why it is important not to misuse that product. Include some ways to avoid misusing health products.

2. If you were inspecting restaurants for cleanliness and safe food preparation, what are some of the things you would check on? Tell why.

3. Think of a health product you would like to buy. List the reasons a wise consumer would give for purchasing this product.

Applying What You Learned

SCIENCE

Research skin cancer using your school library or the public library. Construct a chart that describes the warning signs for skin cancer as well as the steps people should take to lessen their chances of getting skin cancer.

SOCIAL STUDIES

Choose another country and research its health care system. Include in your research how people pay for their health care. Prepare a report describing the advantages and disadvantages of that country's health care system, and present your report to the class.

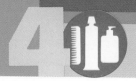
Modified True or False

Write the numbers 1 to 15 in your health notebook or on a separate sheet of paper. After each number, write *true* or *false* to describe the sentence. If the sentence is false, also write a term that replaces the underlined term and makes the sentence true.

1. Anyone who buys or uses a product or a service is a <u>consumer</u>.

2. Advertising is <u>always</u> accurate.

3. A <u>local health department</u> provides screening tests to detect certain health problems.

4. The outer layer of skin is called the <u>dermis</u>.

5. <u>Pimples</u> form when hair follicles become infected.

6. An <u>antiperspirant</u> reduces the amount of perspiration your body releases.

7. <u>Sebum</u> helps strengthen tooth enamel.

8. You should choose a physician when you are <u>ill</u>.

9. You can reduce the expense of serious illness by buying <u>medical insurance</u>.

10. A health professional who does not have a license may be a <u>quack</u>.

11. The <u>higher</u> the sun protection factor of a sunscreen, the more protection it provides from the sun's rays.

12. A <u>regulation</u> is a rule that deals with the details or procedures for enforcing a law.

13. Dandruff occurs when oil from the <u>sebaceous</u> glands in your scalp dries and mixes with dead skin cells.

14. <u>Perspiration</u> is the waste that leaves the body through the skin.

15. Someone who specializes in skin care problems is a <u>quack</u>.

Short Answer

Write the numbers 16 to 23 on your paper. Write a complete sentence to answer each question.

16. How can going to a quack harm your health?

17. What steps should you follow in choosing a family physician?

18. Why should you read product labels?

19. How do consumers learn most of their information about health products?

20. Why is it important to read advertising carefully?

21. How might it be harmful to use a health product for something for which it was not intended?

22. What is the first step you need to take in making an informed consumer choice?

23. How is a quack different from a physician?

Essay

Write the numbers 24 and 25 on your paper. Write paragraphs with complete sentences to answer each question.

24. Describe what you would say to someone who spends money on breath spray but not on toothpaste.

25. Why is medical insurance important?

ACTIVITIES FOR HOME OR SCHOOL

Projects to Do

1. Make a list of five health products your family now has in your home. Include the brands and the sizes. Visit a pharmacy and ask for the current prices of these products. Compare their prices with those of other, similar products.

■ *List some of the health products that you have in your home and make a chart about using them safely.*

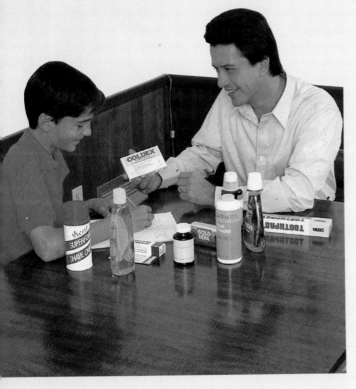

2. Select another five over-the-counter health products in your home. Read the directions carefully. Make a chart to show when and how to use the products. Also, list any warnings or cautions about using the products.

Information to Find

1. Prepare a report for your class about quacks. How does the federal government protect you from quacks? Look in the library for examples of medical quackery in history. Ask someone at your post office how the postal service helps fight quackery and deceptive trade practices.

2. What kind of medical insurance does your parent or guardian have, if any? Does it include insurance for you? Is the medical coverage satisfactory? What changes would be helpful in this health insurance coverage?

3. Find advertisements for five health products. Show each advertisement to several people, and ask them to describe their feelings about the product. Determine whether the advertisement was accurate, misleading, or inaccurate.

Books to Read

Here are some books you can look for in your school library or the public library to find more information about being a wise consumer and taking care of your health.

Bains, Rae. *Health and Hygiene*. Troll Associates.

Kyte, Kathy. *The Kids' Complete Guide to Money*. Knopf.

LuBowe, Irwin I., and Barbara Huss. *A Teenage Guide to Healthy Skin and Hair*. Irvington.

Saunders, Rubie. *The Beauty Book: Head-to-Toe Beauty Tips*. Simon & Schuster.

123

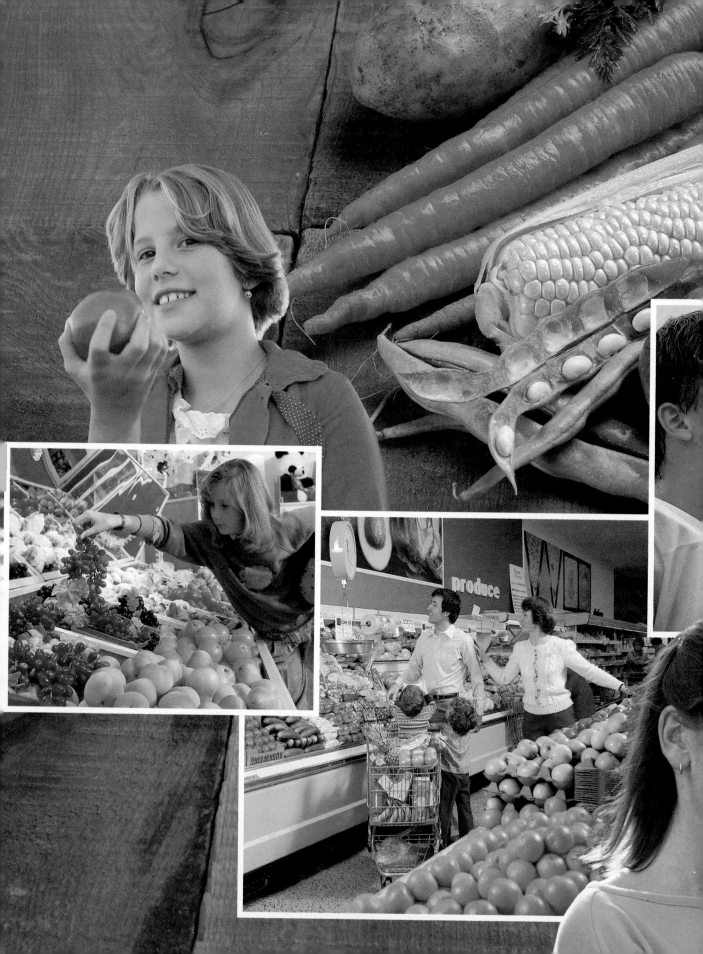

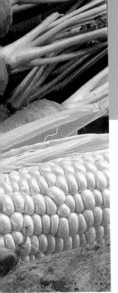

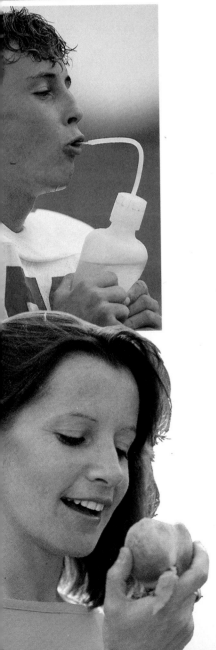

CHAPTER 5

EATING TO BE HEALTHY

Think about some of the things food does for you. Food affects your appearance. Healthy skin and hair, strong teeth and nails, and firm muscles all come from eating well-balanced meals. The food you eat can affect your body size and shape as well. If your diet is low in certain nutrients, you may not reach your fullest possible growth. Too much food or the wrong kinds of food may cause you to become overweight.

Food can affect you in other ways, too. For example, a healthful diet gives you the energy to concentrate and to learn new things. Diet can also affect your emotions. Knowing about good nutrition is important for all people. When you eat healthful foods, you are helping yourself achieve wellness.

GETTING READY TO LEARN

Key Questions

- Why is it important to learn about food?
- How can you develop healthful eating habits?
- How can you learn to make healthful food choices?
- What can you do to take more responsibility for the foods you eat?

Main Chapter Sections

1 Your Nutrient Needs
2 Choosing Healthful Foods
3 Some Reasons for Having Healthful Eating Habits

1 Your Nutrient Needs

Your body needs the right foods to work as it should. But it does not need just any food! To keep your body working properly, you need to eat a variety of foods that, together, contain about 50 different nutrients. These 50 nutrients can be divided into six groups: carbohydrates, fats, proteins, vitamins, minerals, and water. By regularly eating the right amounts of foods containing these nutrients, you should get all the nutrients your body needs so it can grow, repair body cells, and stay healthy.

How Does Your Body Use Carbohydrates?

Carbohydrates are energy nutrients. They provide your body with much of the energy it needs to grow and be active.

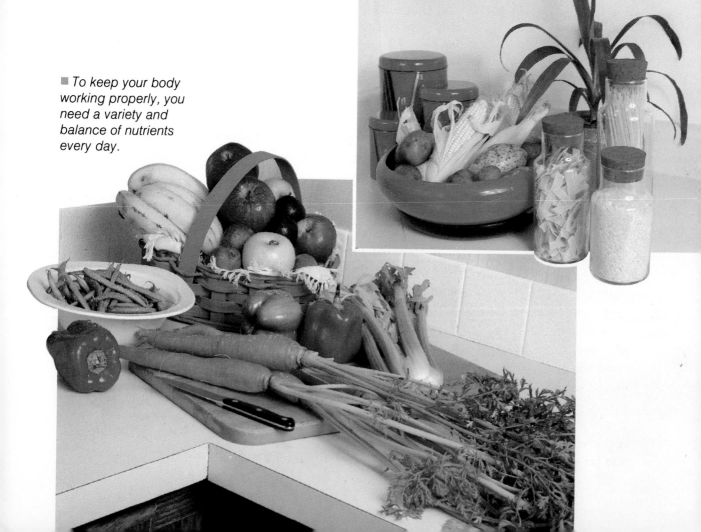

■ To keep your body working properly, you need a variety and balance of nutrients every day.

Two kinds of carbohydrates are found in foods. They are simple carbohydrates and complex carbohydrates. **Simple carbohydrates** are various kinds of sugars. These sugars are found in milk, fruits, vegetables, and sweets. Simple carbohydrates are easy to digest and give quick energy.

Complex carbohydrates are made of many simple carbohydrates that are bound together. Starches and fiber are two examples of complex carbohydrates. Foods such as potatoes, rice, corn, and noodles contain *starch*. Starches take longer to digest than simple carbohydrates. Foods such as bran cereal, whole grains, seeds, and many fruits and vegetables contain the second kind of complex carbohydrate, *fiber*. Although you cannot digest fiber, it helps your digestive system work as it should. Without enough fiber in your diet, wastes can build up in your intestines.

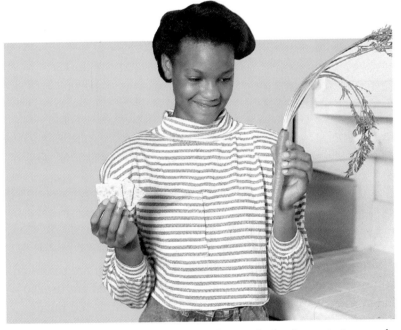

The most important role of nonfiber carbohydrates is to supply the body with energy. Carbohydrates do this by providing the body with calories. **Calories** are units for measuring energy. All foods contain some calories.

As your body digests carbohydrates, it changes them into **glucose,** or blood sugar. The blood carries the glucose to cells where energy is needed. If you eat more carbohydrates than your body can use at one time, the liver changes some of the extra glucose into glycogen. **Glycogen** is a form of glucose stored in the muscles and liver for later use. When your muscles and liver become full of glycogen, any extra glycogen is changed into fat and is stored in your fat cells. Body fat stores energy and

simple carbohydrates (SIHM puhl • kahr boh HY drayts), carbohydrates that are digested easily and give quick energy to the body.

complex carbohydrates (KAHM plehks • kahr boh HY drayts), combinations of simple sugars bound together.

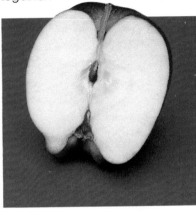

■ *The skin of an apple is a good source of fiber.*

■ *These crackers and this carrot contain the same number of calories.*

calories (KAL uh reez), measurement units for energy in foods.

glucose (GLOO kohs), blood sugar.

glycogen (GLY kuh juhn), a form of glucose stored in the muscles and liver for later use.

helps cushion and protect the internal organs. However, too much body fat caused by eating food with too many calories makes a person overweight.

How Does Your Body Use Fats?

Fats are the most concentrated form of energy found in foods. Fats have more calories than carbohydrates. In fact, an ounce (28.35 grams) of fat yields twice as much energy as a similar amount of carbohydrate. Fats are vital to your health. They help carry other nutrients throughout your body, and they are part of each cell membrane. Fats help your skin stay healthy. They are also used by the body to make necessary chemicals.

■ *Saturated fats found in shortenings and meats may increase blood cholesterol that can clog blood vessels. Unsaturated fats found in some oils do not increase cholesterol levels.*

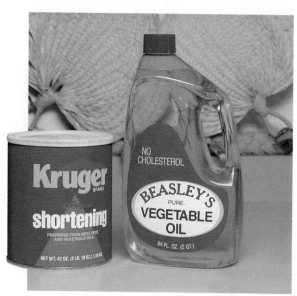

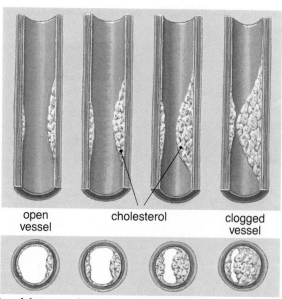

open vessel   cholesterol   clogged vessel

saturated fats (SACH uh rayt uhd • FATS), fats that are generally solid at room temperature.

unsaturated fats (uhn SACH uh rayt uhd • FATS), fats that are usually liquid at room temperature.

cholesterol (kuh LEHS tuh rohl), a waxy substance found naturally in the blood and in some foods.

Two major kinds of fats are found in foods. They are saturated and unsaturated fats. **Saturated fats** are those that are usually solid at room temperature. Animal products such as red meats, milk, cheese, and butter have saturated fats. **Unsaturated fats** are usually liquid at room temperature. Fish oils and plant products such as corn oil, olive oil, and soybean oil contain unsaturated fats. Foods that contain unsaturated fats are thought to be more healthful for the body.

A diet high in certain saturated fats may cause health problems. Saturated fats contain **cholesterol,** a waxy substance made by the body and found in the blood. Eating animal products high in saturated fats—such as red meats and cheese—adds cholesterol to the body's natural level. Too much cholesterol in the blood can clog the blood vessels and lead to heart disease. Plant oils, such as sunflower and soybean, do not contain cholesterol.

For good health, you need to have a balance of the energy nutrients. Energy from any food is always being used and stored. But if you store more energy than you use, you will gain weight in the form of body fat. Everything you eat in excess of your basic needs for energy is turned into fat. Excess fat places extra demands on some of your body systems. Your heart, for example, must work harder to keep the extra fat cells supplied with oxygen. Your muscular and skeletal systems must also work harder to support your heavier body.

How Does Your Body Use Proteins?

Almost every cell in your body contains proteins. Your muscles, hair, and nails are made up chiefly of proteins. To keep your body healthy, you need high-protein foods, such as meat and nuts. These are digested and broken down into the building blocks of proteins, **amino acids.** There are 20 different amino acids that make up proteins. Some amino acids are made by your body, but 8 are not. The 8 are called *essential amino acids.* They must come from the foods you eat.

Proteins are the chief nutrient for building and repairing body cells. As much as 3 to 5 percent of the protein in your body wears out and must be replaced every day. For example, the cells lining your small intestine last only a few days before they need to be replaced. You need amino acids from proteins in food to replace these cells.

amino acids (uh MEE noh • AS uhdz), building blocks of proteins.

■ *The muscle tissue of active people requires a lot of protein for maintenance.*

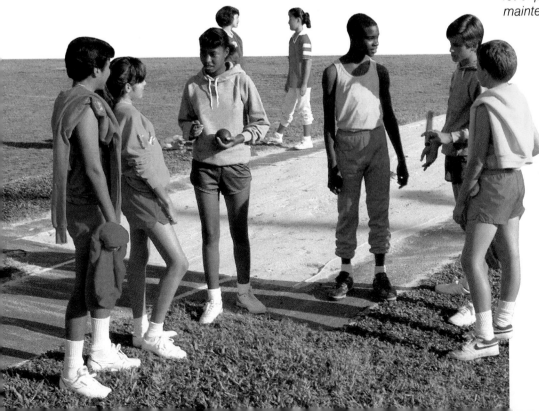

COMBINING INCOMPLETE PROTEINS TO MAKE COMPLETE PROTEINS

Nuts and Grains	Peanut butter sandwich
Vegetables and Nuts	Three-bean salad with pecans
Vegetables and Seeds	Salad topped with sesame seeds

Proteins are classified by whether or not they contain essential amino acids. Foods that have *complete protein* provide all the essential amino acids needed by the body. Good sources of complete protein are red meat, milk, milk products, poultry, and fish. Foods that do not have some essential amino acids are *incomplete protein* sources. Such foods are grains, nuts, and legumes—dried beans and peas, as well as peanuts. A balance of both complete and incomplete protein foods is needed for good health. If you do not eat foods that contain complete proteins, you can combine foods that contain different incomplete proteins to make sure you are getting all the essential amino acids.

How Does Your Body Use Vitamins?

Vitamins are nutrients that your body needs every day to maintain good health. Your body uses vitamins differently from the way it uses energy nutrients. Instead of being digested, vitamins are just released from food. They pass into the blood and are absorbed by the body's tissues. Once inside the tissues, vitamins become part of certain chemicals that help break down other nutrients.

Vitamins do a variety of jobs in the body. Some vitamins help make blood cells, hormones, and certain other substances your body needs. Other vitamins help you use energy nutrients. Most people in the United States could get all the vitamins they need by eating a variety of foods. They do not need to take vitamin pills to get them. Taking too many vitamin supplements can actually be dangerous. Before using vitamin supplements, talk with a parent or guardian, a school nurse, or your physician.

The 13 known vitamins are vitamins A, B-complex (a group of 8 vitamins), C, D, E, and K. Vitamins A, D, E, and K are called *fat-soluble vitamins* because they dissolve in fats. The fats in your diet help carry these vitamins throughout your body. Fat-soluble vitamins can be stored in your body. Because they can be stored, you need a good source of these vitamins every few days rather than every day.

■ *The body does not retain water-soluble vitamins. However, the body can store fat-soluble vitamins for use when needed.*

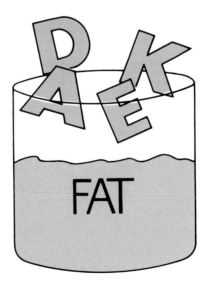

The B-complex and C vitamins are called *water-soluble vitamins* because they dissolve in water. Only small amounts of water-soluble vitamins can be stored in the body. Because of this, it is important to eat foods that are good sources of these vitamins every day.

The table "Some Vitamins Your Body Needs" lists some of the vitamins, their uses in the body, and their food sources.

SOME VITAMINS YOUR BODY NEEDS

Vitamin	Uses in Your Body	Sources
A (retinol)	keeps skin and body membranes healthy; helps you see well at night; keeps bones strong	milk, liver, green leafy vegetables, yellow vegetables
B_1 (thiamin)	helps appetite; keeps nervous system healthy; helps body get energy from food	pork, liver, whole-grain cereals, breads
B_2 (riboflavin)	keeps skin healthy; helps body get energy from food	milk, eggs, liver, green leafy vegetables
B_3 (niacin)	helps keep skin, nervous system, and other tissues healthy; helps body get energy from food	fish, beans, peas, eggs, meat
B_6 (pyridoxine)	helps in forming red blood cells	liver, corn, brown rice, wheat germ, whole grain cereals and breads, bananas
B_{12} (cobalamin)	helps in the normal development of red blood cells	meat, eggs, milk, oatmeal
C (ascorbic acid)	keeps gums healthy; helps wounds heal	citrus fruits, tomatoes, potatoes, dark green vegetables
D	helps body take in and use calcium and phosphorus; keeps bones and teeth strong	milk, eggs, liver; made by skin exposed to sunlight
E	helps form red blood cells and other body tissues	vegetable oils, whole-grain cereals, bread
K	helps the body digest certain foods; helps the blood to clot	egg yolks, cabbage, green leafy vegetables

How Does Your Body Use Minerals?

Minerals are nutrients needed by your body to make special materials for cells. Minerals also build and maintain certain body tissues. The 21 known minerals used by the body can be classified into two groups, based on the amount that the body needs. These two groups are macrominerals and trace minerals.

The minerals your body needs in large amounts are called major minerals, or **macrominerals.** The macrominerals are calcium, phosphorus, magnesium, sodium, potassium, chlorine, and sulfur. Of all these minerals, your body needs calcium and phosphorus in the greatest amounts. They are the major materials of your skeleton and teeth.

Minerals that you need in small amounts each day are called **trace minerals.** Trace minerals include iodine, iron, copper, cobalt, manganese, zinc, and fluorine.

macrominerals (mak roh MIHN uh ruhlz), minerals that your body needs in large amounts.

trace minerals, minerals that are needed in tiny amounts each day.

■ *Milk is a good source of the minerals calcium and phosphorus, which your body needs for healthy bones and teeth.*

133

The table "Some Minerals Your Body Needs" lists the sources and functions of some macrominerals and trace minerals.

SOME MINERALS YOUR BODY NEEDS

Mineral	Uses in Your Body	Sources
Calcium	helps make strong bones and teeth; helps heart and other muscles work; helps nerves send messages	milk and milk products, dark-green leafy vegetables (except spinach)
Copper	helps form red blood cells	nuts, liver, dried beans, whole grains
Fluorine	helps form strong teeth and bones	fish, most animal meats, fluoridated water
Iodine	regulates function of thyroid gland, which controls the body's use of energy	fish and other seafood, iodized salt
Iron	helps blood carry oxygen	liver, egg yolks, green leafy vegetables, dried fruits, whole-grain cereals
Phosphorus	helps make strong bones and teeth; takes part in cell activities	meat, poultry, fish, egg yolks, nuts, cereals, milk products
Potassium	helps muscles contract; helps nerves send messages	orange juice, bananas, meats, peanuts, beans and peas, green leafy vegetables
Sodium	helps nerves function; helps maintain fluid balance in tissues	table salt
Zinc	helps wounds heal; forms part of many enzymes needed for growth	meats, grains, nuts

How Does Your Body Use Water?

Water is sometimes called the "forgotten" nutrient. Actually, water is one of the most important of all the nutrients. You cannot live without it. Every cell in your body contains water. About two-thirds of your body is water.

Water has many important uses in your body. It helps keep your body temperature constant and helps you maintain a proper fluid balance. It helps in body growth and digestion. Because of these important uses, water must be replaced almost as quickly as it is lost. Usually, a person loses about about 2 1/2 quarts (2.4 liters) of water every day in perspiration, urine, and exhaled water vapor. Some of this water can be replaced by drinking. Water can also be replaced by eating high-moisture foods. The table "Water Content in Certain Foods" shows some foods that are high in moisture.

■ *In addition to eating foods that contain a lot of water, you should drink about eight glasses of water a day.*

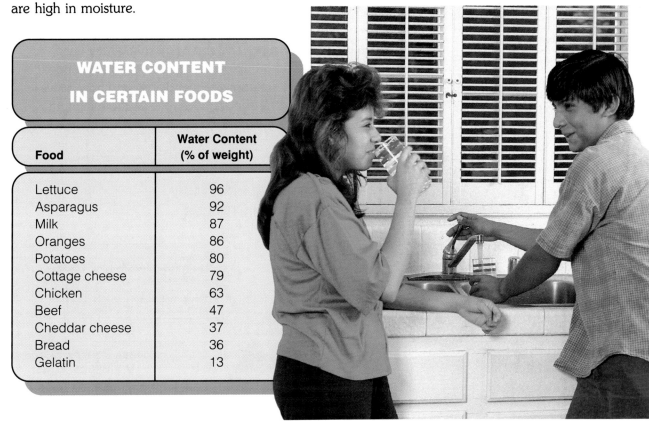

WATER CONTENT IN CERTAIN FOODS

Food	Water Content (% of weight)
Lettuce	96
Asparagus	92
Milk	87
Oranges	86
Potatoes	80
Cottage cheese	79
Chicken	63
Beef	47
Cheddar cheese	37
Bread	36
Gelatin	13

STOP REVIEW SECTION 1

REMEMBER?

1. What kinds of carbohydrates are found in foods?
2. What is an incomplete protein?
3. How are vitamins used by the body?
4. How are minerals used by the body?

THINK!

5. Why is it important to eat a variety of foods?
6. Why is it important to eat meals at least three times a day?

135

2 Choosing Healthful Foods

KEY WORDS

servings
balanced diet

servings (SUR vihngz),
amounts people are
likely to eat of particular
foods during a meal.

Most people can get all the nutrients they need by eating a balanced variety of foods. This balance is gained by eating combinations of foods chosen from the five basic food groups. Amounts of foods are often recommended by nutrition experts in measures called **servings.** The size of a serving may vary depending on the food group. The amount of food you need depends on your age, sex, physical condition, and how active you are. Almost everyone should have at least the minimum number of servings from each food group daily.

Food Guide Pyramid
A Guide to Daily Food Choices

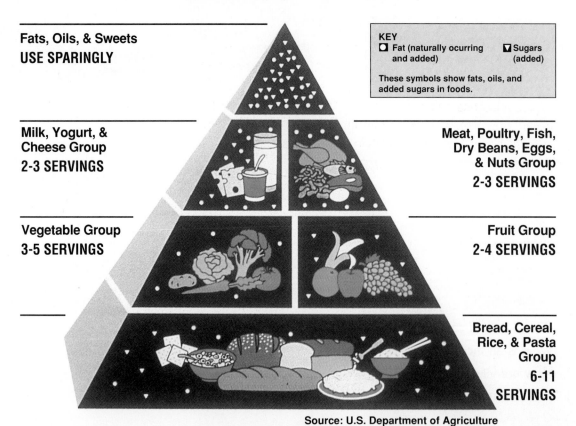

Fats, Oils, & Sweets
USE SPARINGLY

KEY
▢ Fat (naturally ocurring   ▼ Sugars
and added)   (added)

These symbols show fats, oils, and
added sugars in foods.

Milk, Yogurt, &
Cheese Group
2-3 SERVINGS

Meat, Poultry, Fish,
Dry Beans, Eggs,
& Nuts Group
2-3 SERVINGS

Vegetable Group
3-5 SERVINGS

Fruit Group
2-4 SERVINGS

Bread, Cereal,
Rice, & Pasta
Group
6-11
SERVINGS

Source: U.S. Department of Agriculture

How Much Food Do You Need from the Meat, Poultry, Fish, Dry Beans, Eggs, and Nuts Group?

Foods from the *Meat, Poultry, Fish, Dry Beans, Eggs, and Nuts Group* are the body's chief source of proteins. Those with complete proteins are animal products such as beef, fish, poultry, and eggs. Those with incomplete proteins are the plant products such as nuts, grains, and dried beans and peas. People who do not eat animal products can combine legumes and grains with foods from other food groups to form protein sources that are more complete.

Besides being the chief source of proteins, most foods that belong in the Meat, Poultry, Fish, Dry Beans, Eggs, and Nuts Group also contain iron, niacin (vitamin B_3), and thiamin (vitamin B_1). Two to three servings of foods in this group each day usually will supply all the proteins and iron needed to help a person grow and stay healthy.

How Much Food Do You Need from the Milk, Yogurt, and Cheese Group?

Milk and milk products make up the *Milk, Yogurt, and Cheese Group.* Foods in this group contain proteins. In addition, they supply needed fats and the minerals calcium and phosphorus. Some milk is fortified with vitamin D. A teenager's daily food selections should include about two to three servings of milk or milk products.

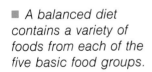
■ A balanced diet contains a variety of foods from each of the five basic food groups.

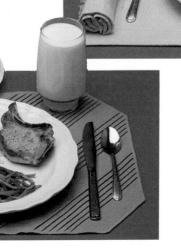

How Much Food Do You Need from the Fruit Group and the Vegetable Group?

The *Fruit Group* and the *Vegetable Group* foods supply carbohydrates, chiefly in the form of simple carbohydrates and fiber. Essential vitamins and minerals are also supplied by these two groups. Along with helping the digestive system, fiber may help prevent some diseases of the large intestine. Your daily food selections should include two to four servings of fruits and three to five servings of vegetables each day.

How Much Food Do You Need from the Bread, Cereal, Rice, and Pasta Group?

The body's chief source of complex carbohydrates is foods in the *Bread, Cereal, Rice, and Pasta Group.* Six to eleven servings from this food group are needed every day. One serving is equal to about one slice of wheat bread, one ounce of dry cereal, or a half cup of cooked rice, pasta, or cereal.

A GUIDE FOR DAILY FOOD CHOICES

Food Group	Number of servings	Examples of servings
Bread, Cereal, Rice, and Pasta	6–11 servings	1 slice bread 1 ounce dry cereal 1/2 cup cooked cereal, rice or pasta
Vegetable	3–5 servings	1 cup raw, leafy vegetables 1/2 cup cooked or chopped raw vegetables 3/4 cup vegetable juice
Fruit	2–4 servings	1 medium-sized apple, banana, or orange 1/2 cup chopped, cooked, or canned fruit 3/4 cup fruit juice
Milk, Yogurt, and Cheese	2–3 servings	1 cup milk or yogurt 1 1/2 ounce natural cheese 2 ounces processed cheese
Meat, Poultry, Fish, Dry Beans, Eggs, and Nuts	2–3 servings	2–3 ounces cooked lean meat, poultry, or fish 1/2 cup cooked dry beans, 1 egg, or 2 tablespoons peanut butter count as 1 ounce lean meat

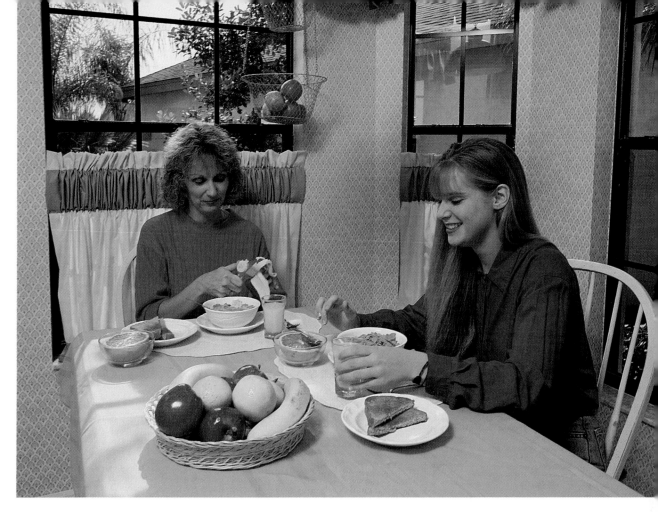

Why Should People Limit Their Sugar and Salt Intake?

The foods you eat each day make up your daily diet. When your diet contains foods from each of the five basic food groups in the right amounts, it is called a **balanced diet.** When people have balanced diets, their bodies get enough of all the nutrients they need.

Two foods often found in a balanced diet are sugar and salt. They are found naturally in many healthful foods. Fresh fruits are rich in natural sugar. Salt can be found naturally in many vegetables. People who eat adequate servings of these foods in their daily diets are able to get all the salt and sugar their bodies need. However, many people add salt they do not need to their diets. They may add salt to foods as they prepare a meal. Or they may sprinkle extra salt on each bite of food they take. Many people also add extra sugar to their diets by making food choices from a sixth food group. This is the *Fats, Oils, and Sweets Group.* Eating extra sugar each day is a bad dietary habit.

balanced diet (BAL uhnst • DY uht), healthful amounts of foods from the five basic food groups.

Excess sugar and salt can produce harmful effects in the body. The calories in extra sugar are stored as body fat. Refined sugar also contributes to tooth decay when eaten too often. Extra salt causes body tissues to hold more water. High blood pressure can develop as a result.

People add sugar and salt to foods to give them more flavor. But if you try, you can think of more healthful ways to make foods more flavorful. For example, you can add seasonings such as herbs and spices or lemon juice.

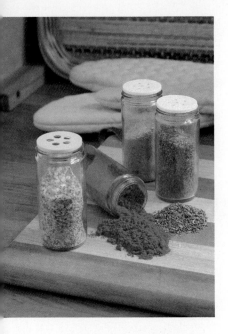

■ *Seasonings other than salt can be added to food to enhance the flavor.*

STOP **REVIEW**
SECTION 2

REMEMBER?

1. What are the main nutrients in each of the five food groups?
2. What is a balanced diet?
3. Why should people limit the amount of sugar and salt in their diets?

THINK!

4. What is one dish that has ingredients from at least four food groups?
5. What foods should be limited in people's diets besides salt and sugar?

Thinking About Your Health

Can You Plan Healthful Meals?

Plan three different breakfast menus that can be prepared in less than ten minutes. Use a variety of healthful foods that your family members enjoy. You may wish to include foods that are not traditional breakfast foods.

If you have trouble planning these meals, talk about this with your parent, guardian, school nurse, or teacher. Or you may wish to contact local offices of the American Heart Association or American Cancer Society for some suggestions.

Health Close-up

Wise Consumer Shopping

You want to get the most value for your money when shopping for food. To accomplish this, you should consider two things: the nutrient density and the unit price. *Nutrient density* indicates the amount of nutrients compared to the number of calories. The *unit price* is the cost per unit (weight or piece) of the food. Nutrient density and unit pricing help you compare foods for best buys.

To determine nutrient density, you need to know the ratio of nutrients to calories that a food supplies. For example, one large baked potato and 12 to 15 potato chips both contain 150 calories. However, the baked potato contains at least twice as much protein, iron, thiamin (vitamin B_1), niacin (vitamin B_3), and vitamin C as the potato chips, even though the potato chips contain much more fat. Therefore, the baked potato is more nutrient-dense than are the potato chips.

Packaged foods sold in the grocery store have food labels that tell you the products' contents. The ingredients are listed in order based on the amount present by weight, from most to least. A box of cereal whose first ingredient is sugar, for example, would not be a good nutritional value. There is more sugar in this product than any other ingredient. Food labels are required to provide accurate nutritional information to help consumers plan healthful meals.

Once you have determined which foods you want to buy, compare prices. How can you determine whether a 2-pound (.9-kilogram) box of cereal at $2.49 is a better buy than a 1 1/2-pound (.7-kilogram) box at $1.99? Even though it costs less, the second box may not be a better value.

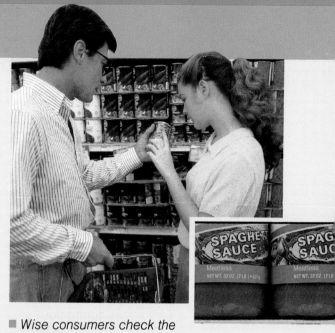

■ *Wise consumers check the nutrition labels and unit prices of products before making a selection.*

Unit pricing can help you compare prices. The unit price is the cost of a product per pound, gram, or other unit of measure. The unit price for a product is often shown on the store shelf. Or you can calculate it by dividing the price by the amount of the product. In this case, the unit prices of the two cereals are $1.25 per pound for the 2-pound box and $1.33 for the 1 1/2-pound box. The larger box is the better buy.

Buying the larger box is not always the wisest choice. You need to be sure you will use all the product so it will not spoil. By understanding the nutrient content and the unit price of the foods you choose, you can be a smart and healthy consumer.

Thinking Beyond

1. Why might someone need to buy a smaller container of food at a higher unit price?
2. Why is it unhealthful to eat a lot of food that is not nutrient-dense?

141

3 Some Reasons for Having Healthful Eating Habits

malnutrition (mal nu TRIHSH uhn), poor health resulting from inadequate nutrients.

■ *Most school cafeteria lunches provide a balanced meal.*

It has been said that people in the United States generally have poor eating habits. Is this true? For each person, the answer depends on what foods he or she chooses to eat every day. **Malnutrition,** a condition of poor health, can result from not getting enough of the nutrients you need. That is why you should make wise choices about the foods you eat.

What Can Happen to You If You Take in Too Little of Some Nutrients?

A balanced diet is important all through your life. A diet that contains nutrients in balanced amounts is *especially* important during your years of rapid growth. Many teenagers get too little

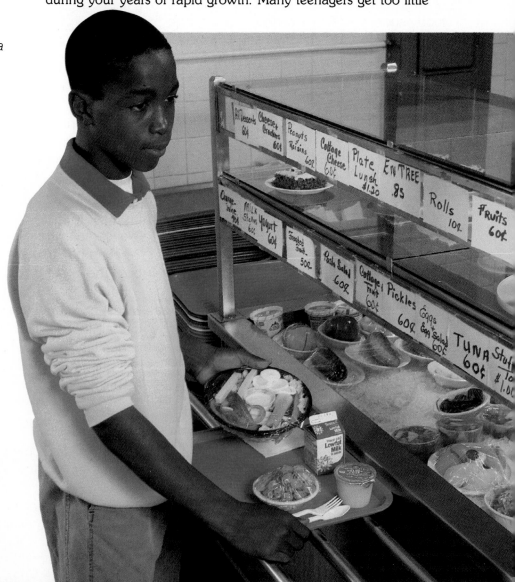

iron, calcium, and vitamins A, C, and B_1 (thiamin). You can do without some nutrients for a few days and not damage your health. But after a longer time, you can develop a **nutritional deficiency.** If a nutritional deficiency continues, you will develop health problems.

nutritional deficiency (NU TRIHSH uhn uhl • dih FIHSH uhn see), a health problem associated with not taking in enough of certain nutrients.

Vitamin Deficiencies. As you know, your body needs vitamins to help maintain wellness. By eating a balance of various foods, you can generally avoid vitamin deficiencies while keeping your calorie intake low. The table "Effects of Some Vitamin Deficiencies on Health" shows some illnesses and symptoms caused by deficiencies. Some of these health problems are very dangerous and should be treated only by a physician.

EFFECTS OF SOME VITAMIN DEFICIENCIES ON HEALTH

Vitamin	Illness Caused by Deficiency	Possible Effects on Health
A	night blindness	rough, dry skin; unhealthy teeth
B_1	beriberi	weak muscles; digestive problems; irritability; depression; difficulty in concentrating
B_2	none	sore, cracked skin; itchy eyes; blurred vision
B_3	pellagra	diarrhea; skin rash
C	scurvy	bleeding gums; sore joints; rough, scaly skin; tendency to bruise easily
D	rickets	soft, weak bones; bones bent out of shape; unhealthy teeth

Protein Deficiencies. Because their cells and tissues are growing rapidly, teenagers need more protein in their diets than adults do. Without enough protein, people can develop a protein deficiency. People with this condition become ill easily because their bodies cannot fight off disease well. A severe kind of protein deficiency is called *kwashiorkor.* In the African language of Ghana,

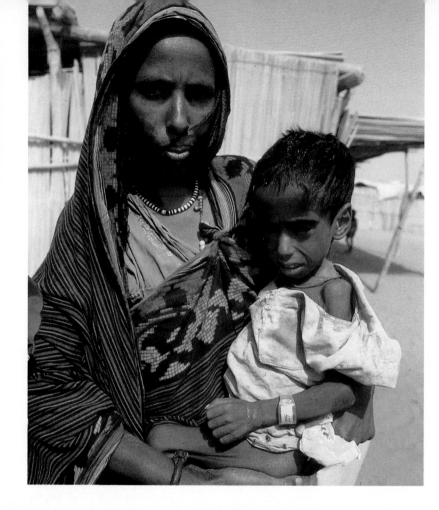

■ *In many parts of the world, people's diets are often deficient in certain nutrients.*

■ *A calcium deficiency can cause weakened bones and teeth.*

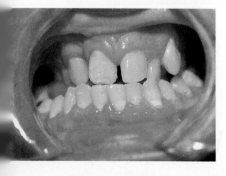

the word *kwashiorkor* means "red child." Kwashiorkor is a serious form of malnutrition seen in infants and children. It affects skin color, growth, and mental ability. It is caused by a diet adequate in carbohydrates but very low in proteins. Kwashiorkor is not common in the United States.

Mineral Deficiencies. The most common forms of nutritional deficiency in the United States are mineral deficiencies. Scientists say that many teenagers have an iron deficiency, although good food sources for this mineral are available. Some teenagers have difficulty absorbing iron from the intestines, and some choose not to eat foods that are rich in iron. Without enough iron, a person may tire easily and become ill.

Other minerals that are low in the diets of many young people are calcium and magnesium. Foods high in calcium are chiefly milk products, which may also be high in fat and calories. However, skim milk and 1- or 2- percent milk and milk products are low in fat and calories. People most likely to show a deficiency of magnesium are those who eat no whole-grain cereals or breads and few vegetables.

What Can Happen When You Take in Too Much of Some Nutrients?

A balanced variety of foods is the key to healthful eating. A balanced diet provides enough, but not too much, of the essential nutrients. Too many calories, usually from simple carbohydrates and fats, can cause a person to gain unwanted weight.

To stay healthy, a person should maintain a desirable weight. A person's **desirable weight** usually falls within a range of weights, depending on his or her age, sex, and body frame size. Use the "Desirable Weights" tables to compare your weight with the desirable range for young people 12 to 17 years old. To determine your frame size, measure the distance around your wrist. If your wrist measures less than 6 inches (15.2 centimeters), you have a small frame. If it measures 6 to 6 1/2 inches (15.2 to 16.5 centimeters), you have a medium frame. If it is more than 6 1/2 inches (16.5 centimeters), you have a large frame.

desirable weight (dih ZY ruh buhl • WAYT), a weight that falls within a range determined to be healthful, depending on age, sex, and frame size.

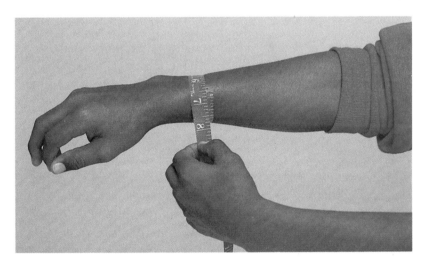

■ *Measuring your wrist can help you determine your frame size.*

How Can You Control Your Weight?

As teenagers grow, their body weight will vary. Most of the time, these gains and losses are normal. Too great a change either way, however, can cause serious health problems.

Sometimes a person gains more weight than is healthy and becomes overweight. Being overweight can affect a person's wellness. The extra weight makes it hard for the body to work efficiently. People who are overweight tend to tire easily.

Many teenagers worry about their weight. They think they are overweight, but often they are not. If you think you have a weight problem, you may want to talk with a parent or guardian, school nurse, or physician.

145

DESIRABLE WEIGHTS FOR GIRLS 12–17 YEARS OLD

Height (barefoot)	Small Frame	Medium Frame	Large Frame
4' 8"	85–91	89–100	97–112
4' 10"	89–97	94–106	102–118
5' 0"	95–103	100–112	108–124
5' 2"	101–109	106–119	114–131
5' 4"	107–116	113–128	122–139
5' 6"	115–124	121–136	130–147
5' 8"	123–133	129–144	138–156
5' 10"	131–141	137–152	146–166

Numbers represent weight in pounds when lightly clothed.
Source: National Dairy Council

How to Lose Weight. Ten to twenty percent of teenagers are actually overweight. Some may have poor eating habits. They may eat snacks that are high in calories but low in nutrients. They may eat when they are worried or bored. Others gain weight because they do not get enough regular exercise.

The best way to lose extra weight is to eat less fat and exercise more. If you think you should lose weight, first talk with a parent or guardian, your school nurse, or a physician. He or she may suggest the amounts and kinds of food that will give you a balanced diet, yet still help you lose weight. You may also get help in planning an exercise program. With a balanced diet and an exercise program, you should slowly lose weight. You will be forming new eating habits that will make it easier for you to control your weight.

How to Gain Weight. Some young people weigh less than they should for their age, sex, and frame size. Being underweight can cause certain health problems. Very underweight people have difficulty building muscle strength or fighting disease as well as people who are at a healthful weight.

If you are underweight, you need more calories than you are taking in. A parent or guardian, your school nurse, or a physician can help you determine if you need to gain some weight. He or she can suggest a balanced diet that will meet your calorie needs and help you reach your most healthful weight.

FOR THE
CURIOUS

About 70 percent of the world's children do not have enough food to eat.

146

DESIRABLE WEIGHTS FOR BOYS 12–17 YEARS OLD

Height (barefoot)	Small Frame	Medium Frame	Large Frame
5' 1"	100–108	105–117	114–129
5' 3"	106–114	112–124	120–136
5' 5"	112–121	118–131	125–144
5' 7"	120–129	125–140	135–154
5' 9"	128–138	134–148	143–162
5' 11"	136–146	142–158	152–172
6' 1"	144–155	150–168	161–182
6' 3"	152–163	160–178	170–192

Numbers represent weight in pounds when lightly clothed.
Source: National Dairy Council

What Are Fad Diets?

Many people try to lose weight too rapidly. They do not eat a balanced diet. They may not take in all the nutrients they need. They may not get enough exercise. Instead they look for diets promising quick weight loss. Many of these are **fad diets.** They are popular for only a short time because they are not possible to maintain. A fad diet often has some kind of gimmick, such as eating only one kind of food. Some fad diets tell people to cut out certain kinds of foods altogether.

Many people who follow fad diets lose weight. But fad diets can threaten wellness. The main purpose of these diets is to produce quick weight loss; they do not attempt to provide good nutrition. They may leave out important nutrients your body needs. Fad diets may not supply much energy. The dieters may feel tired and irritable. In the long run, most fad diets do not work very well. People who lose weight quickly in this way gain it back shortly after they stop dieting. Fad diets may harm your health.

The best way to reach your desirable weight is to develop good eating habits. Knowing about the different kinds of foods your body needs is the first step in this process. You may reach your ideal weight more slowly with a balanced diet than with a fad diet. But you will be more likely to maintain that weight. You will be providing your body with all the nutrients it needs.

fad diets, diets that promise quick weight loss; usually popular for only a short time.

147

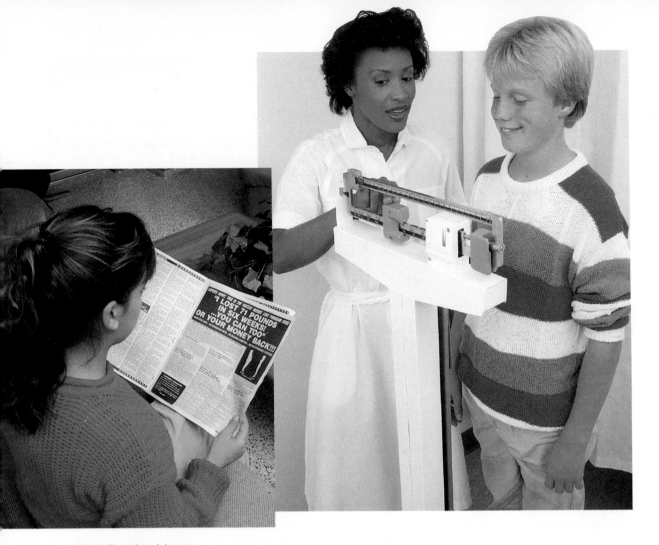

■ A fad diet should not be considered by young people as a way to lose weight. Fad diets can cause harm to a growing body.

Finally, you will be building good eating habits that will help you maintain wellness all through your life.

What Are Eating Disorders?

People often use food to soothe their feelings. Some people eat too much when they face emotional stress. Others develop eating disorders and do not get enough nutrients. They may actually starve themselves to death if they do not get professional help.

Two serious eating disorders are *anorexia nervosa* and *bulimia*. These disorders chiefly occur in young women. Anorexics, people with anorexia nervosa, always think of themselves as overweight, even when they are not. They may actually refuse to eat anything. Bulimia is a disorder that involves extreme overeating. However, the victims then feel guilty and make themselves vomit or use laxatives to rid their bodies of all food.

Anorexia nervosa and bulimia both cause physical problems. People with these disorders become malnourished because they do not get necessary nutrients. Often their hormones get out of balance, they develop heart problems, and they are likely to get infections and other diseases.

Treatment for eating disorders requires the help of an entire health team. A physician usually treats the person's medical problems. A psychologist helps the person work out emotional problems and build self-esteem. A nutritionist helps the person plan a healthful diet. Eating disorders can be cured, but the people must get help before irreversible problems develop.

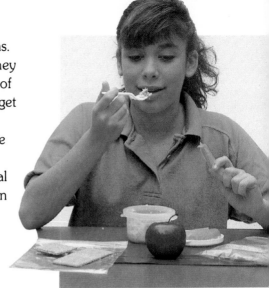

STOP REVIEW
SECTION 3

■ *A balanced diet, with slightly fewer calories than needed to maintain body weight, will enable a person to lose weight slowly and safely. Always talk with a parent first.*

REMEMBER?

1. What are two nutritional deficiency diseases?
2. What is the best way to lose weight?
3. How can fad diets threaten your wellness?
4. What are eating disorders?

THINK!

5. What are some things you can do to maintain your desirable weight?
6. What are two fad diets that are popular with people in your age group?

Making Wellness Choices

On Monday, John and Nathan decided that they wanted to join the wrestling team. They want to be in the 100-pound (45-kilogram) weight class, but both boys weigh slightly over the limit for that class. They would have to lose the extra weight by Friday, when tryouts begin. John has suggested that they stop eating for the rest of the week in order to lose the weight. He also has some pills that he says will help them lose water weight quickly.

 What should Nathan do? Explain your wellness choice.

149

People in Health

An Interview with a Food Scientist

Martha Stone does research with food and teaches about food. She is a food scientist at a university in Manhattan, Kansas.

What does a food scientist do?

A food scientist is a trained person whose goal is to provide a safe, nutritious, and plentiful food supply for the people of our country and of the world. Food scientists work in research laboratories and teach at colleges and universities. They also work for the government and for private companies.

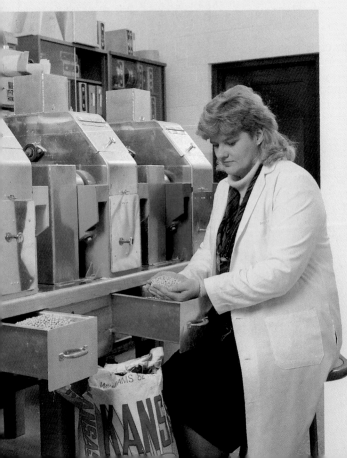

■ *Ms. Stone works in a research laboratory and teaches about nutrition.*

Wherever they work, food scientists share a common goal.

How does the work of a food scientist differ from that of a dietitian or nutritionist?

A food scientist uses chemical and physical information about a food to develop basic understandings about its nature. One specialized job in food science is that of food technologist. A food technologist uses the information provided by the food scientist to develop new and improved food sources, products, or ways of processing food. Food scientists form ideas. Food technologists apply the ideas.

Dietitians and nutritionists are concerned with the nutrients that are in food. They find ways to prepare food so that it is as healthful as possible.

The world's population is increasing, but the land on which to grow crops is not. Are there new sources of food that we might be using in the near future?

Developing new food sources is one of the newest and most exciting areas of food science. But we also are studying new ways to use the food sources that exist. We are looking for ways to use food materials that we have been throwing away in the past. One example of this is whey. Whey is the clear, watery liquid left when the curd is separated from milk in making cheese. Billions of tons of whey have been wasted in the past. Now we realize that whey is an excellent source of protein. Whey is now being used in the production of various food products, such as breakfast bars and some fruit-flavored drinks.

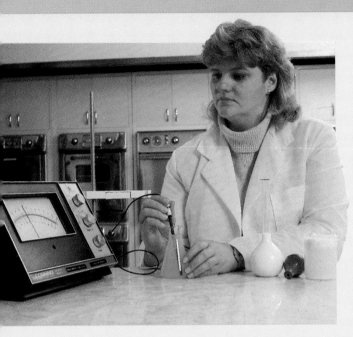

■ *The use of technology may increase the world food supply in the future.*

How will fresh foods be made to last longer in the future?

Irradiation is one process that is already being used to preserve certain fresh foods. It is, however, a controversial process. *Irradiation* means that food is exposed to low levels of radiation for a very short time. This radiation stops or slows biological or chemical changes so that the food stays fresh. I have seen potatoes, for example, that were still fresh after four years. Irradiation does sometimes slightly change the color or taste of the food. But studies indicate that irradiation does not affect the nutrients. Irradiation will help make more fresh foods available to more people.

In what other new ways will foods be preserved?

Another way will be aseptic, or sterile, packaging. This means that the foods will be packaged in an environment totally free of microbes. When there are no microbes in foods, the foods do not spoil. There are foods available now in single-serving packages that have been preserved in this way. Some examples are fruit drinks, yogurts, puddings, and fruits.

What kind of research do you do?

My research is in improving and developing grain products here in the Kansas area. I have done research on the length of time items made from soybeans can be stored safely.

Another area I have studied is how microwave heating affects various foods. I have also done some work with an artificial sweetener called *aspartame*. Aspartame sweetens foods without adding as many calories as sugar. The problem with aspartame is that it breaks down if it is exposed to heat for a long time. I have been trying to find a way to keep it from breaking down so that it can be used in cooking.

What do you like best about your work?

Food science is an exciting field. The world's population continues to grow. That means that more people will need more food. Food scientists are doing something to make sure there will be enough food for everyone.

Learn more about people who work as food scientists. Interview a food scientist. Or write for information to the Institute of Food Technologists, 221 North LaSalle Street, Suite 300, Chicago, IL 60601.

Main Ideas

- Your body needs a variety of nutrients to work properly.

- Your body uses nutrients to provide energy, build and repair cells, make blood cells and hormones, and make special materials for the cells.

- You can get all the nutrients your body needs by eating a balanced variety of foods each day.

- A balanced diet includes recommended amounts of foods from each food group each day, with limited intake of sugar and salt.

- People who do not have a balanced diet may develop a nutritional deficiency. The particular condition that results depends on which nutrients are lacking in the diet.

- Good health includes maintaining a desirable weight achieved through good eating habits and regular exercise.

1. The form of glucose stored in the muscles and liver for later use is called ___?___ .

2. Someone suffering from ___?___ does not get enough of the nutrients needed for good health.

3. The building blocks of proteins are ___?___ .

4. ___?___ are fats that are usually liquid at room temperature.

5. The units for measuring energy in foods are ___?___ .

6. Portions of foods are called ___?___ .

7. Your body needs ___?___ in large amounts.

8. A waxy substance found naturally in the blood is ___?___ .

9. You have a ___?___ if you eat foods from each of the five food groups.

10. Another name for blood sugar is ___?___ .

Key Words

Write the numbers 1 to 10 in your health notebook or on a separate sheet of paper. After each number, copy the sentence and fill in the missing term. Page numbers in ( ) tell you where to look in the chapter if you need help.

calories (127)
glucose (127)
glycogen (127)
unsaturated fats (128)
cholesterol (128)

amino acids (129)
macrominerals (133)
servings (136)
balanced diet (139)
malnutrition (142)

Write the numbers 11 to 17 on your paper. After each number, write a sentence that defines the term. Page numbers in ( ) tell you where to look in the chapter if you need help.

11. simple carbohydrates (127)

12. complex carbohydrates (127)

13. saturated fats (128)

14. trace minerals (133)

15. nutritional deficiency (143)

16. desirable weight (145)

17. fad diets (147)

Remembering What You Learned

Page numbers in ( ) tell you where to look in the chapter if you need help.

1. Why does your body need nutrients? (126)

2. How are carbohydrates used? (127)

3. Why is fiber important in your diet? (127)

4. What are the chief energy nutrients? (128)

5. What are four ways in which fats are used in the body? (128)

6. Why are high levels of cholesterol and saturated fats harmful to the body? (128)

7. Why are proteins important to your diet? (129)

8. Why is vitamin C essential to good health? (132)

9. What kinds of minerals does the body require in very small amounts? (133)

10. What are the macrominerals? (133)

11. Why is water an important nutrient? (134–135)

12. What are the five basic food groups? (136)

13. What is involved in planning a balanced diet, besides choosing foods from each basic group? (139)

14. Name two health problems caused by nutritional deficiencies. (143–144)

15. What happens if you continually take in too much of the nutrients that you need? (145)

16. What is the best way to control your weight? (146)

Thinking About What You Learned

1. Many adults weigh more when they are 40 than they did when they were 20. Why do they gain weight?

2. Why is it unwise to skip meals?

3. What is your desirable weight?

4. What sources of protein are low in cholesterol?

Writing About What You Learned

1. Write a menu plan for your family for one day. You should include foods that will contain all the nutrients necessary for a balanced diet. Then vary your menus to make a plan for one week.

2. Survey your classmates to find out what everyone had for breakfast. Make a list of all those foods. Decide what foods were high in nutrients. Present your results to the class.

3. Make a chart, for use at home, that lists the five food groups, foods in each group, and the recommended numbers of daily servings. Keep the chart in your kitchen as a reminder for your family to eat a balanced diet.

Applying What You Learned

PHYSICAL EDUCATION

Plan a personal exercise routine that you can combine with your daily balanced diet to help maintain your desirable weight. If you need to gain or lose weight, consult a parent or guardian first. Then plan your diet and exercise to fit your needs.

Modified True or False

Write the numbers 1 to 15 in your health notebook or on a separate sheet of paper. After each number, write *true* or *false* to describe the sentence. If the sentence is false, also write a term that replaces the underlined term and makes the sentence true.

1. A <u>serving</u> is a healthful amount of food to eat from a food group at one meal.

2. If you do not get enough of the nutrients you need, <u>nutrition</u> may result.

3. Fiber is a <u>simple</u> carbohydrate.

4. <u>Unsaturated</u> fats are usually liquid at room temperature.

5. Not getting enough <u>iron</u> in your diet may result in a mineral deficiency.

6. Your body needs the minerals calcium and <u>sodium</u> in the greatest amounts.

7. B-complex and C vitamins are <u>water-soluble</u> vitamins.

8. Glucose not used by the body is changed into <u>refined sugar</u>.

9. <u>Fiber</u> helps your body digest food.

10. Every cell in your body contains <u>water</u>.

11. The Meat, Poultry, Fish, Dry Beans, Eggs, and Nuts Group is your chief source of <u>glycogen</u>.

12. Extra <u>salt</u> in the diet causes body tissues to hold extra water.

13. Kwashiorkor is a disease caused by a <u>protein</u> deficiency.

14. A diet to lose weight that involves eating only bananas is an example of a <u>fad diet</u>.

15. <u>Protein</u> is a waxy substance made by the body and found in blood.

Short Answer

Write the numbers 16 to 23 on your paper. Write a complete sentence to answer each question.

16. How can eating foods high in saturated fats be harmful to your health?

17. How are vitamins used by your body?

18. Why does your body need large amounts of calcium and phosphorus?

19. How is the Fats, Oils, and Sweets Group different from the five basic food groups?

20. How can you determine a person's desirable weight?

21. What are three ways in which the body loses water every day?

22. From which food group should you obtain your major supply of carbohydrates?

23. Why is a diet high in refined sugar not a balanced diet?

Essay

Write the numbers 24 and 25 on your paper. Write paragraphs with complete sentences to answer each question.

24. How can it be possible to eat three meals a day and still suffer malnutrition?

25. Describe how different methods of cooking a particular food might change its nutritional value.

ACTIVITIES FOR HOME OR SCHOOL

Projects to Do

1. The labels on food packages show the ingredients that make up the food. Some labels also list the nutrients in the products. Collect and display a variety of food labels that show nutrients. Determine the number of calories and grams of fat that a serving of each food contains.

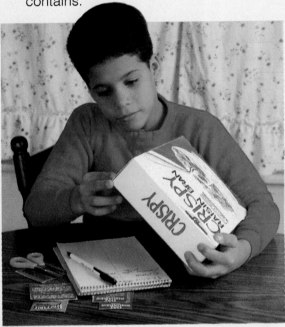

■ *Collect labels from several foods and list the nutrients.*

2. Choose a region of the United States other than where you live. Find out names of foods served in that region. You may want to look in various cookbooks for help. Then plan a nutritious meal that might be served in that part of the country. Try to include something from each of the four food groups in your meal. If you can, prepare the meal for your family.

3. Find a simple recipe for a protein-rich food (fish, cheese, eggs, meat) to discuss with your classmates. What ingredients are needed to prepare the food? What steps are involved in the preparation? If possible, prepare the dish for your family and friends.

Information to Find

1. Vitamin or mineral deficiencies in a person's diet can cause certain diseases. In your school library or public library, find out about beriberi, rickets, or pellagra. In a written or oral report, describe the disease and the discovery of the cure.

2. Scientists are studying ways to grow more nutritious foods to feed the world population. Find articles in books and magazines about some of their discoveries. You may want to look up information about a grain called *triticale,* food "farms" in the sea, or plant products that can be substituted for meats.

Books to Read

Here are some books you can look for in your school library or the public library to find more information about food, nutrition, and your daily diet.

Arnold, Caroline. *Too Fat? Too Thin? Do You Have a Choice?* Morrow.

Perl, Lila. *Junk Food, Fast Food, Health Food: What America Eats and Why.* Houghton/Clarion.

Thompson, Paul. *Nutrition.* Franklin Watts.

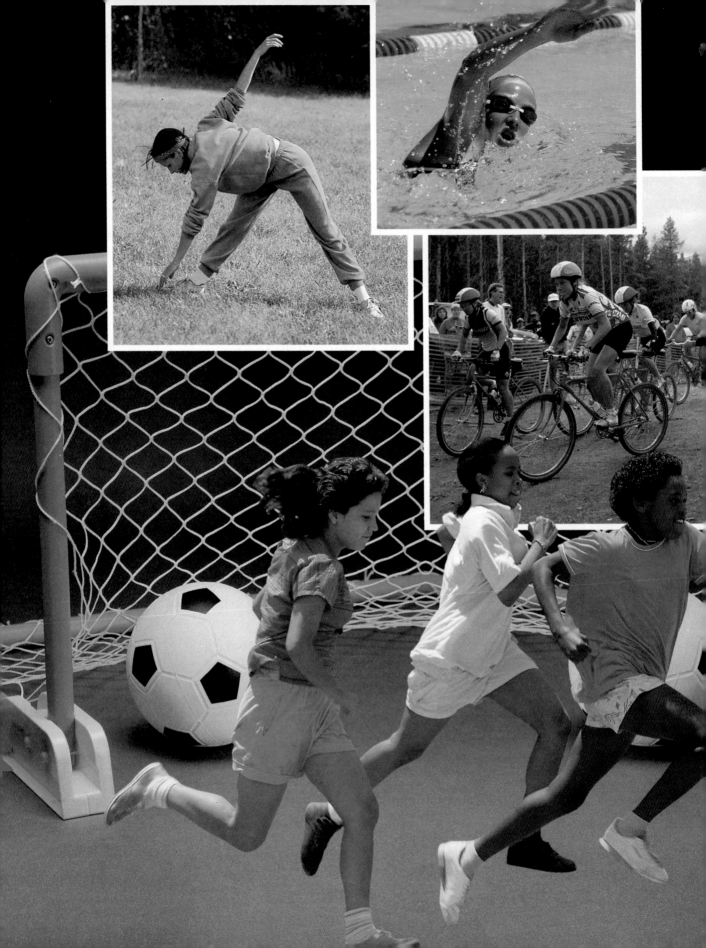

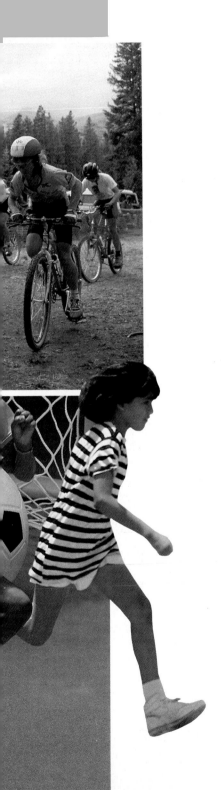

EXERCISE AND YOUR HEALTH

Achieving the goals of feeling good on the inside and looking good on the outside depends a lot on your health habits. Exercise, rest, and sleep can make you strong and give you energy. But you need them in a daily balance that helps you maintain wellness. The amount and kinds of exercise, rest, and sleep that you need may change during your teenage years. When you know how much of each you need, you can start a personal program for wellness. Following such a program can help you develop habits that will benefit you throughout your life.

GETTING READY TO LEARN

Key Questions

- Why is it important to learn about balancing exercise, rest, and sleep?
- How do you feel about the way you now exercise, rest, and sleep?
- How can you take more responsibility for choosing healthful ways to exercise, rest, and sleep?

Main Chapter Sections

1 Exercise and Physical Fitness
2 Planning an Exercise Program
3 Rest, Sleep, and Physical Fitness

1 Exercise and Physical Fitness

KEY WORDS

physical fitness
exercise
aerobic exercise
target heart rate
cardiorespiratory
  system
endurance
muscle fibers
strength
flexibility
posture

physical fitness (FIHZ ih kuhl • FIHT nuhs), a condition in which each of the systems of the body works properly.

exercise (EHK suhr syz), any activity that makes the body work hard.

Like most people today, you probably have an interest in your body's fitness and appearance. You may want to have a firm body or develop the strength to do well in a certain activity. You need to feel energetic to get through a busy day. Taking an interest in your body's fitness now can get you started on a program of fitness activities that will help you throughout your life. Being fit and staying fit are strongly related to health and wellness.

Being physically fit allows you to handle all your usual daily activities with a sense of energy. You are also able to handle extra physical work or stress without too much difficulty. **Physical fitness** is a condition in which each body system works properly. For example, physically fit lungs take in plenty of air each time you inhale. A fit heart pumps plenty of blood each time it beats. It does not have to beat too quickly. Your muscles can work hard without aching or tiring easily.

When you are active, your body works harder than when you are resting. Physical activity is the key to physical fitness. Any activity that makes your body work hard is **exercise.** Swimming, dancing, jogging, hiking, walking, and playing sports are several kinds of exercise. You can probably think of others.

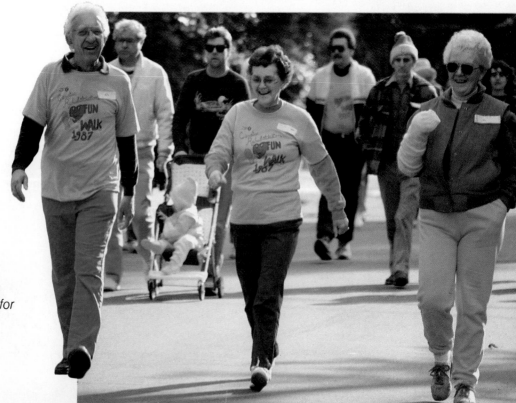

■ No matter what a person's age, regular exercise is important for maintaining physical fitness.

What Happens When You Exercise?

If you watch an experienced jogger from a distance, his or her actions may seem effortless. Inside, however, the person's body is like a power plant pouring out energy. This outpouring of energy is a response to the demands of vigorous exercise. The muscles need extra energy when a person exercises hard for a long time. The lungs respond by supplying more air with each breath. The heart pumps more blood with each beat. More oxygen is carried by the blood to the muscle cells. This oxygen helps "burn" the additional nutrients needed for extra energy.

Warming Up. Before your body can start to use the large amount of energy needed for exercise, you need to warm up. A warm-up, which slowly gets the body ready for vigorous activity, might be stretching and then jogging in place for five minutes. Warm-up exercises are mild exercises, such as stretching, that raise the body's level of functioning. They bring more oxygen into your body and lessen your chances of getting muscle cramps or injury during exercise.

As you warm up, your breathing becomes faster and deeper. You take more air into your lungs. The extra oxygen taken in is carried by your blood to your muscles. The blood vessels in your muscles expand so that more blood can enter.

■ Before doing vigorous exercise, you need to warm up your body with mild exercise, such as stretching.

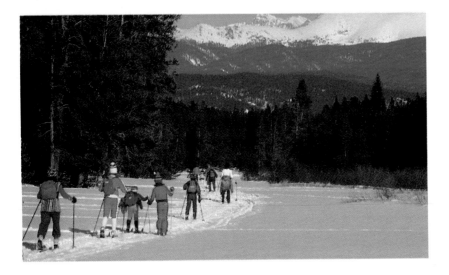

■ Cross-country skiing is one of many kinds of aerobic exercise.

Aerobic Exercise. Once you have warmed up, you are ready for vigorous exercise. Exercise that makes the body use a lot of oxygen is **aerobic exercise.** Swimming, cross-country skiing, jogging, bicycling, brisk walking, and skipping rope are all forms of aerobic exercise. Any game that involves continuous running or other movement may also be aerobic exercise.

aerobic exercise (air OH bihk • EHK suhr syz), any kind of exercise that makes the body use a lot of oxygen.

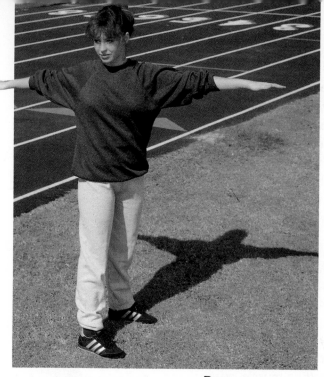

■ *After vigorous exercise, your body needs to slow down. Cooling down with mild exercise allows your muscles to relax gradually.*

An aerobic exercise is done to keep your heart at its target heart rate. A **target heart rate** is the rate at which a person's heart needs to beat to ensure that the cardiorespiratory system is working hard enough to benefit from the exercise. The **cardiorespiratory system** is the combination of the circulatory and respiratory systems, which work together.

During a warm-up, a person's heart rate may increase from about 80 to over 120 beats per minute within two to three minutes. During aerobic exercise, it may further increase to 150 beats per minute and level off. To get the most benefit, the person should exercise at his or her target heart rate for at least 20 minutes three times per week. Before you start exercising, be certain that you are healthy enough to exercise vigorously. Check with your physician before beginning an exercise program.

target heart rate, the rate at which your heart needs to beat so that your cardiorespiratory system works hard enough to benefit from exercise.

cardiorespiratory system (KAHRD ee oh RES puh ruh tohr ee • SIHS tuhm), the combination of the circulatory and respiratory systems.

Cooling Down. After a session of aerobic exercise, you need to gradually slow your activity. By stretching and doing other mild exercises, you allow your muscles to gradually relax. This prevents the extra blood supply in your leg muscles from being trapped there by the too-sudden narrowing of your blood vessels. If you stopped right after aerobic exercise, this pooling of blood could cause painful muscle cramps. Cool-down exercises allow blood vessels to narrow gradually. Then the extra blood from your leg muscles goes back to your heart, to be made available again to other body systems, such as the digestive system.

How Does Exercise Improve Physical Fitness?

The real benefits of exercise come after you have been exercising regularly for several weeks or months. When the body has been exercised, it can adapt more readily to a need for more oxygen and a higher heart rate. Your improved physical fitness provides increased endurance, strength, and flexibility, as well as other benefits.

Exercise Builds Endurance. The ability to perform an activity for a long time is **endurance.** Muscle endurance and cardiorespiratory endurance are both important parts of physical fitness. They let you work or play hard for a long time without becoming overly tired. When you exercise, your body needs more nutrients and oxygen. As your cell activity increases, your body also needs to get rid of more waste products. Therefore, your endurance depends on the efficiency of your circulatory and respiratory systems. Exercise that makes your heart and lungs work harder increases your endurance.

endurance (ihn DUR uhns), the ability to perform an activity for a long time.

Exercise Builds Strength. Muscles consist of bundles of long muscle cells, called **muscle fibers.** When a part of your body moves, muscle fibers contract. Normal movement involves only some of the fibers in a muscle. When you exercise vigorously, however, you use more muscle fibers. Regular periods of exercise will cause these bundles of fibers to grow thicker and stronger. Your muscles' **strength,** or the amount of force they can apply, increases.

muscle fibers (MUHS uhl • FY buhrz), bundles of long muscle cells.

strength, the amount of force muscles can apply.

■ *Regular exercise causes muscle tissue to grow thicker and stronger.*

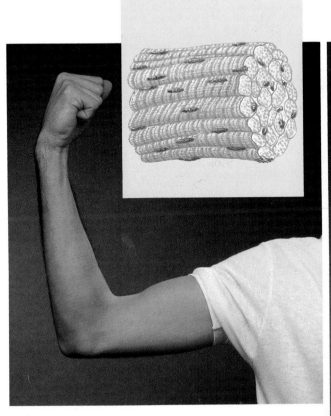
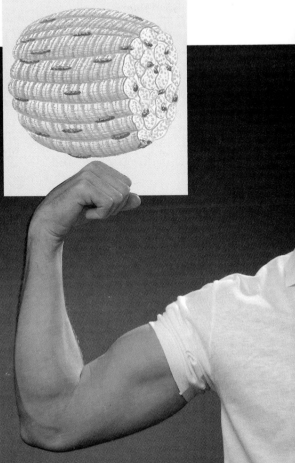

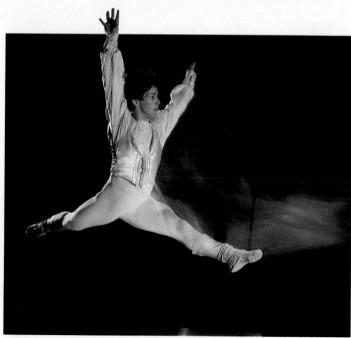

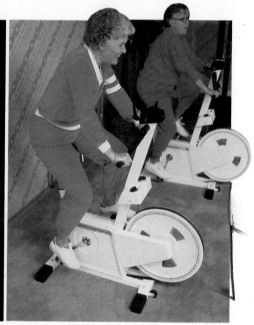

■ *Certain exercises, left, help develop flexibility. Other exercises, right, improve cardiovascular fitness.*

flexibility (flehk suh BIHL uht ee), the ability to move joints freely and smoothly.

Exercise Builds Flexibility.   Another sign of fitness is the ability to move freely and smoothly. The ability to move this way is called **flexibility.** To be flexible, you must be able to move your joints freely. Your muscles must be capable of stretching.

Dancing and gymnastics are two forms of exercise that increase flexibility. Because they involve stretching and bending, they help lengthen and loosen muscles. This in turn allows greater movement of your joints.

Exercise Builds Cardiovascular Fitness.   With regular vigorous exercise, the heart works to capacity and the blood vessels expand to carry more oxygen and nutrients. The muscles can then become stronger and able to work for a longer time without tiring. As a person continues to exercise, the body responds by becoming more efficient. The heart of an average adult male beats about 60–80 times a minute when resting. A strong, fit heart will beat only about 60 time a minute. The fit heart can pump the same amount of blood in fewer beats. It does the same work with less effort and more efficiency.

Cardiovascular fitness is very important because cardiovascular diseases are the number one killer of adults. The most common cardiovascular problems include heart attack, stroke, and high blood pressure. They are caused in part by poor health habits such as overeating, smoking, and lack of regular exercise. By improving your circulation, you lower your blood pressure and reduce your risk of a stroke caused by a blocked blood vessel in the brain.

Exercise Helps Your Posture. Your **posture** is the way you hold your body as you sit, stand, or walk. Regular exercise can improve your posture by strengthening your muscles. Strong abdominal and back muscles enable you to hold your body straight without conscious effort. Good posture keeps you from slumping and slouching and developing aches and pains. All this certainly helps your appearance.

If you find you tire easily when you sit at your desk for a long time, you may need to improve your posture. Try sitting with your back straight and your shoulders back. When you lean forward, lean from your hips. These suggestions may help you avoid neck and back pains.

Posture is also important for doing hard physical work without damaging your body. For example, if you were to pick up a heavy box of books from the floor simply by leaning over and straightening up, you could hurt your back. You can avoid back injuries by keeping your back straight and bending your knees instead. Grasp the load close to your body. Then push up with your thighs to straighten your knees and stand up. By using this method, you lift the load with the strong muscles of your legs. Using this safe posture when lifting is a good habit for home, school, and work.

posture (PAHS chuhr), the way a person holds the body to sit, stand, and walk.

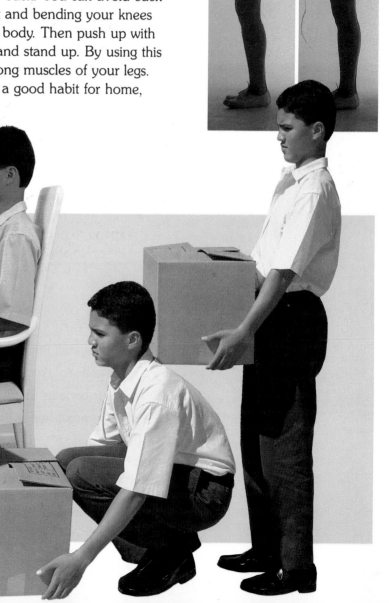

■ *Proper posture means more than just standing up straight. It means sitting and lifting properly, too.*

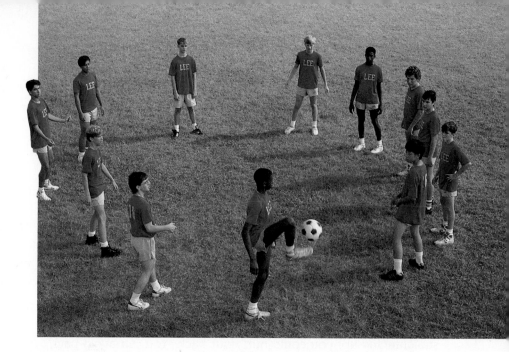

■ *Some forms of exercise provide the opportunity to meet new people and make new friends.*

Exercise Helps Your Emotional Health.   Looking your best and mastering new activities can improve your self-esteem as well as your physical fitness. Exercise activities can also provide a chance to meet other people who share your interests. Playing games or sports with others can give you a sense of belonging. It can help you develop positive attitudes and improve your ability to get along with other people.

Exercise can also help you relieve tension and worry. After exercising, you may feel calm and relaxed. Feeling this way will help you handle the demands of your daily activities.

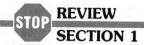 **REVIEW**
SECTION 1

REMEMBER?

1. What is physical fitness?
2. What role does oxygen play in aerobic exercise?
3. State four benefits of exercise.
4. What is a target heart rate?

THINK!

5. How can exercise relieve stress?
6. Why are warm-up and cool-down periods necessary parts of an exercise workout?

Health Close-up

Physical Fitness and Physical Disabilities

People with physical disabilities have the same fitness needs that other people have. Good physical health, good emotional health, and the ability to cooperate with others are important to everyone's well-being. Physical-fitness programs can be developed to fit the special needs of people with physical disabilities. These programs can be designed around any person's abilities and interests.

Conditioning. Exercises adjusted to a person's special needs may be selected to increase flexibility, strength, and endurance. Muscles that are not used or stretched tend to become weak and stiff. A program involving weight machines or simple movements can help people keep their bodies in the best shape possible.

Swimming. Swimming is an excellent activity for people confined to wheelchairs or for people who may not have the use of an arm or leg. Since water helps support the body's weight, swimming places less strain on the body than other kinds of exercise.

Sports. Many sports, with minor rule or equipment changes, can be enjoyed by people who have disabilities. Blind people can take part in a sprint race by skimming their hands along a string while running. Wheelchair-bound people can play basketball. Sports may be more fun than straight exercising for those who like being part of a team.

Dance. People who have physical disabilities can enjoy many forms of dance. Learning to dance improves a person's control of body movements. It offers a special sense of achievement to a person with a physical disability. Dancing builds relationships with others and lets people express themselves.

Thinking Beyond

1. What physical fitness needs do all people have?
2. Give an example of a particular physical disability. Develop an activity regimen that includes a warm-up, various kinds of exercise, and a cool-down.

■ *Aerobic exercise, including swimming and basketball, benefits people who exercise regularly.*

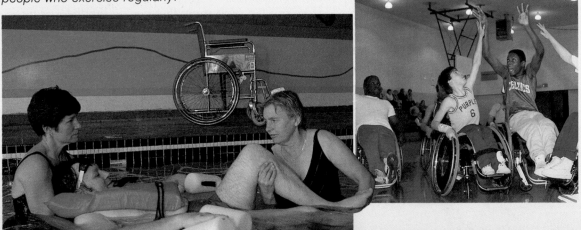

2 Planning an Exercise Program

In order to maintain good cardiovascular health and fitness, it is necessary to establish a lifetime habit of regular exercise. The benefits of exercise are quickly lost if an exercise program is not maintained. Therefore, it is important to plan an exercise program that you like and will continue to follow. Many people say that they want to follow good health habits and intend to start an exercise program. Unfortunately, many people never actually get started. Others start but soon drop out of their own programs because they lose interest and motivation. Choose an activity you enjoy, and avoid becoming a dropout.

■ *In order to be successful, an exercise program needs to include activities that are enjoyable.*

MYTH AND FACT

Myth: Once you are in good physical condition, you can stop exercising.

Fact: The benefits you get from regular exercise do not last for more than a month after you stop. The benefits of exercise cannot be stored; you must do it regularly.

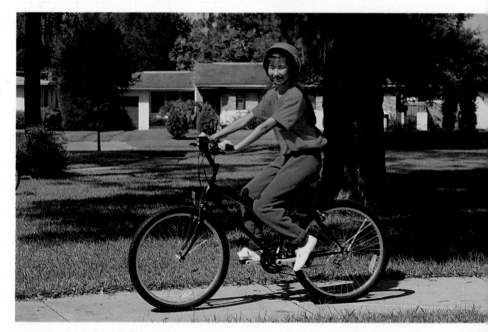

What Makes Up an Exercise Plan?

You may think that you do not have time to exercise. To develop an exercise plan, you must first decide that exercising is important. It must become part of your regular activity. How can you find time to exercise? Planning is essential.

You can plan for exercise by setting aside a certain time for it during your day. Perhaps the best time for you to exercise is in the morning before going to school. Many people find that early morning is a good time for exercise since there is less interruption than later. They find that they begin the day feeling more energetic after exercising.

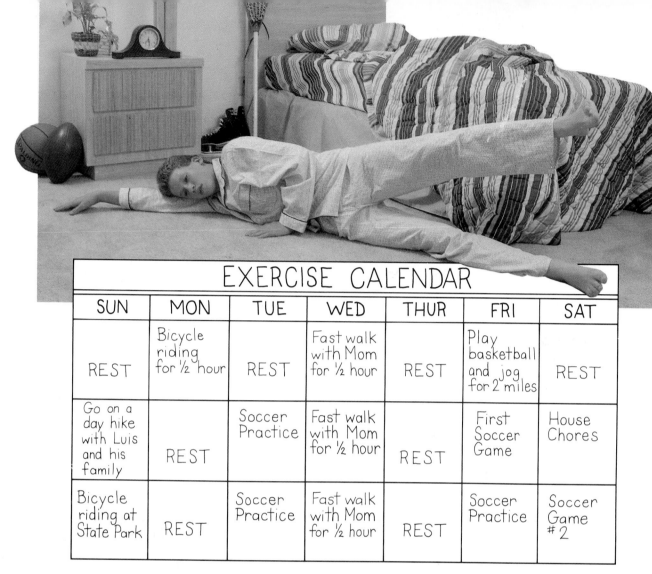

EXERCISE CALENDAR

SUN	MON	TUE	WED	THUR	FRI	SAT
REST	Bicycle riding for ½ hour	REST	Fast walk with Mom for ½ hour	REST	Play basketball and jog for 2 miles	REST
Go on a day hike with Luis and his family	REST	Soccer Practice	Fast walk with Mom for ½ hour	REST	First Soccer Game	House Chores
Bicycle riding at State Park	REST	Soccer Practice	Fast walk with Mom for ½ hour	REST	Soccer Practice	Soccer Game #2

Others prefer vigorous exercise right after a day of school or work. Then they feel not only more relaxed, but also more energetic during the evening. Students feel more alert for doing homework. Vigorous exercise is usually not best just before you want to sleep. The body is more ready to work than sleep after vigorous exercise.

By developing a plan and a habit of exercise, you will find it easier to continue. You should plan to do aerobic exercise *at least* three times a week. Less than that will not give you enough cardiorespiratory and strength benefit. As you progress, you may want to keep your workout periods short but increase them to four or five a week.

The kind of activity you choose may determine when and where you exercise. The time and place may not always stay the same. Perhaps there are certain sports and activities that you enjoy at different times of the year.

■ Exercising at the same time each day is not as important as exercising at least three times each week.

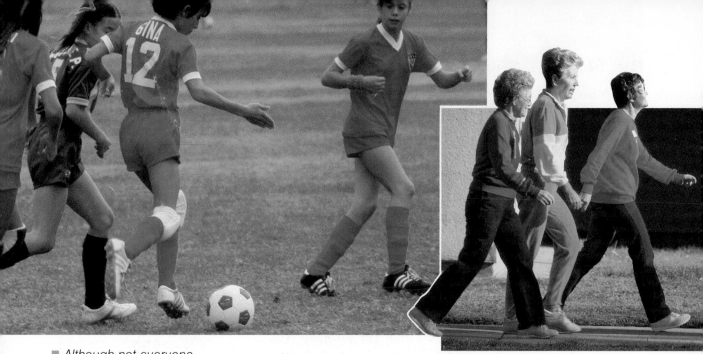

■ *Although not everyone can do the same kinds of exercise, regular exercise needs to be a part of everyone's life.*

Why Should You Vary Your Exercise?

To develop fitness, it is important to do exercises for strength, flexibility, and endurance. However, there are many ways to stretch or strengthen your muscles. You may become bored by doing the same exercises over and over. One important decision for you to make is what kind of aerobic exercise you like best at a given time. You are more likely to continue exercising if you enjoy the activity. It may be helpful to try a new activity when you grow tired of what you are doing.

For example, aerobic dance has become very popular. Many people find it especially enjoyable when done to music. But they may enjoy jogging, cycling, or swimming as variations. You do not have to do the same kind of exercise every day. By varying the aerobic exercise you do, you will stay interested.

Another part of making exercise choices is recognizing that your aerobic activities may need to change as you grow older. It is important to select an activity that you will be able to continue to do. Perhaps you like playing basketball with your friends or on a school team. Later, as an adult, you may find it difficult to get enough friends together for a game. Sports played in pairs, such as tennis and racquetball, may be easier to arrange. For this reason, you may need to consider a pair sport.

The most important thing to remember is that you need to continue some form of aerobic exercise for a lifetime. If you do, you will continue to enhance your fitness.

How Should You Begin an Exercise Program?

Most people your age can begin nearly any exercise program. Your physical education teacher can help you set up a plan based on your interests and your current fitness level. If you have had medical problems with your heart, breathing, muscles, or bones, ask a parent or guardian to check with your physician. Your physician will help you set any needed limits on your exercise. There are also several steps you can take when you begin to exercise that will help you stay safe.

Set Achievable Goals. Start your exercise plan by knowing your fitness limits. Then set goals for yourself that are realistic. Once your body has become used to regular exercise, you will want more vigorous exercise. Gradually increase the amount of time you spend and the amount of muscle work needed. You may feel a little sore, but a gradual increase in time and work should not cause pain.

Avoid Certain Conditions. There are several conditions that can make exercising outdoors unsafe. High air-pollution levels can make outdoor exercise unsafe for your lungs. High temperatures can also be a problem. If it is more than 90 degrees Fahrenheit (32 degrees Celsius) or if the humidity is 80 percent or more, you should not exercise outdoors. Modify your exercise to fit your environment.

A combination of high heat and humidity is the most dangerous. Heat and humidity can prevent your body from cooling itself quickly enough. Exercising in these conditions can cause heat exhaustion. **Heat exhaustion** occurs when the body loses too much fluid because of sweating. The symptoms of heat exhaustion include clammy skin, headache, extreme weakness, and nausea.

heat exhaustion (HEET • ihg ZAWS chuhn), an illness that occurs when the body loses too much fluid because of sweating.

■ *On hot, humid days, you should exercise in the evening or in the morning, when it is cooler.*

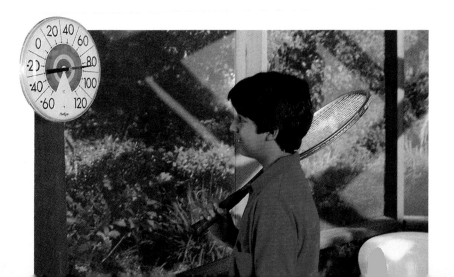

169

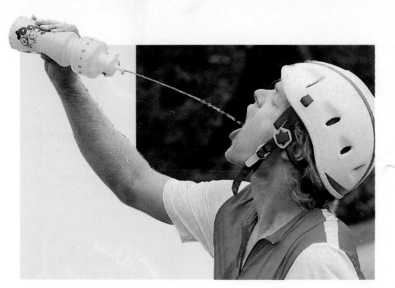

Drink Plenty of Water.

Drinking water before, during, and after exercise is an important safety precaution. Your body must have plenty of water to work properly. If you sweat a lot during exercise, you must replace the water you lose. Drinking enough water regularly will help keep you healthy and ready for exercise.

■ *Be sure to drink plenty of water when exercising in hot weather.*

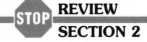

REVIEW
SECTION 2

REMEMBER?

1. How often should you exercise?
2. Why is variety important in exercise?
3. How is safety involved in planning your exercise program?

THINK!

4. How can you continue to exercise if it is hot and humid outdoors?
5. What are some benefits of exercising with other people?

Making Wellness Choices

Joan and Alex like to go jogging three times a week. They enjoy exercising together and plan to go jogging today. While Alex is on his way over to Joan's home, Joan hears on the radio that the temperature is 90 degrees Fahrenheit (32 degrees Celsius) and the humidity is 95 percent. When Alex arrives, Joan tells Alex the news. Alex says they can go ahead and jog anyway because they are already physically fit.

 What should Joan do? Explain your wellness choice.

170

3 Rest, Sleep, and Physical Fitness

When you are physically fit, you can work or play long and hard without tiring. Still, enough hard work will make even the most physically fit person tired. This tired feeling is known as **fatigue.** Physical fatigue can occur when the body's cells have used up available energy supplies and have built up waste materials that need to be removed.

The fatigue that comes after exercise can be a pleasant feeling. Too much exercise, however, can make your muscles feel weak and shaky. They may even cramp, or fail to relax properly. Cramps can occur when muscles do not get enough blood to supply oxygen and nutrients and carry off wastes.

Sometimes inactivity can cause fatigue. After a long bus ride, for example, you may be tired and your muscles may be stiff because you have had to sit for several hours. Your neck and back may ache.

Strenuous mental activity can also bring on fatigue. Studying all day or worrying a lot about a problem can be tiring. You can develop tense muscles and even headaches.

Why Do You Need to Rest?

Fatigue is a signal from your body to stop what you are doing and rest. Rest gives your body a chance to restore energy to your cells. It also allows your body to get rid of the waste materials produced by your cells.

fatigue (fuh TEEG), tired feeling.

■ *Even for people who are physically fit, hard work causes fatigue.*

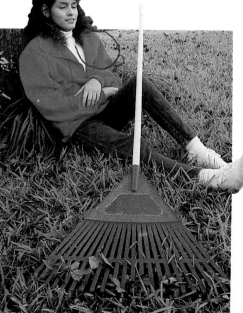

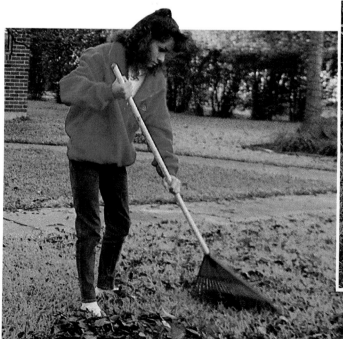

Sometimes a short period of relaxation will take care of your fatigue. One way of relaxing is to change what you are doing. Simple activities, such as games or hobbies, can help you relax after hard mental work. Walking with a full arm swing or doing a few easy exercises can also be relaxing. You can loosen up stiff muscles by stretching. Breathing deeply and slowly can also help relax your whole body.

What Is Sleep?

Sleep is a special kind of rest. About one-third of your life is spent asleep. During sleep your body carries out certain activities that are vital to your health.

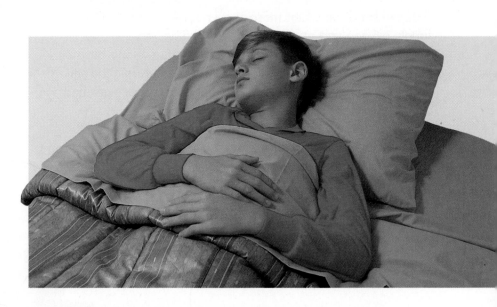

■ *Sleep is vital to your well-being. Lack of sleep affects you physically and mentally.*

Scientists still do not know everything that happens during sleep, but they do know that sleep is absolutely necessary. People's behavior changes after several days without sleep. They become unpleasant and unfriendly. They cannot talk or think clearly or even carry out simple tasks. They may begin to see and hear things that do not exist. Once these people begin to sleep regularly again, their behavior returns to normal.

What Happens When You Sleep?

If you have ever watched someone sleep, you may have noticed that he or she moved and turned many times without waking up. There are also changes that occur during sleep that cannot be seen. During sleep your body gives off less heat and your temperature drops about one degree. Your heart rate and breathing rate slow down, and your blood pressure drops.

Your blood flows more slowly. Moving during sleep helps keep blood flowing smoothly throughout your body. Muscle relaxation during sleep helps you recover from the fatigue of the day.

While you sleep, your mouth and nose produce less mucus and saliva. That is why sleep may lessen many cold symptoms. Other secretions of the body increase during sleep. The pituitary gland, for example, sends out more growth hormone. The extra growth hormone speeds up cell growth and repair.

Sleep dulls your senses. Usually you do not hear noises unless they are very loud. You do not smell things that you would if you were awake. Your brain, while remaining active, shifts into special sleep activities.

All these changes occur in stages. Scientists have identified four different stages of sleep. During each stage, certain activities take place. Each activity is essential to your well-being.

■ *During an average night's sleep, a person may change position 40 to 70 times.*

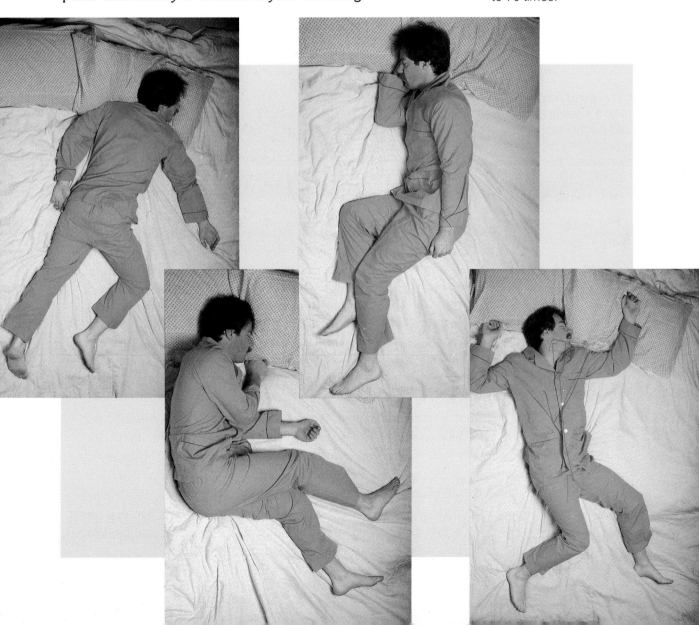

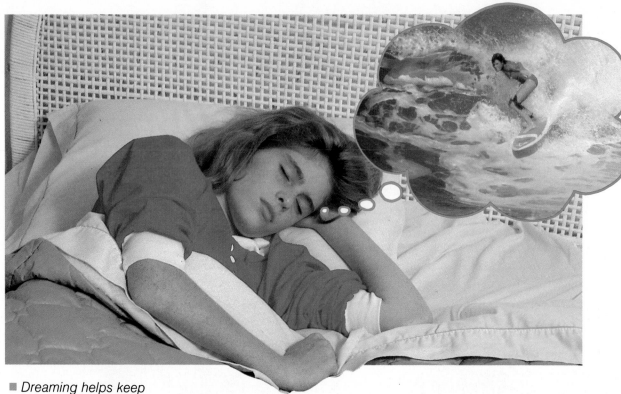

■ *Dreaming helps keep people healthy. It may help people work through their problems or learn about their hidden wishes.*

What Are Dreams?

Among the most puzzling mysteries of sleep are dreams. Everyone talks about having dreams, yet scientists have not discovered what causes them.

Scientists do know, however, that everyone needs to dream. In one study, volunteers were awakened every time they entered rapid eye movement (REM) sleep, the stage during which dreaming occurs. Researchers wanted to find out what would happen to people who were prevented from dreaming. They discovered that after several days without dreaming, the volunteers became upset and irritable. They became hungry more often and ate more than usual. When they were then allowed to sleep normally, they skipped the other stages of sleep and went straight to REM sleep. It seemed as if they needed to catch up on the dreaming they had missed.

You dream several times every night, although you may not always remember your dreams. Researchers believe that your most intense period of dreaming occurs during REM sleep just before you are ready to wake up.

Dreams take place in certain parts of your brain. While some parts of your brain are at rest during sleep, others become more active. It is in these parts, many scientists believe, that the images and events called dreams are created.

Dreams can take many different forms. Some seem as real as everyday life, while others have a magical, make-believe quality. Dreams can be pleasant or disturbing. When dreams are very frightening and upsetting, they are called nightmares.

Although scientists believe dreaming helps keep people healthy, they are not sure exactly what purpose it serves. Dreaming may be a safe way of exploring certain thoughts and feelings. They may help you "dream up" solutions to problems in your life. Sometimes, scientists feel, you may become comfortable with new experiences by dreaming about them.

STAGES OF SLEEP

Stage	Characteristics	Brain-Wave Activity
1	Sleep is very light. Your thoughts wander. You begin to fall asleep. You could be awakened at this point and not know you had fallen asleep.	
2	Sleep becomes deeper. Under your eyelids, your eyes slowly roll. Your body temperature and blood pressure drop.	
3	Sleep is deep and calm. Your heart rate, body temperature, and blood pressure drop to their lowest points. Your muscles are completely relaxed. During this stage it would be difficult to awaken you.	
Rapid Eye Movement (REM) Sleep (similar to stage 1)	Dreams take place. Under your eyelids, your eyes roll and move rapidly. You may toss and turn, and the muscles in your arms and legs may twitch. Your breathing and heart rate speed up.	

After REM sleep, you return to the second and third stages and then enter another period of REM sleep. During the night, you may go through this sleep cycle four or five times.

How Much Sleep Should You Get?

Not everyone requires the same amount of sleep. Babies often sleep 16 hours a day. During your teenage years, you need about 8 hours of sleep every night. As you grow older, you may need less sleep. Some elderly people need only 5 to 6 hours of sleep each night. When you are ill, you may sleep more. Your body cells are working extra hard to fight your illness. Being especially active can also increase your need for sleep.

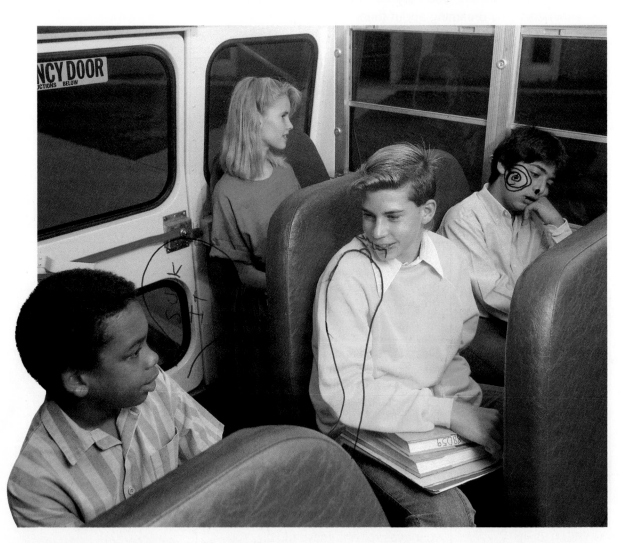

■ *People who do not get enough sleep at night may find themselves falling asleep at quiet moments during the day.*

Your body has ways of telling you whether you are getting enough sleep. If you have little trouble staying awake and alert during the day, you are probably getting enough sleep. If you often feel tired or sleepy during the day, you may need more. Going to bed an hour earlier can give you the extra sleep you need. A comfortable bed and a quiet, dark room will also help.

Rest and sleep, like exercise, are important to your physical fitness. Finding out how much exercise, rest, and sleep your own body needs is important to maintaining your personal wellness.

STOP **REVIEW**
SECTION 3

REMEMBER?

1. What is fatigue?
2. How much sleep do most young people need every night?
3. What are the four stages of sleep?

THINK!

4. How is relaxing different from sleeping?
5. Why might your need for sleep affect your exercise schedule?

Thinking About Your Health

Do You Have Healthful Fitness Habits?

How do you know if you are developing healthful exercise and fitness habits? Ask yourself whether each of the following statements applies to you. If you say no to any of them, you might need to improve your habits. You should talk about this with your parent, guardian, school nurse, or teacher.

■ You have enough energy to get through the day.

■ You exercise vigorously for 20 to 30 minutes at least three times each week.

■ You use exercise to relieve tension and worry.

■ When lifting something heavy, you use your legs and arms, not your back.

■ You practice good posture when you stand, sit, and walk.

■ You do different kinds of exercises to improve your endurance, strength, and flexibility.

■ You find a quiet time each day to relax.

■ You get at least 8 hours of sleep every night.

People in Health

An Interview with a Fitness Instructor

Tim Volk knows about the importance of physical fitness and aerobic exercise. He is a fitness instructor in Cheyenne, Wyoming.

What is a fitness instructor?

A fitness instructor is a person who teaches a group of people safe and effective ways to exercise. A fitness instructor helps motivate and educate people in all areas of physical fitness, including aerobic exercise.

How is your fitness class organized?

I begin each class with a series of warm-up activities. These help raise the body's level of functioning and prepare it for more vigorous exercise. Contracting and stretching the muscles not only warms them but also prevents injuries. After the warm-up section of class, I demonstrate low-impact movements.

What are low-impact movements?

Low-impact movements are those in which one foot is kept on the ground at all times. If both feet leave the ground at the same time, certain parts of the body feel an *impact,* or force, upon landing. Keeping one foot on the ground helps reduce the impact on the body. An example of a low-impact movement is a marching step in which the knees are raised and lowered with no bouncing movement.

Are low-impact movements aerobic?

Yes, low-impact movements can be aerobic if they are done correctly. I instruct the class to add arm movements and keep their arms above the heart. These movements make the heart work harder and faster. For members of the class who want to do something a little different from the low-impact movements, I demonstrate high-energy movements. An example of a high-energy movement would be jumping jacks.

■ *Mr. Volk teaches low-impact movements to an aerobics class.*

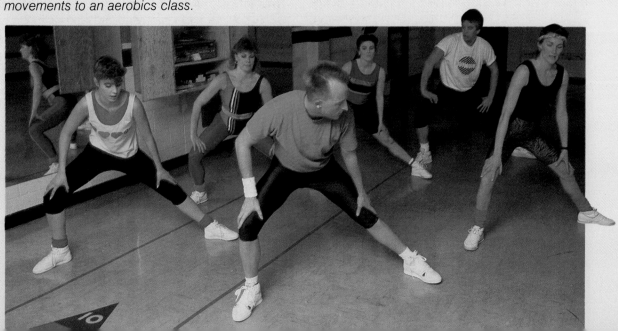

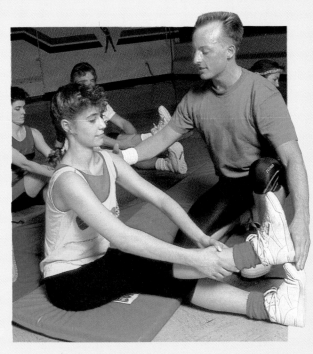

Stretching increases flexibility, helping to prevent injuries during vigorous exercise.

What do you do after the aerobics section of the class?

After the aerobics section, class members cool down by walking around the room, moving their arms above their heads, and taking deep breaths. Then it is time to do exercises that work specific muscle groups, such as those in the abdomen and legs. Next, I lead the class in stretching exercises to increase flexibility and to prevent soreness. Finally, I ask everyone to count his or her pulse for 10 seconds. By multiplying by 6, it is possible to determine whether the heartbeat has returned to its normal rate.

Do you have people take their pulse at any other time during the class?

At certain times during the class, I ask members of the class to check their pulse. Each person is working toward a different level of fitness. Using specific calculations based on age and fitness, I can determine the safest and most beneficial heart rate each should maintain during exercise. This is referred to as the target heart rate. Exercising beyond that target heart rate might make a person feel faint. When a member of the class is working too hard, I have him or her gently run in place or walk around the room.

Do you use music in your fitness class?

Yes. Music gives members of the class a consistent beat to follow. Also, when people have music to exercise to, they are able to take their minds off the hard work they are doing. I play the kinds of music people want to listen to so that they enjoy their exercising more.

What are some of the benefits of exercise?

In addition to improving physical fitness, exercise promotes mental health. For example, after I exercise, I feel good about myself. Exercising promotes self-confidence and self-esteem and helps people feel better and perform better in all areas of their lives.

Learn more about people who work as fitness instructors. Interview a fitness instructor. Or write for information to the American College of Sports Medicine, P.O. Box 1440, Indianapolis, IN 46206.

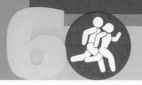

Main Ideas

- You can maintain physical fitness through regular aerobic exercise.

- Physical fitness includes endurance, strength, flexibility, cardiovascular fitness, and good posture.

- An exercise program with a variety of activities will be more likely to maintain your interest.

- You should not exercise outdoors in very hot, humid weather or in areas with heavy air pollution. Modify exercise to fit your environment.

- Drinking plenty of water will help prevent heat exhaustion.

- An important health habit is getting enough sleep and rest.

- There are four stages of sleep; most dreaming occurs during the REM stage.

Key Words

Write the numbers 1 to 12 in your health notebook or on a separate sheet of paper. After each number, copy the sentence and fill in the missing term. Page numbers in ( ) tell you where to look in the chapter if you need help.

physical fitness (158)

exercise (158)

aerobic exercise (159)

target heart rate (160)

cardiorespiratory system (160)

endurance (161)

muscle fibers (161)

strength (161)

flexibility (162)

posture (163)

heat exhaustion (169)

fatigue (171)

1. Someone who can exercise for a long time without getting tired has ___?___ .

2. You feel ___?___ when you have used up the available energy in your body's cells.

3. ___?___ is a condition in which each body system works properly.

4. If you lose too much body fluid because of sweating, you may suffer ___?___ .

5. Exercise that makes the body use a lot of oxygen is ___?___ .

6. Long muscle cells arranged in bundles are ___?___ .

7. Any activity that makes the body work hard is ___?___ .

8. People who have ___?___ can move their bodies freely and smoothly.

9. To make sure that your cardiorespiratory system is working hard, you need to reach your ___?___ .

10. The way you hold your body is your ___?___ .

11. The circulatory and respiratory systems working together make up the ___?___ .

12. The amount of force that muscles can apply is their ___?___ .

Remembering What You Learned

Page numbers in ( ) tell you where to look in the chapter if you need help.

1. Why is physical fitness important? (158)

2. What is aerobic exercise? (159)

3. What information does your target heart rate give you? (160)

4. Why is it important to cool down after you exercise? (160)

5. How can you tell if you are increasing your endurance? (161)

6. How can you improve your flexibility? (162)

7. What are three problems of the cardiovascular system? (162)

8. How does physical fitness affect posture? (163)

9. Why do people sometimes get heat exhaustion in hot, humid weather? (169)

10. What safety precautions should you take when exercising? (169–170)

11. How does sleeping help reduce fatigue? (173)

12. How is REM sleep different from the other stages? (174–175)

Thinking About What You Learned

1. Why is it important to know what your target heart rate should be before you begin exercising?

2. Why is dreaming important?

3. How does variety in exercise improve your chances of continuing your exercise program?

4. Why would you not want to exercise outdoors if there was a smog alert in your area?

5. What are the benefits of setting reasonable goals when you begin exercising?

Writing About What You Learned

1. Plan a schedule of exercise suitable for someone who is just beginning to exercise. Explain the choices you make.

2. Interview six people about their sleep patterns. Find out how much sleep they normally get and whether or not they remember their dreams. In a paragraph or two, write what you learn about sleep patterns.

Applying What You Learned

SOCIAL STUDIES

Consider how landscape and climate influence exercise habits. Find examples of sports and activities that seem to be adapted to the conditions of different regions of the United States.

LITERATURE

Find a story that uses dreams as a major theme. Present an oral report to the class describing how dreams were used in the story.

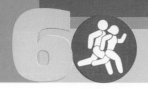
Modified True or False

Write the numbers 1 to 15 in your health notebook or on a separate sheet of paper. After each number, write *true* or *false* to describe the sentence. If the sentence is false, also write a term that replaces the underlined term and makes the sentence true.

1. Cross-country skiing is a form of <u>aerobic</u> exercise.

2. After you exercise, you should <u>warm up</u>.

3. Good <u>posture</u> helps keep your weight evenly balanced.

4. Clammy skin, headache, and nausea are all symptoms of <u>fatigue</u>.

5. You dream during <u>REM</u> sleep.

6. To get the most benefit from an aerobic exercise, you must do it for at least <u>20</u> minutes three times per week.

7. Dancing and gymnastics improve <u>muscle strength</u> through stretching.

8. A strong, physically fit adult heart beats about <u>85</u> times each minute.

9. Improving cardiovascular fitness can lower your <u>blood pressure</u>.

10. Strenuous mental activity can cause <u>heat exhaustion</u>.

11. Cold symptoms may <u>lessen</u> while you sleep.

12. You might not know you had been sleeping if you were awakened during <u>stage 1</u> sleep.

13. Older people may need <u>more</u> sleep than younger people.

14. If you can exercise for a long time without tiring, you have good <u>flexibility</u>.

15. Your body temperature goes <u>down</u> when you sleep.

Short Answer

Write the numbers 16 to 23 on your paper. Write a complete sentence to answer each question.

16. How does relaxing help reduce fatigue?

17. How can a person improve flexibility?

18. Why should you drink plenty of water when you exercise?

19. What are some reasons why people stop exercising?

20. How does aerobic exercise improve cardiovascular fitness?

21. What are the four stages of sleep?

22. Why should you always warm up before you exercise?

23. What happens to people when they do not get enough sleep?

Essay

Write the numbers 24 and 25 on your paper. Write paragraphs with complete sentences to answer each question.

24. Explain what happens inside the body during an exercise session, from the time you begin warming up to the time you finish cooling down.

25. Write a letter to a young person who has trouble relaxing because of stressful conditions—a noisy home or serious illness in the family. What advice could you give to help this person relax enough to get adequate rest and sleep?

ACTIVITIES FOR HOME OR SCHOOL

Projects to Do

1. With a group of your classmates, make up an exercise routine. Each of you should choose one or two simple exercises to do, such as jumping jacks or sit-ups. Choose music to accompany your routine. Perform your exercise routine, and teach it to the rest of the class.

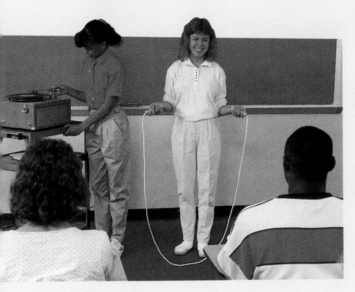

■ *Teach your class an exercise set to music.*

2. Collect advertisements for exercise equipment and use them to make a display. Read each advertisement to see what it claims the equipment will do. Do you think a person could get the same health benefits by exercising without the equipment? Why or why not?

3. On a sheet of paper, list three sports or physical activities that you enjoy. Plan a regular exercise program in which you participate in all three activities. Predict how your exercise program will contribute to your wellness.

Information to Find

1. Choose an athlete or dancer whom you admire. Find out about this person from books, magazines, or newspaper articles. Find out at what age the person became interested in his or her field, whether the person had to overcome any disadvantages or handicaps to achieve success, and how the person stays physically fit. Report this information to the class.

2. Backache is one of the most common physical ailments people have. There are many causes and treatments for backache. Find out what exercises and simple home treatments are often recommended to prevent or help types of common backache (types not caused by illness, injury, or bone problems). Your physician, local health department, or library may have information that can help you. Prepare a written or oral report about what you find out.

Books to Read

Here are some books you can look for in your school library or the public library to find more information about exercise, rest, and sleep.

Cosgrove, Margaret. *Your Muscles and Ways to Exercise Them.* Dodd, Mead.

Fodor, R. V., and G. J. Taylor. *Growing Strong.* Sterling.

Lyttle, Richard B. *The New Physical Fitness.* Franklin Watts.

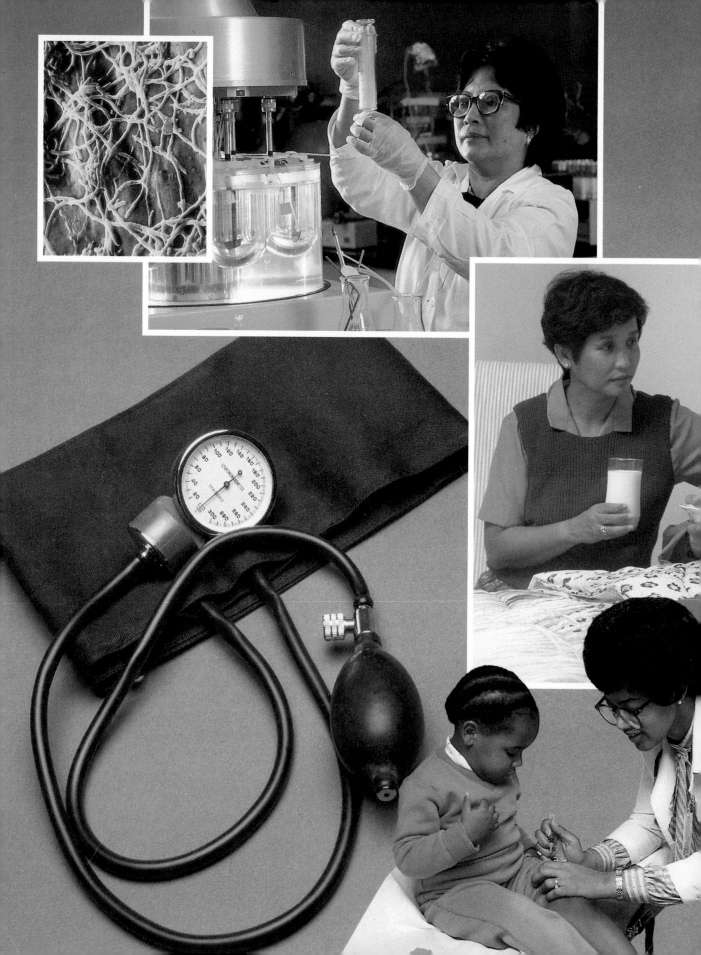

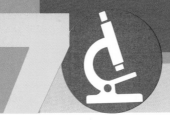

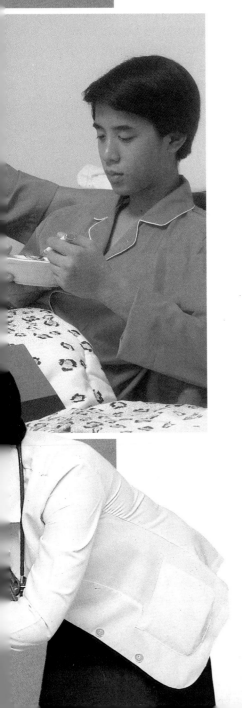

PROTECTING YOURSELF FROM DISEASE

What causes disease? Why do people get certain diseases? What can people do to keep from becoming ill? Why do some illnesses end quickly and others last a lifetime?

Learning the causes of disease is a first step in protecting yourself against it. Responsible health habits you begin now can help you maintain wellness.

GETTING READY TO LEARN

Key Questions

- Why is it important to learn about disease?
- Why is it important to know how to avoid those things that cause disease?
- What healthful habits can you develop to protect yourself from disease?
- How can you become more responsible about not spreading disease?

Main Chapter Sections

1 Communicable Disease
2 Some Common Communicable Diseases
3 Your Body's Defenses Against Communicable Disease
4 Noncommunicable Disease
5 Some Common Noncommunicable Diseases

1 Communicable Disease

communicable diseases (kuh MYOO nih kuh buhl • dihz EEZ uhz), diseases that can be passed from person to person.

■ *Communicable diseases, such as colds and influenza, are caused by microbes that spread from person to person.*

You probably know what it feels like to have a cold. Your body aches and your nose runs. You may even have a fever. A disease can cause you to feel ill and uncomfortable. *Disease* means "not at ease." Your body is not working easily and normally.

Many diseases can be passed from person to person. These are known as **communicable diseases.** Communicable diseases are caused by tiny organisms called *microbes*. Microbes are everywhere, although most of them are too small to be seen without a microscope. Microbes float in water and drift through the air. They are present in the soil. Plants and animals, as well as people, have microbes in and on them. If you were to look at the palm of your hand under a microscope, you would see millions of microbes. Most microbes are harmless, and some are actually necessary for a healthy body.

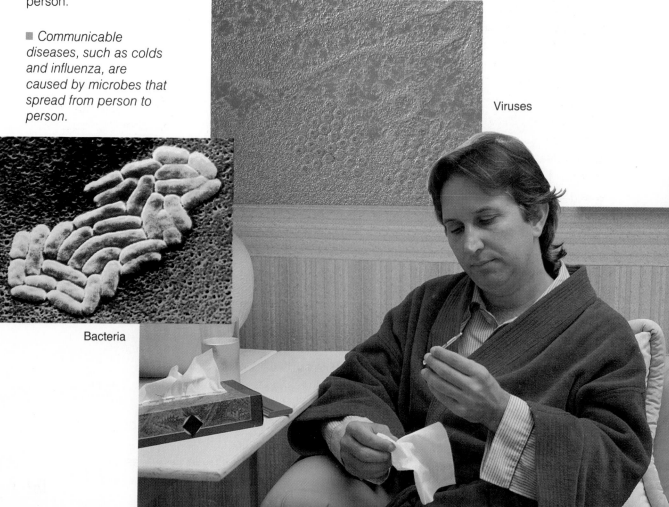

Viruses

Bacteria

Whenever you breathe, eat, or drink, you are taking microbes into your body. They can enter your body through a cut as well. If they are harmful microbes, they may cause disease. Microbes that cause disease are called **pathogens.**

What Microbes Cause Communicable Disease?

There are several kinds of pathogens. **Bacteria** are the most common. Bacteria are single cells, and they can have many shapes. Some are rod-shaped, others are round, and still others look like corkscrews. Like the cells of your body, they reproduce by dividing in two. In warm, dark, moist places, bacteria can reproduce quickly.

Many diseases are caused by bacteria. Strep throat is caused by round bacteria living in the throat. Tuberculosis bacteria cause damage in the lungs.

Viruses are another kind of pathogen. Viruses are so tiny that many of them can fit inside one bacterium. Some scientists feel that viruses may not be living things. It is known that viruses can reproduce only inside a living cell. When viruses enter your body, they go into some of your cells. These cells then help the viruses reproduce instead of following their normal activity. When a cell is full of viruses, it bursts. These new viruses spread to other cells in your body. Then these steps are repeated. Colds and influenza are diseases caused by viruses.

Like bacteria, **protozoa** are single-celled microbes that can cause disease. Protozoa can grow only where there is enough water for them to live. Some live in salt water, and others live in fresh water. Some live in wet soil, and others live in people and animals. Many protozoa that cause disease are found in tropical places. They multiply quickly in the warm, humid climate. Malaria and some kinds of diarrhea are caused by protozoa.

Fungi are a fourth kind of pathogen. Some fungi, such as mushrooms, are large. Others, such as molds and yeasts, can be seen only with a microscope. Fungi are found in warm, moist places. They get their food from living and nonliving things around them. Only certain kinds of fungi can cause disease. Athlete's foot is a disease caused by fungi.

How Does Communicable Disease Spread?

A communicable disease spreads when pathogens go from a person who is ill to one who is not ill. There are many ways pathogens can get to humans. By knowing some of the ways communicable diseases are spread, you can make responsible decisions that will avoid risks to yourself and others.

pathogens (PATH uh juhnz), harmful microbes that can cause disease.

bacteria (bak TIHR ee uh), single-celled microbes that vary in shape and reproduce by dividing in two; some bacteria are pathogens.

viruses (VY ruhs uhz), tiny microbes that can cause disease; they reproduce only inside of living cells.

protozoa (proht uh ZOH uh), single-celled microbes that grow wherever there is enough water for them to live; some protozoa are pathogens.

fungi (FUHN jy), organisms that get food from living and nonliving things; some fungi are pathogens.

Contact with a Person Who Is Ill.   Many pathogens can be spread by *direct contact*, such as touching a person who is ill. Some can be spread by *indirect contact*, such as handling unwashed dishes, clothes, towels, or other objects used by a person who is ill. Pathogens are often present in saliva and body wastes. When a person coughs or sneezes, tiny water droplets are sprayed into the air. If the person is ill, these droplets can contain pathogens. If other people breathe in these droplets, they may become ill, too.

Sometimes people have pathogens in their bodies and do not feel or look ill. Because these people "carry" the microbes, they are known as *human carriers*. They are not affected, but they can pass the microbes to others, who then may become ill.

■ *Pathogens that cause some communicable diseases can be passed directly from one person to another in a crowd.*

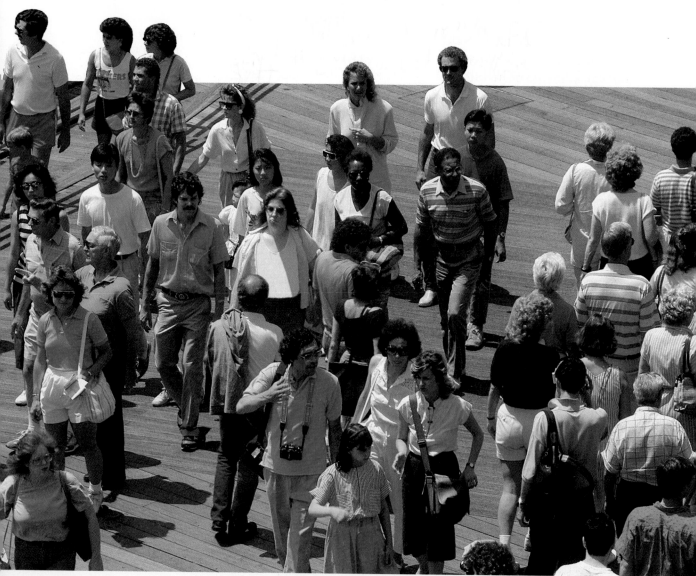

188

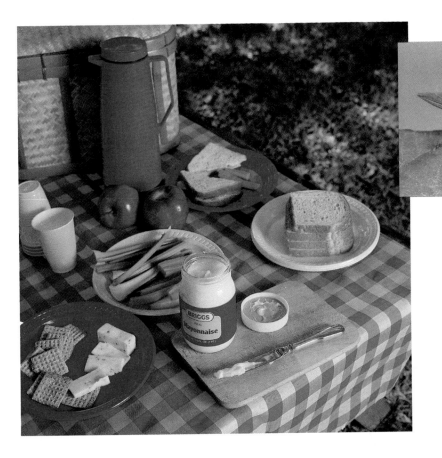

■ *Some communicable diseases can be spread indirectly through spoiled food or by insects.*

Pathogens in the Environment.   Many microbes can live in water for a long time. Drinking this water can make you ill. You can also get ill from swimming in this water. Pathogens in water can enter your body through cuts in your skin or through your eyes, nose, mouth, or ears.

Pathogens can also be on or in food. Food can spread communicable diseases in two ways. If a person who is ill has touched it, the food may carry pathogens. You can become ill by eating this food. Pathogens can also grow from within food. Bacteria grow quickly in certain foods, such as mayonnaise. This is especially true if the food is not kept cold. The food then goes bad, or spoils. If eaten, the bacteria or their wastes can make you ill.

Sometimes animals spread disease. Rabies is an animal disease caused by a virus. It can be present in an infected animal's saliva. If a person is bitten by an animal with rabies, the rabies virus enters the person's body and causes an infection in the nervous system. The disease is fatal unless the person gets a series of injections after being bitten.

Insects also carry certain pathogens. The microbes seldom affect the insects. However, people who are bitten by the infected insects or have their food contaminated by them can become ill.

FOR THE
CURIOUS

One of the most famous human disease carriers was Typhoid Mary. Once physicians determined that Mary was a carrier of typhoid fever, she was isolated from other people for the rest of her life.

189

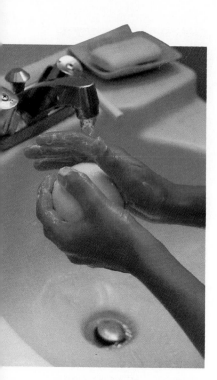

For example, houseflies spread disease by walking on food. They leave microbes on the food.

How Can You Protect Yourself from Pathogens?

You can help protect yourself from pathogens by following these simple health tips:

- Wash your hands before handling food for yourself or others.
- Wash cuts and scrapes with soap and warm water, and keep them clean.
- Make sure food is covered and kept refrigerated, if it should be. Packaged foods that need to be kept cold are identified on their labels.
- Wash all fresh fruits and vegetables before you eat them.
- Wash your hands after using the toilet.
- Do not pet stray or wild animals.
- Keep garbage and trash in closed containers.
- Make sure the water you drink does not contain pathogens. For example, when camping, boil or chemically treat your drinking water.
- Avoid close contact with people known to have communicable diseases.
- Wash your hands well after changing a baby's diaper.
- Avoid sharing eye makeup.
- Use disposable tissues for covering coughs and sneezes. Wash your hands after covering coughs and sneezes.

■ Washing your hands before preparing food for yourself or others can help stop the spread of certain diseases.

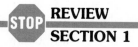

**REVIEW
SECTION 1**

REMEMBER?

1. What are communicable diseases?
2. What four kinds of microbes can cause disease?
3. What are six ways communicable diseases can be spread?

THINK!

4. How can knowing how communicable diseases are spread help keep you healthy?
5. Explain how washing your hands before eating can help protect you against some communicable diseases.

2 Some Common Communicable Diseases

There are hundreds of serious communicable diseases. Many are not as threatening as they once were. Improved sanitation methods keep many diseases from spreading. Personal actions such as handwashing habits help to prevent the spread of pathogens. Some diseases, such as smallpox, have been eliminated because of vaccines. New medicines can often help a person with a communicable disease recover rapidly.

■ *Colds can be spread by water droplets from a cough or sneeze.*

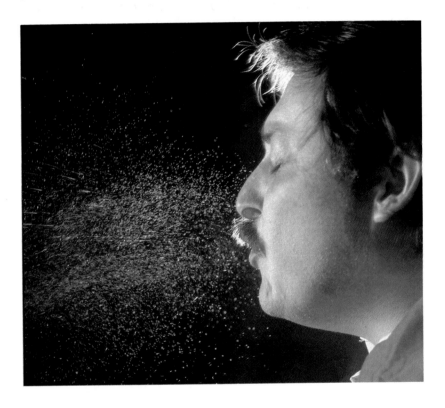

MYTH AND FACT

Myth: You should feed a cold and starve a fever.

Fact: Whether you have a cold or fever, you need to get extra rest, drink plenty of water and fruit juices, and eat healthful foods. You should talk to your parents or guardian and let them decide whether or not you should see your physician.

What Are Colds?

Colds are the most common communicable disease. A cold can be caused by any one of more than 100 different kinds of viruses. A cold attacks the upper respiratory system. Symptoms of a cold may include sneezing, a runny or stuffy nose, a sore throat, and coughing.

Colds spread easily from person to person. Cold viruses can be passed by unwashed hands. People may "catch" colds by breathing in droplets of water coughed or sneezed into the air by others who have colds. For this reason, it is a good idea to stay away from people who have colds.

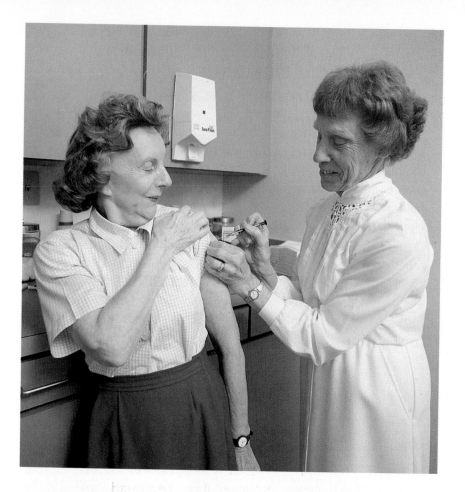

Influenza can be very serious for some older people. "Flu shots" often prevent people from getting the disease.

Colds cannot be cured medically. But the symptoms of a cold can be treated. If you have a cold, you should rest, stay warm, and drink plenty of water and fruit juices. Colds most often last about seven to ten days.

What Is Influenza?

Like colds, "flu" is caused by many different kinds of viruses. The most common kind of influenza is an infection of the nose, throat, and air passages. Symptoms of influenza include fever, chills, headache, sore throat, coughing, and muscle aches.

Like colds, influenza is very contagious. Influenza viruses are carried on water droplets that are coughed or sneezed into the air by a person who is ill. Influenza can be very serious in babies, children with other health problems, people who smoke or have diabetes, and very old people. If you get influenza, you can help yourself recover more quickly if you rest, avoid chills, and drink extra water and fruit juices. Young people should not be given aspirin during an illness caused by a virus, such as a cold or influenza. Aspirin could cause health problems worse than influenza.

What Are Sexually Transmitted Diseases?

Some communicable diseases are transmitted, or passed, by intimate sexual contact. These diseases are called **sexually transmitted diseases** (STDs). Most STDs are caused by specific viruses and bacteria. STDs are a serious health problem because they can cause permanent damage, sometimes before people know they have an infection. Physicians and trained health department workers try to make sure that all persons who have had contact with someone who has an STD get care even if they do not have signs of an infection.

Sometimes symptoms go unnoticed and an STD remains undiagnosed. As a result of some STDs, people can become sterile. This means that they lose their ability to produce babies. A pregnant woman who has an STD often passes it to her developing fetus, who can then be born seriously ill.

A common STD caused by a virus is *herpes simplex type 2*. This disease may cause painful blisters and sores on the external reproductive organs. Although the herpes blisters can be treated, the disease cannot be cured. The sores can always return.

Chlamydia is another common STD. In most cases, infected people have no symptoms. The disease is caused by a chlamydial microbe, not by a bacterium or virus. If untreated, the disease can damage the internal reproductive organs of a woman. Like a bacterial infection, it can be treated with antibiotics.

Syphilis is an STD caused by certain bacteria. If untreated, syphilis can be a very dangerous lifelong disease. Syphilis can be cured if it is caught in its early stages. The use of an antibiotic such as penicillin is usually an effective treatment for this disease.

The first symptom of syphilis is an open sore on the reproductive organs. This sore appears where the bacteria entered the body. As the bacteria reproduce, they can spread and attack nerve tissue and cause paralysis, blindness, and even death.

Gonorrhea is another STD caused by certain bacteria. Symptoms of gonorrhea include pain at the site of the infection and a discharge of pus. If gonorrhea is not treated, it can spread through the blood to other parts of the body. It can cause damage to the reproductive organs, including scars that can prevent a person from having babies. Physicians treat gonorrhea with an antibiotic such as penicillin.

STDs are diseases a person can get again and again. Serious health problems caused by these diseases can be avoided by getting immediate medical treatment by a physician. STDs can be prevented by abstaining from sexual contact.

sexually transmitted diseases (SEHKSH uh wuhl ee • tranz MIHT uhd • dihz EEZ uhz), STDs; communicable diseases spread by intimate sexual contact.

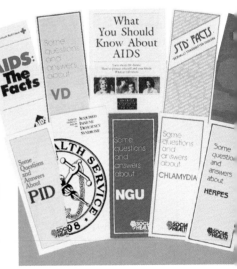

■ *Certain diseases are passed through sexual contact.*

193

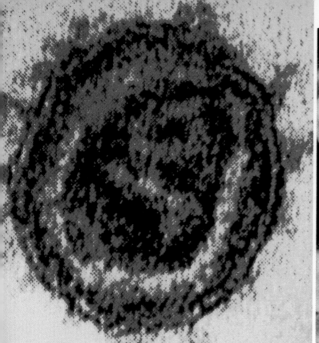
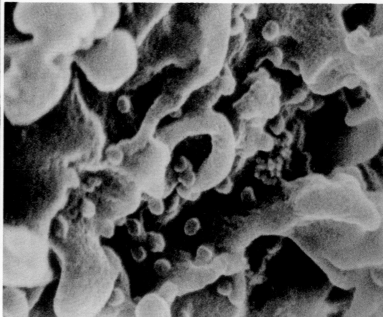

■ *HIV, left, causes AIDS. It attacks and destroys cells of the human immune system.*

human immunodeficiency virus (HYOO muhn • ihm yuh noh dih FIHSH uhn see • VY ruhs), the virus that causes AIDS.

The Spread of HIV

- Males who have had sexual contact with other males—over 60 percent
- People who use needles to inject illegal drugs—about 20 percent
- People who have sexual contact with an infected person of the opposite sex—5 percent
- People who have received blood transfusions—3 percent
- Babies born to infected mothers—1 percent

What Is AIDS?

AIDS stands for *acquired immunodeficiency syndrome*. It is an STD caused by a **human immunodeficiency virus** (HIV). HIV can damage the brain and destroy the body's ability to fight off other diseases. HIV does not kill by itself. It weakens the body's immune system. Then when other pathogens infect the body, the diseases they cause are not resisted. The result is AIDS. People with AIDS often die of infections that healthy people do not get. HIV is transmitted to people in three main categories:

1. those who have sexual contact with an infected person
2. those who share drug needles with an infected person
3. babies who are born to an infected mother

In the past some people became infected with HIV through receiving blood transfusions. Now, however, all blood donations are screened and tested so that the blood supply is safe.

Human carriers can spread HIV even though they do not feel or look ill. Sometimes many years go by before a person with HIV has any symptoms of AIDS.

No one gets HIV easily. A person cannot get HIV by casually touching someone who is infected. Neither can a person get HIV by being in the same room with an infected person or by donating blood. No person has ever been infected with HIV by an insect bite. People cannot get HIV by casual contact in schools, at parties, in swimming pools, in stores, or at workplaces.

People are afraid of HIV, AIDS, and other STDs because they do not understand that they have control over their own risks. People can choose their own behaviors. They can avoid placing themselves at any risk for STDs, HIV, and AIDS. Knowing how to handle pressures to become sexually active will help you gain self-respect as well as avoid the risk of STDs. Resisting pressure to use injected drugs is also a way to avoid HIV infection and AIDS.

STOP REVIEW SECTION 2

REMEMBER?

1. How can influenza be treated?
2. What causes sexually transmitted diseases?
3. How is HIV transmitted?

THINK!

4. How can your family or your physician help you learn to resist pressures that would cause you to risk a sexually transmitted disease?
5. How could you avoid catching a cold or getting influenza?
6. How are HIV and AIDS similar to herpes? How are they different?

Making Wellness Choices

Robert and Meredith plan to drop off some homework to their friend Samantha after school today. Samantha has missed several days of school because she is ill with the flu. She wants to try and catch up with her work so that she will not be too far behind. When they arrive, Samantha's brother George answers the door. While they are talking with George, Samantha calls down from upstairs. She invites them to come and visit with her. She says she is bored of being alone. She also says she has some snacks to eat. Both Meredith and Robert are very hungry.

 What could Robert and Meredith do? Explain your wellness choice.

Health Close-up

Disease Detectives

For many years, Carlos Juan Finlay, a Cuban physician, had wanted to know what caused the spread of yellow fever, a communicable disease caused by a virus. In the summer of 1900, an epidemic of yellow fever raged through Havana, Cuba. Dr. Finlay shared his ideas with a young United States Army surgeon, Walter Reed, and the search was on.

For many weeks, Finlay and Reed tried to find out how yellow fever was passed from person to person. They first thought that the disease was spread by direct contact with an infected person. But experiments showed this did not spread the disease. The two physicians then thought that the disease might be spread by indirect contact, that is, by using something that had been used by an infected person. The physicians asked volunteers to wear the pajamas and sleep in the beds of people who had yellow fever. The volunteers did not get the disease. Finlay and Reed therefore concluded that yellow fever was not spread by indirect contact.

After several weeks of study, Dr. Finlay came up with the idea that yellow fever was spread by mosquitoes. He noticed that yellow fever appeared only in those places where mosquitoes were present. With the help of Dr. Reed, Dr. Finlay asked for volunteers. The volunteers allowed themselves to be bitten by mosquitoes that had also bitten people with yellow fever. Within a few days, all of the volunteers came down with yellow fever. Dr. Finlay's idea was proved correct. Yellow fever is spread by mosquitoes.

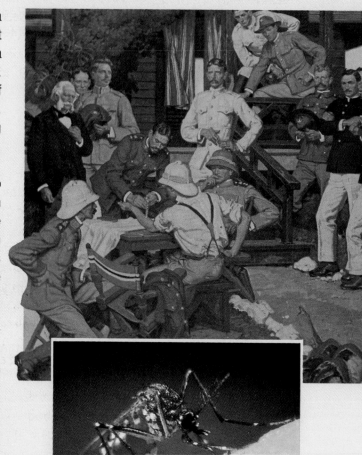

■ Drs. Finlay and Reed allowed volunteers to be bitten by mosquitoes that carried yellow fever.

Thinking Beyond

1. What can you do to prevent the spread of a disease like yellow fever?
2. What diseases other than yellow fever might be spread by insects?

3 Your Body's Defenses Against Communicable Disease

You are surrounded by microbes that can cause disease. Therefore, you may wonder why you do not become ill more often. The answer lies in your behaviors and in your body's natural defenses against disease. When you maintain wellness, your body's defenses usually are strong enough to fight off disease microbes.

What Are Your Outer Defenses?

Some of your body's defenses prevent pathogens from getting inside your body and entering your blood. These are called your body's *outer defenses.* Your most important outer defense is your skin. Unless you cut or burn your skin, it keeps out most pathogens. Skin also produces sweat, which kills some microbes.

A layer of special skin cells lines the inside of your nose, mouth, and throat. These skin cells, which make up a **mucous membrane,** form mucus. Mucus can trap pathogens and keep them from getting into your body systems. Once trapped in the mucus, microbes are prevented from going any farther into the body by hairs in the trachea. These hairs move in a wavelike motion to push mucus up toward the throat and away from other body systems.

Your body has other outer defenses as well. Coughing and sneezing help push microbes out of your body. Tears can wash them out of your eyes. Acids in your stomach kill many microbes before they can get into your blood. Blood flowing from a cut helps wash away some microbes.

KEY WORDS

mucous
  membrane
antibodies
antigens
vaccine
toxins
toxoid

---

mucous membrane
(MYOO kuhs • MEHM brayn), a layer of skin cells that produce mucus.

■ Unbroken skin, mucous membranes, and tears, left, are part of the body's outer defenses against the many microbes that try to invade the body, right.

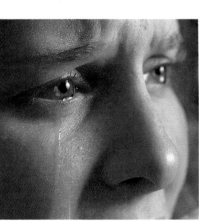
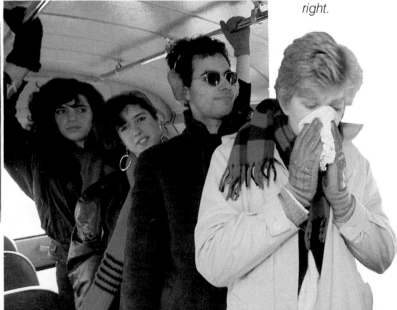

197

What Are Your Inner Defenses?

If a large number of pathogens do get by your body's outer defenses, they may enter your blood and cells. When pathogens are present in your blood and cells, your body's *inner defenses* go to work to fight them. Blood itself contains certain cells that fight infection. These are the white blood cells, which squeeze through the walls of blood vessels and move to infected areas. They surround the pathogens and kill them.

■ *White blood cells, which surround and kill pathogens, are part of the body's inner defenses.*

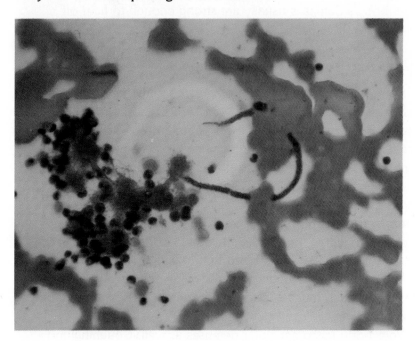

Fever. Normal body temperature may range from 96 to 99.9 degrees Fahrenheit (35.6 to 37.7 degrees Celsius). When microbes begin to multiply inside your body, your temperature may rise. When it is higher than normal, you have a fever. A fever may slow down the speed at which microbes can multiply. Fever is a reflection of the increased energy your cells are generating to battle the microbes. A fever can be a good sign that your body is fighting an infection. A fever over 104 degrees Fahrenheit (40 degrees Celsius) or any fever that lasts several days needs medical attention. Otherwise, let a fever do its work. Help your body by drinking extra water and eating healthful foods.

Lymphatic System. Another inner defense is your lymphatic system. Lymph is a fluid that moves through your body picking up harmful bacteria. When the lymph passes through your lymph nodes, the bacteria are screened out. White blood cells in the lymph nodes then surround and kill the harmful bacteria.

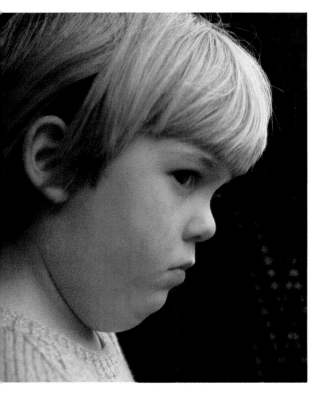

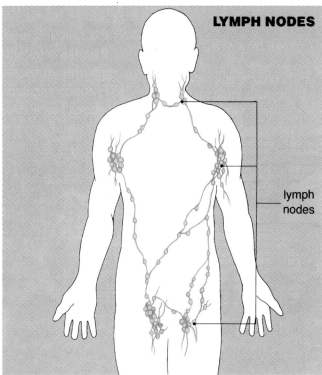

LYMPH NODES

lymph
nodes

■ *Some of the body's lymph nodes, right, become swollen when a person has an infection such as mumps, left.*

Your lymph nodes may become sore and swollen when you have an infection. This is a sign that the lymph nodes are working to help you regain your health.

Immunity. You may have heard people say they are immune to a certain disease. This means that they will not become ill if the pathogens that cause the disease enter their bodies.

Your body's ability to develop immunity is an important part of its defenses against disease. An immunity to a certain disease comes from substances in your body called **antibodies.** White blood cells make antibodies against each kind of pathogen that gives you an infection. After you get well, some of these antibodies stay in your blood. They keep you from getting the same diseases again. For example, if you have had mumps, and the mumps viruses enter your body years later, your immune system "recognizes" the pathogens. The body can then immediately send mumps antibodies to kill the viruses before you become ill. You probably will never get mumps again. For some diseases, however, immunity does not last a lifetime.

Microbes contain proteins that are called **antigens.** Antigens cause your white blood cells to make antibodies. Each disease has its own antigen, which in turn causes the immune system to form a certain antibody. An immunity to one disease, such as chicken pox, will not give you immunity to other diseases.

antibodies (ANT ih bahd eez), substances in your blood that provide immunity to certain disease microbes.

antigens (ANT ih juhnz), proteins in microbes that cause your white blood cells to make antibodies.

199

How Can You Protect Yourself Against Communicable Disease?

vaccine (vak SEEN), a substance that protects people from a certain disease by causing the blood to make antibodies.

toxins (TAHK suhnz), poisons produced by certain kinds of microbes.

You do not always have to get ill to develop an immunity. You can become immune to some diseases by receiving a vaccine. A **vaccine** contains an antigen that causes your body to form antibodies without making you ill. There are vaccines for many diseases, such as polio, measles, mumps, and influenza.

Another kind of vaccine works against poisons formed by certain kinds of microbes. These poisons are called **toxins.**

HOW CERTAIN DISEASES CAUSE IMMUNITY

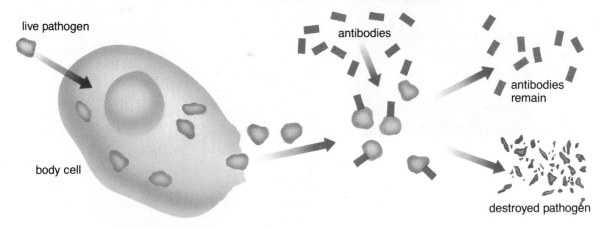

live pathogen

antibodies

antibodies remain

body cell

destroyed pathogen

HOW VACCINES CAUSE IMMUNITY

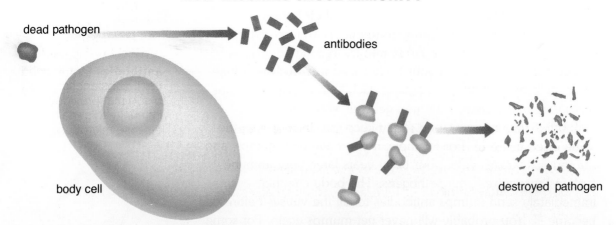

dead pathogen

antibodies

body cell

destroyed pathogen

■ While your body fights certain diseases, top, antibodies are made to produce immunity. Receiving vaccines, bottom, for certain diseases produces immunity against these diseases.

200

A vaccine that helps your body form an immunity to toxins is called a **toxoid.** A toxoid is a toxin that has been treated so that it does not make you ill. However, it still causes your body to make antibodies against the toxin. For example, tetanus is a disease caused by bacteria that make a toxin. The bacteria that cause tetanus can enter the body through a puncture wound or deep cut. People who have these kinds of injuries should get a vaccine against tetanus. The vaccine against tetanus has the tetanus toxoid in it. It causes your body to make antibodies against the tetanus toxin for several years. Boosters are needed periodically to keep your immunity to tetanus active.

There are other ways you can guard against communicable disease. Washing your hands before handling food and before touching your face is a good protection from many diseases. You can increase your ability to resist disease by eating healthful meals. Daily habits of regular exercise and adequate rest and sleep also help resistance. Together, these actions help prevent disease. You can also get regular medical checkups. A physician or nurse can often spot health problems before they become serious. By getting early treatment, you may avoid serious illness and more costly health care.

Finally, you can help yourself stay healthy by knowing the signs of disease. Some common symptoms of communicable disease are fever, headache, rash, and muscle aches. A sudden tiredness or weakness can also be a symptom of disease. If symptoms continue, you should see a physician. Your physician will know how serious your problem is and can help you become well again.

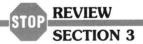

REVIEW
SECTION 3

REMEMBER?

1. What is your body's most important outer defense against communicable disease?

2. What are three other outer defenses against disease?

3. How do your white blood cells defend your body against disease?

4. In what other ways can you fight disease?

THINK!

5. Why might your body not be able to fight an infection?

6. What are some diseases to which you might be immune?

toxoid (TAHK soyd), a toxin that has been treated so that it does not make you ill; causes your body to produce antibodies against the toxin.

REAL-LIFE
SKILL

Checking Your Temperature

Clean the thermometer with rubbing alcohol. Shake down the clean thermometer to below 96 degrees Fahrenheit or 36 degrees Celsius. Place it under your tongue for four minutes. Do not bite the thermometer; it is glass and may break. Remove and turn the thermometer until you see a line inside. The point on the scale where the line stops is your temperature.

4 Noncommunicable Disease

Diseases that cannot be passed from person to person are called **noncommunicable diseases.** They are not caused by pathogens. You cannot form an immunity to these diseases. Noncommunicable diseases can affect any system of your body.

Many noncommunicable diseases can be treated to relieve the symptoms. But they cannot be completely cured. As a result, people may live with a noncommunicable disease for all or most of their lives. Such long-lasting diseases are called **chronic diseases.** You may have heard of some—hypertension, diabetes, asthma, and bronchitis.

What Causes Noncommunicable Disease?

Some noncommunicable diseases are inherited. Others come from conditions in the environment. The diseases may be caused by poor health habits or by exposure to harmful substances. Some start because of people's choices about their behavior. Physicians do not always know why people get some noncommunicable diseases. They know that many diseases start to develop long before any symptoms appear. Research has shown that certain factors affect your likelihood of becoming ill.

KEY WORDS

noncommuni-
cable diseases
chronic diseases

noncommunicable diseases (nahn kuh MYOO nih kuh buhl • dihz EEZ uhz), diseases that are not caused by pathogens and cannot be passed from person to person.

chronic diseases (KRAHN ihk • dihz EEZ uhz), diseases that last a long time.

■ *Noncommunicable diseases may be chronic. That is, they may last a very long time.*

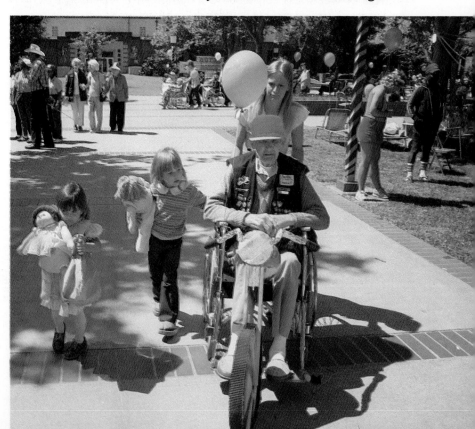

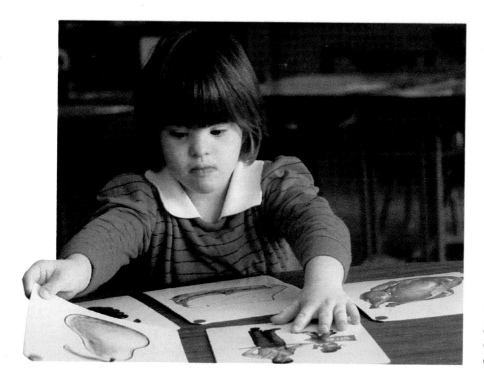

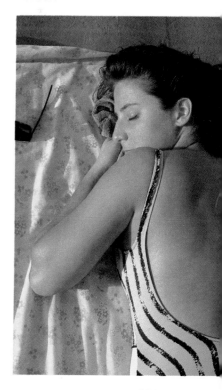

■ Down syndrome is an inherited condition caused by an extra chromosome.

■ Too much exposure to the sun's rays can cause certain kinds of skin cancer.

Heredity. Some noncommunicable diseases come from inherited traits. These diseases are inherited by a child from his or her parents. Two such disorders are cystic fibrosis and Down syndrome. Cystic fibrosis is a glandular disorder. It causes respiratory and digestive problems. Down syndrome is a condition caused by an extra chromosome. It results in physical and mental growth problems.

It may also be possible to inherit a tendency to develop a certain disease. For example, some studies show that compared to other children, the children of parents with heart disease have a greater chance of developing heart disease themselves.

Environment and Life-style. Poor health habits and exposure to harmful substances in your environment can add to your chance of getting a noncommunicable disease. Too much sun, for example, may cause skin cancer in some people. Motor vehicles and some factories release chemical gases that can cause lung diseases.

How you live, or your life-style, can also affect the chance of your getting a noncommunicable disease. Smoking leads to diseases of the lungs, heart, and blood vessels. Poor eating habits, lack of exercise, and too much stress in your life can lead to high blood pressure, heart disease, and stroke.

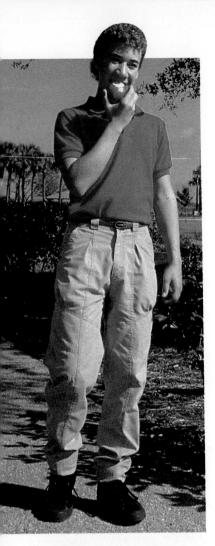

■ *Developing and keeping good health habits now may prevent noncommunicable diseases later.*

How Can Noncommunicable Disease Be Prevented?

Inherited noncommunicable diseases cannot be prevented. Nor can you change an inherited trait that adds to your chance of getting a certain disease. However, the effects of some inherited diseases can be controlled by proper treatment. Also, by developing wise health habits now, you may be able to avoid some noncommunicable diseases when you are older.

Eating a balanced diet, getting regular exercise, managing stress, and getting adequate rest and sleep can add to your resistance to disease and help you maintain wellness. You need to maintain a desirable weight. Being overweight may add to your chance of getting some diseases, such as heart disease.

You can guard against many chronic diseases by not using tobacco, alcohol, and other drugs. Studies have shown that these substances can damage parts of your body and lower your resistance to disease.

Regular medical examinations can reveal early warning signs of diseases. If found early, many noncommunicable diseases can be stopped or controlled.

STOP **REVIEW**
SECTION 4

REMEMBER?

1. What are noncommunicable diseases?
2. What are two causes of noncommunicable disease?
3. What are two ways you may be able to prevent some kinds of noncommunicable diseases?

THINK!

4. What noncommunicable disease symptoms could be treated?
5. How can you tell whether your life-style is increasing or reducing your chance of developing a noncommunicable disease?

204

5 Some Common Noncommunicable Diseases

You may have heard about some noncommunicable diseases, such as cancer and heart disease. There are many other noncommunicable diseases as well. Physicians believe that your future wellness and general level of health are affected by actions you take now and maintain throughout life.

KEY WORDS

hypertension
insulin

What Is Cancer?

Cancer is a disease in which body cells change and begin to multiply more rapidly than normal cells. They reproduce so quickly that they crowd out normal cells. They keep the affected body systems from working properly.

Physicians do not know why cancer cells begin to grow. But they have identified certain factors that add to the risk of getting some kinds of cancer. For example, cigarette smoking adds to the risk of getting throat and lung cancer. Long-time exposure to the sun can lead to certain kinds of skin cancer. Contact with certain chemicals also may cause cancer.

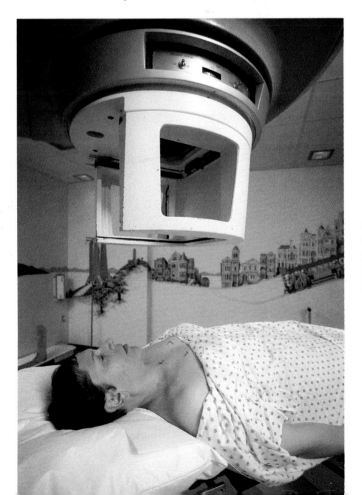

Possible Warning Signs of Cancer

- Changed bowel or bladder habits
- Any kind of sore that does not heal
- Unusual bleeding or discharge
- Thickening or lump in any part of the body
- Indigestion or difficulty in swallowing
- Obvious change in a wart, mole, or birthmark
- Nagging cough or hoarseness in the throat

■ *Some cancer cells can be destroyed by radiation.*

205

hypertension (HY puhr tehn chuhn), high blood pressure.

Cancer can occur in almost any part of the body. Some of the most common areas where cancers form in adults are the skin, lungs, breasts, stomach, and large intestine. If found early, most kinds of cancer can be successfully treated. Cancer cells may be removed by surgery or killed with radiation treatments. Some kinds of cancer cells can be destroyed by medicines in a treatment called *chemotherapy*. Cancer cells must be prevented from spreading to healthy parts of the body. If they do spread, cancer cells may begin to grow there, too.

What Are Some Common Circulatory Diseases?

Diseases of the heart and blood vessels are called *cardiovascular diseases*. Some are brought on by a person's way of living.

One of the most common diseases of the circulatory system is chronic **hypertension,** or high blood pressure. Hypertension occurs when the pressure of the blood on the walls of blood vessels increases to more than normal. Regular blood pressure screenings are a way to detect hypertension early. Untreated hypertension may cause other diseases.

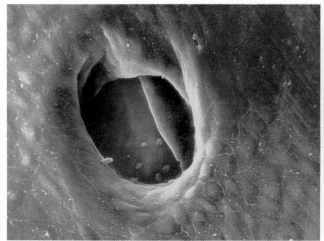 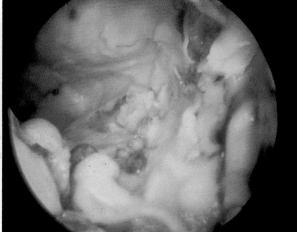

■ *Sometimes the interior wall of an artery, left, can become narrow because of fatty deposits, right.*

Sometimes fat builds up on the inner walls of arteries. In time the fat deposits become hard. They can narrow the arteries and make the artery walls hard. Then the heart must exert itself to pump blood throughout the body. This condition is called *atherosclerosis*. It often appears in old age, although it may have started much earlier. Some physicians believe that cholesterol contributes to this disease. Cholesterol is formed by your body. It is also found in animal fat in red meat, cheese, and butter. Too much fat in the diet can contribute to cholesterol buildup in the arteries.

206

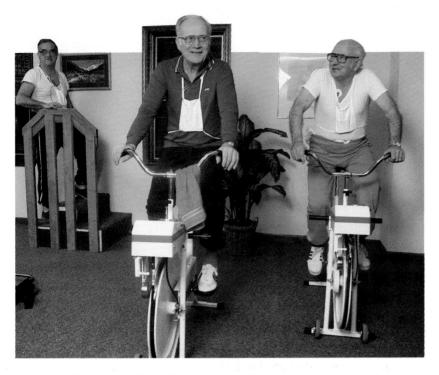

A condition in which the heart itself does not get enough blood is known as *coronary heart disease*. The cause may be blood clots in the small arteries of the heart. These clots can form when red blood cells become damaged as they flow over rough deposits of fat in arteries. Clots can slow or completely stop the flow of blood to the heart tissue. When this blood supply is too low or stopped completely, a *heart attack* can occur. If the heart attack causes the entire heart to stop pumping, the person can die. If the damaged part of the heart is small, a person who has a heart attack can live. Many people who have had heart attacks have recovered and gone on to lead normal, active lives. Most of them must make some changes in diet and exercise habits, and those who smoke must quit.

The conditions that cause coronary heart disease can also occur in the brain, causing a *stroke*. A blocked artery in the brain can keep brain cells from getting enough oxygen, so that they die. A stroke can also be caused by a break in an artery wall. Escaping blood can put pressure on the brain. This also causes cells to die.

What Diseases Affect the Respiratory System?

Diseases of the lungs and bronchial tubes are called *respiratory conditions*. They make it hard to breathe and can affect the supply of oxygen to the body. This in turn makes other body systems work harder. People with respiratory conditions cannot always be as active as they would like to be.

FOR THE
CURIOUS

The danger point of cholesterol buildup in the arteries is reached at 60 percent blockage.

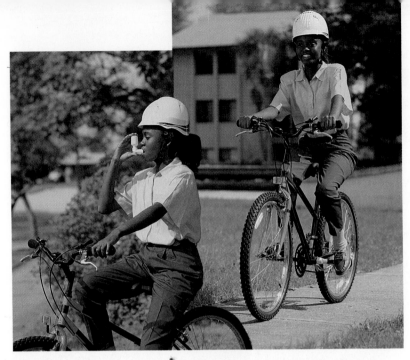

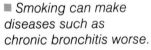

■ *People with asthma sometimes have to inhale certain medicines to help them breathe, left. However, most people with asthma can still enjoy activities involving exercise.*

■ *Smoking can make diseases such as chronic bronchitis worse.*

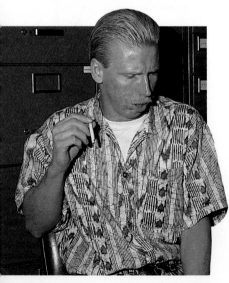

Asthma.   Asthma is an allergic disease that causes breathing difficulty. A person may wheeze and gasp for breath during an asthma attack. Asthma attacks occur when the tiny air tubes in the lungs narrow. This narrowing can be caused by a swelling of the membranes lining the tubes. It also is caused by mucus blocking the tubes or by the tubes squeezing together. When asthma attacks are frequent or long-lasting, they can be frightening. They can cause death if treatment is neglected.

Pathogens infecting the nose and throat can sometimes trigger asthma. But an asthma attack may also be caused by an allergic reaction. The reaction might be to smoke, dust, certain foods, and even medicines such as aspirin. Someone with asthma should see a physician to learn how to control his or her condition. Some ways include recognizing and avoiding whatever sets off attacks and maintaining cardiorespiratory fitness through regular exercise. There are also medicines and breathing methods that can help a person control asthma problems.

Chronic Bronchitis.   Chronic bronchitis is a disease of the bronchial tubes and smaller air tubes in the lungs. The mucous membranes lining these tubes become irritated and infected. Cilia, the hairlike structures that help keep these tubes free of dirt and excess mucus, may be destroyed. Without cilia, the only way to get rid of mucus is by coughing. Frequent coughing is the most common symptom of chronic bronchitis.

The disease is treated by curing the infection and removing the cause of irritation. Two common causes of irritation are tobacco smoke and air pollution.

What Is Diabetes?

Diabetes is a condition in which the blood sugar is too high. Blood sugar is controlled by **insulin,** a hormone made by a special group of cells in the pancreas. Insulin makes blood sugar enter muscle, fat, and liver cells. If insulin is not made or if the cells do not take in the sugar, then the sugar in the blood rises. Symptoms of diabetes include frequent urination, excessive thirst, difficulty in healing, blurred vision, dizziness, and weight loss.

insulin (IHN suh luhn), a hormone made in the pancreas that carries sugar in the blood into the cells of the body.

■ *Insulin is made by certain cells inside the pancreas.*

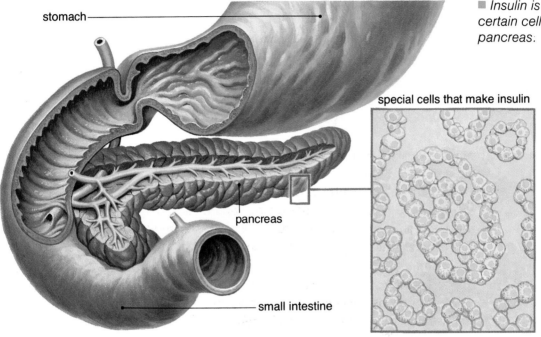

stomach

special cells that make insulin

pancreas

small intestine

There are two major types of diabetes: Type I and Type II. In addition to maintaining a proper diet and regular exercise, people with Type I diabetes need daily injections of insulin. People with Type II diabetes may not need to take insulin. Sometimes they can control their diabetes with regular exercise, proper diet, and medicine. Type I diabetes affects primarily children and young adults. Most older adults with diabetes have Type II diabetes.

Diabetes seems to be common in some families. That is, there is a tendency for diabetes to be hereditary, especially Type II diabetes. Your physician should be told if there is a history of diabetes in your family. Not all people with diabetes show symptoms. The disease can be detected only with medical tests.

Diabetes cannot be cured, but it can be controlled. In mild cases, a special diet may help. Most people who have diabetes, however, must take prescribed medicine or insulin injections daily. Control of diabetes is necessary to remain healthy.

What Are Some Diseases of the Nervous and Muscular Systems?

Diseases of the nervous system are called *neurological diseases*. They can affect the brain, the nerves, or both. Diseases of the muscular system can affect a person's ability to move.

Multiple Sclerosis. Multiple sclerosis destroys the coverings on the nerves of the brain and spinal cord. Without this covering, messages from the brain do not reach the proper muscles. The messages may be stopped or weakened. Loss of muscle control is the chief symptom. Symptoms differ from person to person because the damage can be at different places on the nerve covering. The symptoms of the disease may remain mild for 20 to 30 years. Then they may suddenly get worse. In some people, the disease symptoms never get worse.

■ *Multiple sclerosis causes a loss of muscle control. However, a person who has multiple sclerosis can still do and enjoy many activities.*

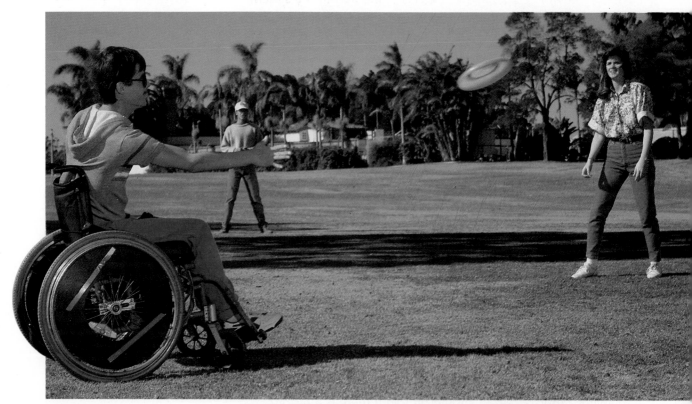

Physicians do not know the cause of multiple sclerosis. Some think that it may be caused by a kind of virus. Others think it may be due to problems with the fatty tissue that makes the nerve covering. There is no way to prevent the disease. However, people with the disease often live productive lives for many years.

Muscular Dystrophy. Muscular dystrophy is an inherited disease in which the body's muscles slowly weaken. People become weaker and weaker as muscle tissue is destroyed. They eventually cannot stand, walk, or breathe without special equipment. It most commonly affects boys. Physicians do not yet know enough about the cause of this disease to prevent it.

STOP | **REVIEW**
SECTION 5

REMEMBER?

1. What happens to cells when a person gets cancer?
2. What is hypertension?
3. What body functions are affected by respiratory conditions?
4. Name and describe two diseases of the respiratory system.

THINK!

5. What are some problems people with asthma might have?
6. What health habits will help you decrease the chance that you will get a circulatory disease?

Thinking About Your Health

Do You Know Your Health History?

Do you know what communicable diseases you have had? Do you know what communicable diseases and chronic noncommunicable diseases members of your family have had? Knowing this information can help keep you healthy. You should be able to answer the following questions about your health. Talk about this with your parents, guardian, school nurse, or family physician in order to have an accurate record of your health history.

■ Do you know what childhood diseases you have had, such as mumps, chicken pox, and measles?

■ Do you know if any members of your family have a history of a chronic noncommunicable disease, such as heart disease, diabetes, muscular dystrophy, cancer, or multiple sclerosis?

■ Do you eat a balanced diet and get plenty of rest, sleep, and exercise?

People in Health

An Interview with a Pathologist

> *Franklin C. Imm studies how diseases develop and how they affect people. He is a pathologist in Tuskegee, Alabama.*

What is a pathologist?

The word *pathology* means "the study of the nature of diseases." A pathologist is concerned with diseases and their impact on people. A pathologist, however, does not treat people who have diseases. It is unlikely that you would ever have a medical appointment with a pathologist.

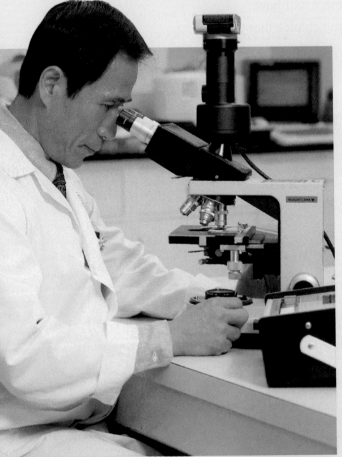

What does a pathologist do?

A pathologist helps other physicians to diagnose their patients' illnesses. He or she might work to determine whether a certain illness was caused by bacteria, viruses, or some other kind of microbe. That is why a pathologist is sometimes called "a doctor's doctor."

How does a pathologist test for specific diseases?

A pathologist might test for cancer by studying a small slice of a tumor under a microscope. Seeing how the cells react can tell a pathologist whether they are cancerous or not. For AIDS, a pathologist might study a person's blood to see the activity of the antibodies. Studying antibodies in the blood is also a way pathologists test for other diseases, such as chicken pox and measles.

How have pathologists helped prevent or control disease?

Pathologists have identified the natures and causes of polio and tetanus, for example. With that information, other scientists were able to develop vaccines for those diseases.

What is your job as a pathologist?

I am the chief of the laboratory services at a large hospital. The department in which I work tests patients' blood and tissue. We test both before and after surgery and share what we learn with the patient's own physician.

■ *Dr. Imm, a pathologist, helps find the causes of patients' diseases.*

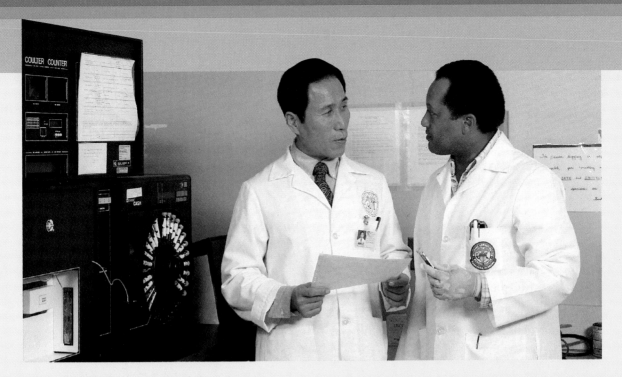

■ *Pathologists use special equipment to study diseases.*

How do you help a patient?

We provide physicians with some very important information about a patient. The physician uses this information to make decisions about how to care for that patient. We also teach physicians about newly developed tests that can be used to diagnose disease. This helps physicians provide up-to-date care for their patients.

What kinds of equipment do pathologists use in their work?

The basic equipment includes a standard microscope, an electron microscope, and various machines that analyze blood cells and body chemicals. [An electron microscope can magnify an object up to 200,000 times its real size.]

How is the field of pathology changing?

One important area of change involves the constant improvement of equipment. Most hospital laboratories are now equipped with computers. Before this, tests had to be done by hand. It was a slow process. Now test results are available in far less time. That means the physician can make treatment decisions sooner. The time we save will save lives.

Another ongoing change involves the continual increase of knowledge about disease. By the time today's young teenagers become adults, pathologists will know the causes and cures of many diseases that are incurable today.

Pathologists are always on guard for new diseases that we do not know about today. The job of the pathologist is always changing.

> *Learn more about the nature of diseases. Contact a hospital and interview a pathologist. Or write for information to the College of American Pathologists, 5202 Old Orchard Road, Skokie, IL 60077.*

Main Ideas

- Communicable diseases can be spread from one person to another.
- Your body fights communicable diseases with its inner and outer defenses.
- Good health habits can protect you from communicable diseases.
- Noncommunicable diseases are not caused by pathogens.
- Noncommunicable diseases are caused by heredity, environment, and life-style.
- Some noncommunicable diseases can be prevented by practicing good health habits.

Key Words

Write the numbers 1 to 18 in your health notebook or on a separate sheet of paper. After each number, copy the sentence and fill in the missing term. Page numbers in ( ) tell you where to look in the chapter if you need help.

communicable
   diseases (186)
pathogens (187)
bacteria (187)
viruses (187)
protozoa (187)
fungi (187)
sexually
   transmitted
   diseases (193)
human
   immunodeficiency
   virus (194)

mucous
   membrane (197)
antibodies (199)
antigens (200)
vaccine (200)
toxins (200)
toxoid (201)
noncommunicable
   diseases (202)
chronic diseases
   (202)
hypertension (206)
insulin (209)

214

1. Disease-causing microbes that get food from both living and nonliving things are ___?___ .

2. Communicable diseases that spread by intimate body contact are ___?___ .

3. Disease-causing microbes are ___?___ .

4. A layer of skin cells that form mucus is a ___?___ .

5. Diseases that you cannot get from other people are ___?___ .

6. A ___?___ is a toxin that has been treated so that it does not make you ill.

7. Another name for high blood pressure is ___?___ .

8. Tiny, disease-causing microbes that grow only inside living cells are ___?___ .

9. Proteins that cause your white blood cells to produce antibodies are ___?___ .

10. Single-celled microbes that grow where there is enough water for them to live are ___?___ .

11. A ___?___ is a substance that causes your body to form antibodies.

12. The poisons formed by certain kinds of microbes are ___?___ .

13. Formed by your white blood cells, ___?___ are substances that give you immunity to certain diseases.

14. The most common pathogens are ___?___ .

15. Long-lasting diseases are ___?___ .

16. ___?___ is produced by the pancreas.

17. Diseases that are passed from person to person are ___?___ .

18. ___?___ damages the immune system and causes AIDS.

Remembering What You Learned

Page numbers in ( ) tell you where to look in the chapter if you need help.

1. What causes communicable diseases? (186)

2. What are three ways microbes can enter the body? (188)

3. What is one way the body uses outer defenses to keep harmful microbes from entering the blood? (197)

4. Why are white blood cells one of the body's inner defenses? (198)

5. Why do you sometimes get a fever when you are ill? (198)

6. What can happen to the body if syphilis and gonorrhea are not treated? (193)

7. How can HIV be transmitted from person to person? (194)

8. How does a vaccine make you immune to certain diseases? (200)

9. What are some ways to guard against communicable diseases? (200–201)

10. What are two noncommunicable diseases that can be passed on from parent to child through heredity? (203)

11. How do cancer cells cause disease? (205–206)

12. What is hypertension? (206)

13. Why do some physicians suggest that people limit the amount of cholesterol in their diet? (206)

14. What part of the body is affected by a stroke? (207)

15. What causes diabetes? (209)

Thinking About What You Learned

1. Explain why it is safe to attend school with and have normal social contact with a person infected with HIV.

2. In what three ways are colds and influenza similar?

3. Explain why it will be hard for scientists to make a vaccine against the common cold.

4. Explain why it is important to keep garbage in covered containers.

Writing About What You Learned

1. Many state laws require students to have had certain vaccines before they can attend school. Write a paragraph explaining why most schools require vaccinations.

2. Write a paragraph describing five ways in which you personally can prevent the spread of communicable diseases.

3. Write a paragraph explaining how you can plan your life-style to keep from having a noncommunicable disease later in life. Give specific examples in your paragraph.

Applying What You Learned

ART

Design a creative chart or pamphlet that identifies ways to protect yourself against harmful microbes. Illustrate each step with a diagram. Share the chart or pamphlet with your classmates.

Modified True or False

Write the numbers 1 to 15 in your health notebook or on a separate sheet of paper. After each number, write *true* or *false* to describe the sentence. If the sentence is false, also write a term that replaces the underlined term and makes the sentence true.

1. <u>Chlamydia</u> is a common STD.

2. When your brain does not get enough oxygen, you may have a <u>heart attack</u>.

3. Some physicians believe that atherosclerosis is due to too much <u>cholesterol</u>.

4. <u>Noncommunicable</u> diseases are caused by heredity, factors in the environment, and life-style.

5. Bacteria that cause disease are <u>toxoids</u>.

6. The inside of your mouth is lined with <u>mucous membrane</u>.

7. Your white blood cells make antibodies when they come into contact with <u>pathogens</u>.

8. A diet high in cholesterol may cause <u>STDs</u>.

9. Emotional stress may increase your chance of getting a <u>noncommunicable</u> disease.

10. A fluid in your body that picks up harmful bacteria is called <u>lymph</u>.

11. If you have a <u>fever</u>, you may have an infection.

12. A <u>toxin</u> is a poison formed by a microbe.

13. Using the same towel as someone who has a communicable disease is <u>indirect contact</u>.

14. Molds and yeasts are <u>protozoa</u>.

15. <u>Diabetes</u> occurs when the body does not make enough insulin.

Short Answer

Write the numbers 16 to 23 on your paper. Write a complete sentence to answer each question.

16. How are HIV and AIDS different from other STDs?

17. How is a cold different from influenza? How is it similar?

18. What are three common shapes of bacteria?

19. How can keeping garbage and trash in closed containers protect you from pathogens?

20. What are three ways in which HIV can be transmitted?

21. What are two signs that you might have an infection?

22. What is the difference between an antigen and a toxin?

23. How can knowing the symptoms of a disease help keep you healthy?

Essay

Write the numbers 24 and 25 on your paper. Write paragraphs with complete sentences to answer each question.

24. Describe the route a pathogen might take from the time it enters your body to the time it is killed.

25. Compare how the environments and life-styles in urban and rural areas affect the people who live there.

ACTIVITIES FOR HOME OR SCHOOL

Projects to Do

1. Collect newspaper or magazine articles about HIV and AIDS and the advances made toward finding a vaccine or cure for the diseases. Make a display or scrapbook of the articles you find.

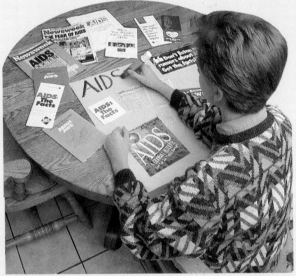

■ *Make a display with current information about AIDS.*

2. With your family, make a list of health practices you can follow to prevent the spread of communicable diseases. Discuss ways that these practices can be included in your family's daily life.

3. Ask a physician or your school nurse to show you how to measure blood pressure. Then find out the normal blood pressure for a person of your age and size.

Information to Find

1. An epidemic is the rapid spread of a disease. Some epidemics have infected hundreds or thousands of people. Check with your local or state Department of Health to find out if and when epidemics have affected your community. Also find out what disease was involved, when the epidemic took place, and how many people were affected. Find out how future epidemics of the same disease are being prevented. Share your information with the class.

2. Ask what your school's policy is on helping a student with HIV or AIDS to attend school. What kind of educational program is available for families of students who attend school with a student or a teacher who has HIV or AIDS?

3. Leukemia is a kind of cancer that affects the blood. Ask a physician to explain the symptoms and treatments for this type of cancer. Also ask the physician about the causes of leukemia.

Books to Read

Here are some books you can look for in your school library or public library to find more information about diseases and their causes.

Burns, Sheila L. *Allergies and You.* Messner.

Hyde, Margaret O., and Laurence E. Hyde. *Cancer in the Young.* Westminster.

Kipnis, Lynne, and Susan Adler. *You Can't Catch Diabetes from a Friend.* Triad Scientific Publishers.

Nourse, Alan E. *Your Immune System.* Franklin Watts.

Patent, Dorothy Hinshaw. *Bacteria, How They Affect Other Living Things.* Holiday House.

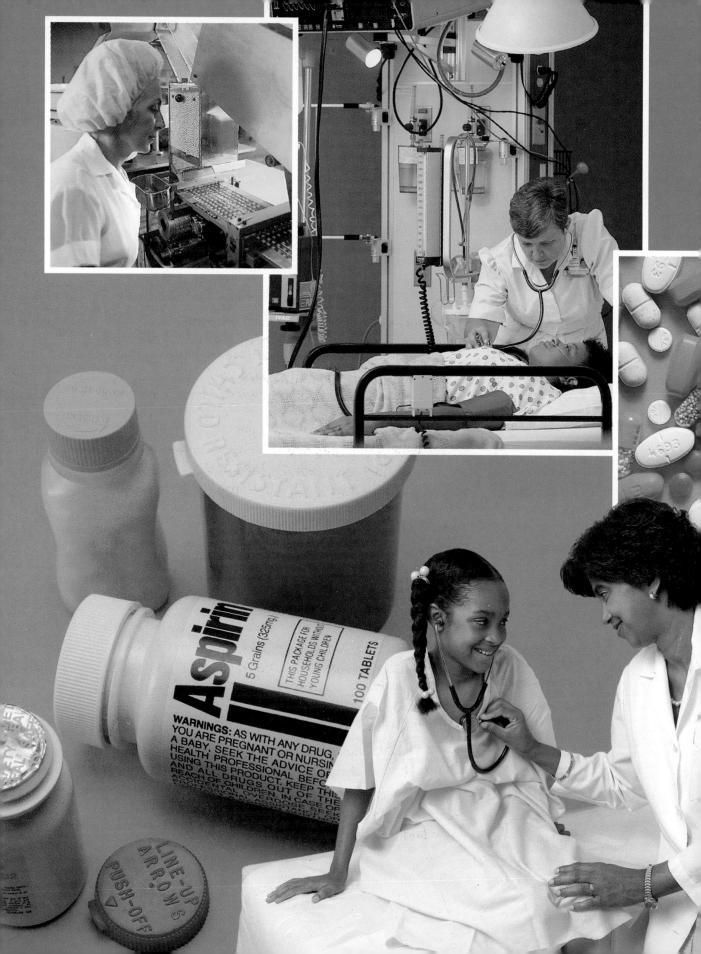

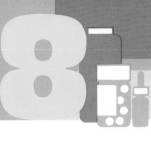

CHAPTER 8

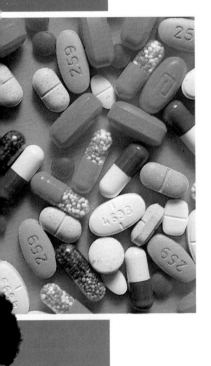

MEDICINES

Medicines have been prepared for years to help treat or cure a great variety of diseases or symptoms. Scientists, nurses, pharmacists, and physicians save lives and relieve discomfort with helpful medicines used safely. However, they know that any medicine can also harm a person's health.

In order to make wise decisions about the use of medicines, you should first understand what medicines do and when they are needed. You also must know how they are used safely and why their misuse or abuse is dangerous. Medicines can contribute to your wellness only when used responsibly.

GETTING READY TO LEARN

Key Questions

- Why is it important to learn about medicines?
- How can you learn to use medicines safely?
- Why is it important to know how you feel about using medicines safely?
- How can you take more responsibility for your health in using medicines?

Main Chapter Sections

1 About Medicines
2 How Medicines Affect the Body
3 Using Medicines Safely

1 About Medicines

drug, any substance, other than food and water, that causes changes in a person's body.

medicine (MEHD uh suhn), a drug that is used for the purpose of treating or curing a health problem.

Any substance, other than food and water, that causes changes in a person's body is a **drug.** Some drugs affect a person's nervous system, speeding it up or slowing it down. Others affect a person's heart or other organs.

When a drug is used to treat or cure an illness or to reduce pain or other symptoms, it may also be called a **medicine.** All medicines are drugs because they cause changes in a person's body. However, not all drugs are medicines. Medicines can be divided into two categories: prescription medicines and over-the-counter medicines.

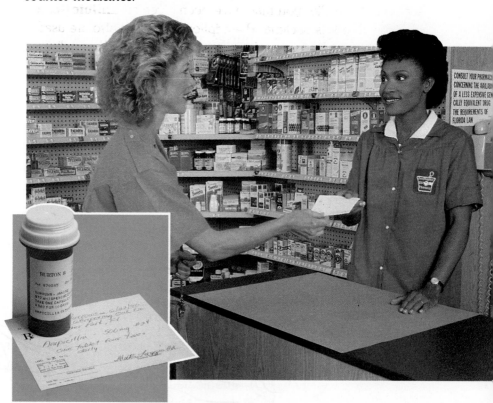

■ Physicians write prescriptions that can be filled for patients at pharmacies.

What Are Prescription Medicines?

There may be times when you need to see a physician because you are feeling ill. After examining you, the physician may write a prescription for you to take to a pharmacy. This **prescription** is an order for a certain medicine that will treat or cure your illness.

prescription (prih SKRIHP shuhn), an order for a medicine given by a physician or other authorized prescriber.

Prescription medicines can be ordered only by a physician or other authorized prescriber. The prescription directs a pharmacist to prepare a certain medicine following certain instructions. The prescription also allows the pharmacist to give the medicine to the patient. Most prescriptions have the following information:

- the physician's name and address
- the patient's name and address
- the letters *Rx*, which stand for "take"
- the medicine's name and the amount to be given
- instructions to the pharmacist about the amount of medicine to be given
- instructions about the proper use of the medicine
- the physician's signature

Think about the kinds of illnesses for which you have taken prescription medicines. You may have had an infection caused by bacteria. If you did, you may have been given an **antibiotic,** a medicine that kills bacteria. Prescription medicines also are used to treat chronic diseases such as diabetes, cancer, and heart disease.

Certain medicines can be prescribed to block or relieve pain. Perhaps you have had your appendix or tonsils removed or have had other surgery. You may remember that a physician or nurse in the operating room gave you a medicine to block the pain of the surgery. This kind of medicine, which acts on your nervous system, is an **anesthetic.** One form of anesthetic, which is used

antibiotic (ant ih by AHT ihk), a medicine used to fight a bacterial infection.

anesthetic (an uhs THEHT ihk), a medicine that acts on the nervous system to numb feeling, including pain.

■ Before surgery a patient may receive a general anesthetic, left, or a local anesthetic, right.

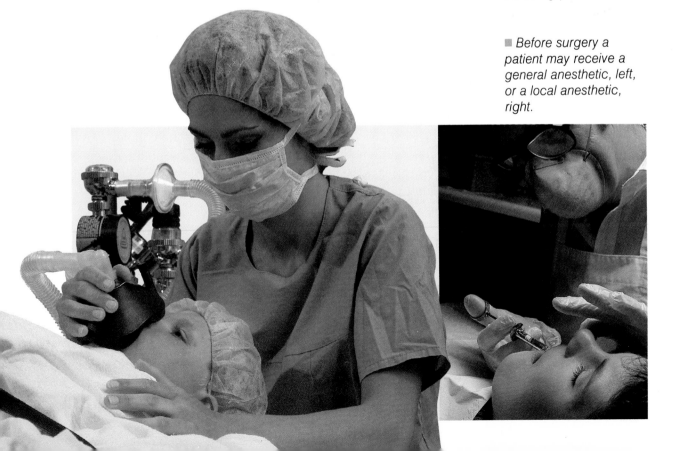

for major surgery, is a general anesthetic. A *general anesthetic* acts on your nervous system, causing you to become unconscious. A second form of anesthetic, which is used for minor surgery and dental work, is a local anesthetic. A *local anesthetic* numbs feeling in just the part of your body that would feel pain.

After surgery, the person will usually have some pain or discomfort when the anesthetic wears off. The physician or dentist may prescribe an **analgesic,** or pain reliever, to make the person feel less uncomfortable.

analgesic (an uhl JEE zihk), a medicine used to relieve pain.

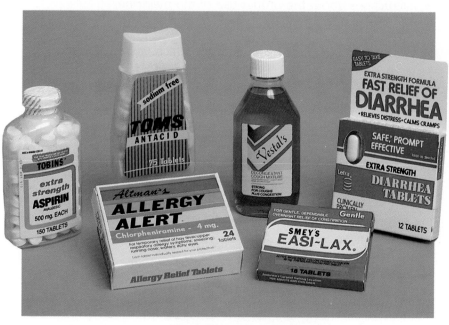

■ *A variety of medicines can be bought without a prescription.*

What Are OTC Medicines?

Some medicines do not require a prescription. These medicines are called **OTC medicines,** or over-the-counter medicines. OTC medicines can be bought at most pharmacies and food stores. OTC medicines are considered to be safe if used according to directions. **Decongestants** are a kind of OTC medicine that can relieve the stuffiness of a cold by shrinking blood vessels in the lining of the nose. Certain other OTC medicines can help stop coughing, relieve aches, and reduce fever.

OTC medicines can be used to relieve the symptoms of other minor illnesses and conditions. For example, laxatives can relieve constipation. Antidiarrheal medicines can relieve diarrhea. However, medicines are not meant to be substitutes for good health habits. Often problems such as constipation and diarrhea can be prevented by wise food choices.

OTC medicines, medicines that do not require a prescription and are considered safe if they are used responsibly and according to directions.

decongestants (dee kuhn JEHS tuhnts), medicines used to relieve a stuffy nose by shrinking blood vessels in the lining.

222

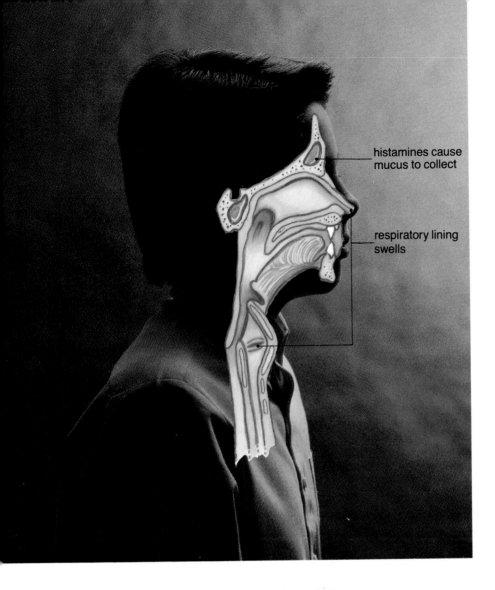

histamines cause
mucus to collect

respiratory lining
swells

*Histamines cause
swelling and an increase
in the production of
mucus in the lining of the
respiratory system.*

Perhaps the coldlike symptoms a person experiences are not caused by a cold. They may be the effects of an allergy to plant pollen. When someone has an allergy to something, such as pollen, certain cells release chemicals called *histamines*. Histamines cause various reactions in the body. In the skin, they may cause itchy rashes or perhaps swelling. In the nose and lungs, histamine causes increased mucus production. These symptoms can be uncomfortable. But they can be relieved with antihistamines. **Antihistamines** are medicines that counter the effects of histamines. They reduce itching, swelling, and mucus production.

The number of OTC medicines available for any one problem is often so great that it can make choosing the proper medicine challenging. For this reason, you can ask a pharmacist to recommend an OTC medicine to relieve your symptoms. A pharmacist can recommend a medicine that will help you.

antihistamines (ant ih HIHS tuh meenz), medicines used to relieve the effects of histamines, which can cause itchy skin, or swelling and increased mucus in the respiratory system.

223

One OTC medicine, aspirin, can relieve pain and reduce fever and swelling. However, aspirin should never be given to a young person who has a viral illness, such as a cold, influenza, or chicken pox. Check OTC medicine labels carefully. Any medicine with aspirin in it, when used to treat viral infections, may cause a very serious and sometimes fatal condition known as Reye's syndrome.

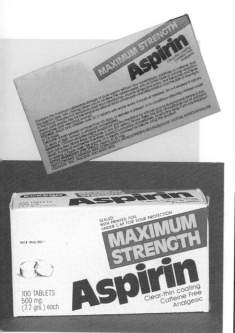

■ Although it is one of the most widely used OTC medicines, aspirin should not be given to a young person with a viral infection.

PURPOSES OF SOME OTC MEDICINES

Medicines	Symptoms to Be Relieved
Analgesics	headache, body aches, and other pain
Antacids	indigestion
Antidiarrheals	diarrhea
Antihistamines	itching, swelling, and mucus production associated with allergies and cold symptoms
Anti-inflammatories	swelling, redness, and heating of tissues
Antipyretics	fever
Antitussives	dry cough
Decongestants	stuffiness of a cold
Expectorants	mucus in the bronchial passages
Laxatives	constipation

How Are Medicines Prepared and Tested?

Making a new medicine is the responsibility of research chemists. The medicine may be a new chemical compound, or it may come from some natural source. Very often medicines are compounds of substances that are found in plants or animals. Other medicines, such as some antibiotics, have been made from organisms found in soil.

Once a new medicine is made, it must be tested before it can be sold. This takes years. Hundreds of laboratory experiments must be carried out to test the safety and effectiveness of the medicine. The company that makes the new medicine sends the information about its laboratory tests to the United States Food and Drug Administration (FDA) and asks for permission to conduct tests on people.

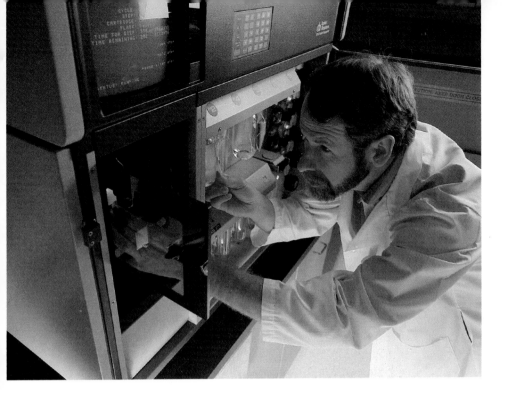

The results of these tests give researchers the information they need to make the medicine in a safe, easy-to-use form. After all the testing is done, the FDA decides whether the medicine should be approved for sale to the public. The FDA also decides whether the medicine should be sold as an OTC medicine or by prescription only. Once approval is given, the company is allowed to make the medicine and offer it for distribution.

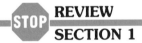 **REVIEW**
SECTION 1

REMEMBER?

1. What is the difference between a drug and a medicine?

2. Explain how prescription and OTC medicines are different.

3. What is the difference between an antihistamine and a decongestant?

THINK!

4. How might it be possible to misuse medicines such as analgesics?

5. Why is it important that new medicines be tested before they can be prescribed or sold over the counter?

Health Close-up

Generic Medicines

People often refer to an OTC or prescription medicine by its trade name. The trade name is the name the manufacturer gives the medicine. This is the name you see in advertising on television and billboards and in newspapers and magazines. Physicians and pharmacists, however, also use a medicine's generic name. The generic name is the name of the medicine's active ingredient, or the ingredient whose action improves the condition of the person taking the medicine.

Many people buy certain trade-name medicines because of advertising they have heard or seen. However, it is becoming more popular to buy medicines by their generic names. This is because they are just as effective as trade-name medicines but often cost less.

Advertising cost is one of the major reasons that trade-name medicines are more expensive than generic medicines. Each time a manufacturer advertises or provides educational materials for

■ *Generic medicines can be less costly than trade-name medicines.*

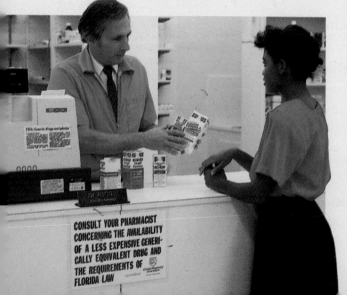

physicians and nurses, the cost is passed on to the people who buy the product. Generic medicines are usually not advertised; thus there is less cost to be passed on.

Another reason trade-name medicines cost more is research. Many times the manufacturer of a trade-name medicine has done the testing. Creating and testing a medicine is a costly, time-consuming job. The trade-name medicine may cost more to cover the expense of development. Once the trade-name medicine has been developed and approved, generic versions are quick and inexpensive to make. The packaging of a trade-name medicine can also increase its cost. Generic medicines are packed in plain containers with labels that give only the name of the medicine, its dosage, and any warnings. The manufacturer's packaging cost is therefore low.

Although generic medicines are less expensive than trade-name medicines, their active ingredients are exactly the same. All medicines must meet the same strength and purity requirements set by the federal Food and Drug Administration. Some states even have laws that allow a pharmacist to substitute a generic medicine for a trade-name medicine that is prescribed. A pharmacist is allowed to do this only if the generic medicine works as effectively.

Thinking Beyond

1. Why do some people prefer trade-name medicines to generic medicines?
2. Write one paragraph describing the advantages of generic medicines.

2 How Medicines Affect the Body

When you are ill and taking medicine, how long is it before the medicine starts to make you feel better? Perhaps you have noticed that some medicines make you feel better quickly because they relieve the symptoms of your illness. Other medicines, which seem to take longer to make you feel better, may be fighting the illness itself. Have you ever thought about how your body and a medicine work together? In order to understand how a medicine works, you first have to understand what happens to a medicine when it enters your body.

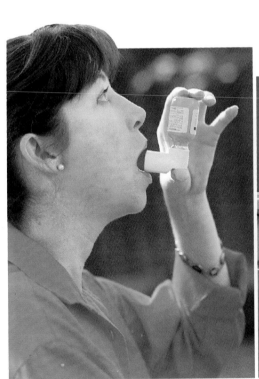
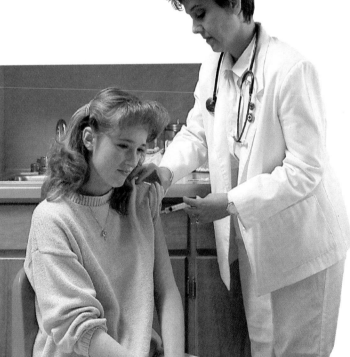

How Do Medicines Move Through the Body?

Medicines can be given in several different ways. You may have taken tablets or liquids, or you may have received medicine by way of an injection or by inhaling it. Unless a medicine is put directly on the affected area, it must enter your circulatory system before it can have an effect.

When you swallow a medicine, for example, it enters your digestive system and from there goes into your circulatory system. This route means a delay before there is any effect.

■ *The medicine that this woman is taking, left, relieves the symptoms of asthma. The medicine being given to the girl, right, destroys disease microbes.*

227

intravenous (ihn truh VEE nuhs), describes injections administered directly into the circulatory system.

intramuscular (ihn truh MUHS kyuh luhr), describes medicines injected directly into a muscle.

side effects, unwanted reactions a person has to a medicine.

■ *Commonly used OTC medicines may have side effects. You need to read all the directions and warnings before taking any medicine.*

If you are injected with a medicine, it enters your circulatory system more rapidly. Some injections produce an effect faster than others. Injections that are **intravenous,** or injected directly into the circulatory system, work very quickly. Those that are **intramuscular,** or injected into a muscle, must first be absorbed from the muscle tissue by the circulatory system. Once in your circulatory system, a medicine is carried throughout your body and does its work.

How Can Medicines Cause Problems?

Most medicines must enter the circulatory system to work. Therefore, they affect all organs and systems of the body, not just those with the illness. Medicines that are used to treat certain illnesses or symptoms may also cause unwanted reactions. These unwanted reactions are **side effects.** They include problems such as sleepiness, nausea, vomiting, hair loss, and temporary vision loss. You should always ask your physician about possible side effects when he or she prescribes a medicine. When you use an OTC medicine, you should read the label so that you are aware of the possible side effects.

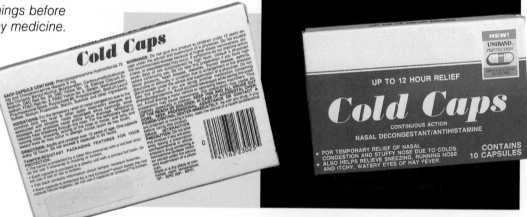

overdose (OH vuhr dohs), an amount of medicine greater than the recommended dosage.

Have you ever known someone who took a medicine in an amount larger than that prescribed or recommended? Maybe the person thought that the larger amount would help to make him or her well faster. Perhaps the person did not understand the prescription or directions. Whatever the reason, taking too much of any medicine is irresponsible and very dangerous. Any amount greater than the prescribed amount is an **overdose.** Too much of some medicines can produce dangerous effects such as abnormal breathing, irregular heart rhythm, bleeding, low or high blood pressure, and even death. Too much of other medicines can cause dizziness, nausea, vomiting, fever, skin rash, vision loss, or hearing loss.

Medicines can also cause problems if they are taken under certain conditions. For example, a woman who is pregnant should not take any medicines without her physician's consent. Medicines taken during pregnancy may cause birth defects in the baby.

Sometimes a medicine causes a reaction that cannot be predicted. Do you know anybody who has allergies? Perhaps you have an allergy to a substance such as pollen, dust, or animal hair. Your immune system can produce an allergic reaction to a foreign substance entering your body. Medicines can be thought of as foreign substances. When taken as directed, most medicines do not cause problems. But for some people, certain medicines set off allergic reactions. Symptoms of an allergic reaction may be mild, involving itchiness, swelling, or a rash. Strong allergic reactions to a medicine can lead to respiratory difficulty and death. Penicillin and aspirin are two medicines to which some people are commonly allergic.

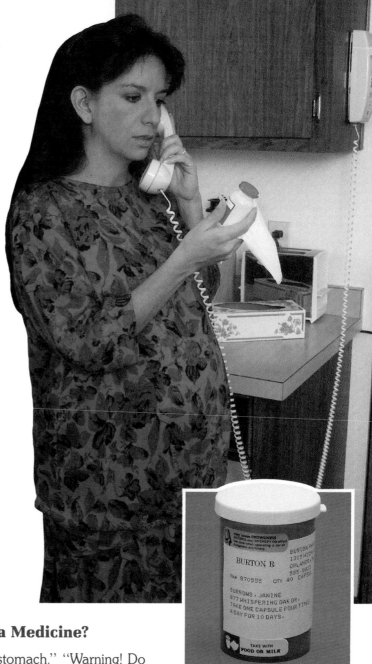

■ A pregnant woman needs to talk with her physician before taking any medicine.

What Can Change the Effect of a Medicine?

"Warning! Do not take on an empty stomach." "Warning! Do not take with milk!" Have you ever seen warnings like these on medicine labels? Some medicines should not be taken on an empty stomach or with certain foods. For example, taking certain medicines on an empty stomach can lead to nausea and ulcers. Some antibiotics, if taken with fruit juice or dairy products, lose their effectiveness. Eating some green leafy vegetables can block the ability of certain medicines to thin the blood.

Certain medicines taken together can also cause problems. In some cases, one medicine blocks the effect of the other. For example, the antibiotic tetracycline should not be taken along with any vitamin tablet or food with iron or calcium in it.

POSSIBLE EFFECTS OF MIXING MEDICINES

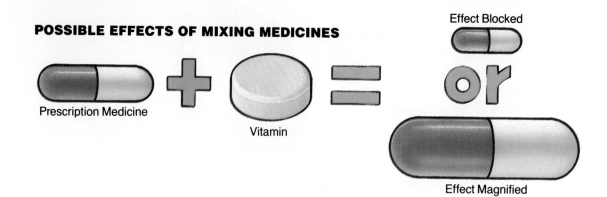

Prescription Medicine + Vitamin = Effect Blocked or Effect Magnified

■ *Mixing medicines may cause serious side effects or change the effectiveness of the medicines. Ask your physician or pharmacist before combining medicines.*

The iron or calcium would decrease the effect of the antibiotic. In other cases, one medicine magnifies the effect of the second.

Despite their possible dangers, medicines are a valuable tool in treating and curing many illnesses. Medicines have been made that will treat symptoms or illnesses of every system of the body. The lives of many people depend upon certain medicines. If a medicine must be used, care must be taken to use it responsibly and only for the purpose for which it is intended.

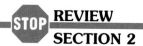 **REVIEW SECTION 2**

REMEMBER?

1. What are some ways in which medicines can be given?
2. Why must most medicines enter the circulatory system before they can work?
3. Why do medicines sometimes cause side effects?

THINK!

4. A person is in the hospital with a life-threatening infection. What might be a good way to give an antibiotic? Why?
5. Bananas have potassium in them. Why might it be a bad idea to eat bananas while taking certain antibiotics?

3   Using Medicines Safely

You have a cold. You are achy, and your nose is stuffy. And now your ear is starting to hurt. You remember that last year when you had a cold, you got an ear infection. Your physician prescribed an antibiotic. You also remember that some of that antibiotic is still in the refrigerator. Should you take some of the antibiotic to fight what you believe is another ear infection? If you do, you are not using medicine responsibly or safely. Not using all of the antibiotic when it was first ordered was also irresponsible.

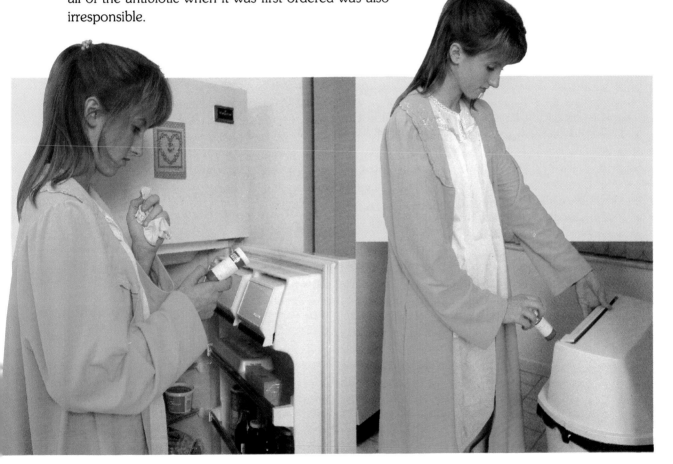

What Can Cause Medicines to Become Unsafe?

The strength of medicines can change over time. A medicine may become either stronger or weaker as it sits on a shelf. Often a medicine label gives an expiration date. After that date, the medicine may have become too strong or too weak to be effective. If it has become too strong, it may be dangerous. If it has become too weak, it may not be helpful.

■ *Taking an old medicine, even for the same illness that you had earlier, is unsafe. Time may have changed the effectiveness of the old medicine.*

231

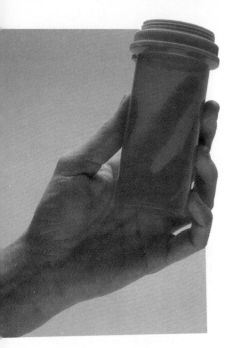

■ *Brown plastic containers prevent light from chemically changing a medicine.*

Medicines also change for reasons other than age. Have you ever noticed that medicines are often packaged in colored containers? The color screens out bright light that could chemically change the medicine. For this reason, medicines should always be stored in the containers in which they were bought. Safety is another reason why medicines should be stored in their original containers. A medicine stored in the wrong container can be taken by mistake, causing poisoning or an allergic reaction.

Medicines can also be affected by extremes of temperature and humidity. Some medicines need to be kept cold, and others are damaged by the cold. The moisture in a humid environment may damage a medicine. Always store a medicine according to the directions on the label and in its original container.

What Are Some Guidelines for Taking Medicines Safely?

Even the mildest medicine should not be taken unless a responsible decision is made that it is necessary. Young people see a lot of advertising, and they sometimes see adults reaching for medicine at the first sign of discomfort. Mild discomfort can often be put up with for a day or two. If a decision is made that it is necessary to take a medicine, it should be taken with caution and only under adult supervision.

Medicines change the way your body works. They are chemicals that mix with other chemicals in your body. Your body chemistry is slightly different from that of other people. Therefore, a medicine may not have exactly the same effect on you as it has on others.

Making Wellness Choices

Sean has been painting the outside of his parents' house. Just as he is about to finish one window, he loses his balance on the ladder and falls to the ground. When he tries to stand, he finds that he has twisted his ankle. It hurts very badly. Sean's older brother Mike, who has been working on another ladder, helps Sean into the house. By now, Sean's ankle is hurting more. Mike goes to the medicine cabinet and comes back with a bottle of prescription medicine.

 What should Sean do? Explain your wellness choice.

For the safe use of prescription and OTC medicines, there are certain guidelines everyone should follow. By following these guidelines, you can benefit from needed medicines without harming yourself.

Take Only for Its Intended Purpose. If you are taking a prescription medicine, ask your physician what its purpose is. Sometimes he or she will ask the pharmacist to put this information for you on the label. OTC medicine labels list the symptoms or illnesses for which the medicine is to be used. If a medicine is to be used to treat certain conditions, you should not use it for any other purpose. Using a medicine for anything else may hide the signs and symptoms of illness. This may make it hard for a physician to make a proper diagnosis. Using a medicine for a purpose for which it is not intended is medicine abuse.

Take Only in the Directed Amount. The label on prescription or OTC medicine explains how it should be taken. The information about the amount to be taken at one time and how often to take it is called the **dosage.** A label may list the size of the dosage in numbers of tablets, teaspoonfuls, drops, or some other kind of measurement. For a medicine to work, a person must follow the recommended dosage. Any amount below that may not treat the illness. Any amount greater than the recommended dosage is an *overdose.* An overdose can result in a dangerous reaction or even death.

Take Only As Often As Directed. The label on a prescription or OTC medicine explains how often the medicine should be taken. Timing is important in getting the greatest benefit from the medicine. Spreading the doses out over time may help maintain the appropriate level of the medicine in your body. The label may also tell you not to take more than a certain amount in a 24-hour period. If the label tells you to take a certain amount "as needed," it allows you to use your judgment in taking the medicine.

Take Only in the Directed Manner. Medicines may have unpleasant effects or no effect when they are not taken as directed. The label may direct you to take the medicine on an empty stomach, with food, after a meal, or with water. It may need to be chewed or swallowed whole. In some cases, the label may direct you to avoid taking the medicine with certain foods or drinks. By following the directions on the label, you are making sure that your body properly absorbs the medicine. If you do not know how the medicine should be taken, ask your physician or pharmacist for written directions.

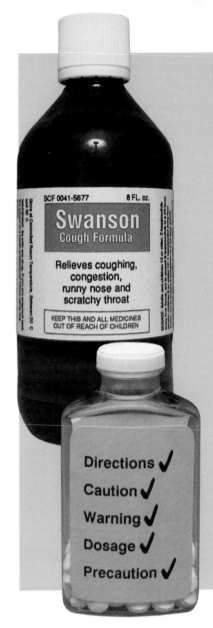

■ *Before taking any medicine, read the label.*

dosage (DOH sihj), the amount of a medicine to take at one time and how often to take it.

233

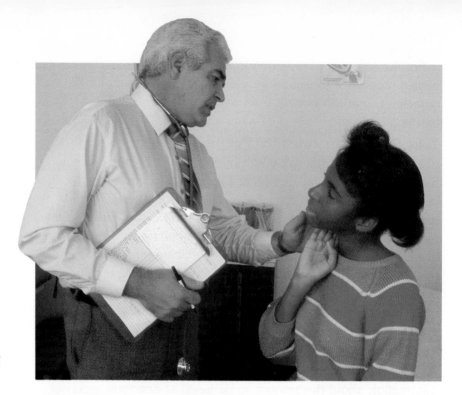

■ *A physician can decide what medicine you need to take. Do not decide on your own.*

Take for As Long As Directed. Follow the label or your physician's directions about how long you should take a medicine. If you stop taking the medicine as soon as you feel better, the illness may return. Often the symptoms of an illness will go away before your body is rid of the cause.

Read the Warnings on All Labels. A medicine label may carry a warning. This usually follows the word *caution*, *precaution*, or *warning*. Some medicine labels warn about dangerous combinations of food and medicine. A label may tell of possible side effects or of the danger of giving the medicine to children under a certain age. It may also list the hazards of taking the medicine if you have another illness or health condition at the same time.

Avoid Mixing Medicines. Taking more than one medicine at the same time can be dangerous, unless prescribed by a physician. In some cases, it can lead to death. Some combinations may cause bleeding, trouble with breathing, headache, dizziness, nausea, vomiting, or high blood pressure.

Do Not Self-Medicate. When you are ill, you may believe you know exactly what is wrong. The illness may seem just like an illness you had before. You may think some leftover prescription medicine could be used to treat your present illness. Self-medication with prescription medicines can hide the symptoms of a serious problem that needs other treatment. This may make your illness difficult to diagnose when you do see your physician.

STOP — REVIEW SECTION 3

REMEMBER?

1. What are some factors that cause medicines to change?
2. Why should you take a medicine for as long as directed even if you have begun to feel better?
3. Why is it dangerous to use a prescription medicine from a previous illness to treat a similar illness?

THINK!

4. Taking a prescribed dose of a medicine helps make you feel better. Why should you not think about taking a larger dose the next time you feel ill?
5. If a prescribed medicine worked in treating an illness, why should you not give that medicine to a friend who you believe has the same illness?

Thinking About Your Health

Checking Medicines in the Home

Use the following questions to help yourself check medicines in your home. These questions should guide you in using and storing medicines.

- Are there prescription medicines that are no longer being taken on a physician's advice?
- Are there medicines that are not in their original containers?

- Are there medicines with missing or hard-to-read labels?
- Are there medicines that have changed color or odor?
- Is any medicine stored within reach of small children?

If you answer yes to any of these questions, what should you do with the medicines? How can your actions help you and your family?

235

People in Health

An Interview with a Hospital Pharmacist

Barbara Sorrell knows about medicines and their safe use. She is the head pharmacist at a hospital on an Indian reservation in Zuni, New Mexico.

How is a hospital pharmacist different from a pharmacist who works in a neighborhood pharmacy?

Hospital pharmacists dispense medicines for patients in a hospital. They generally have little professional contact with people outside the hospital. They work closely with physicians and nurses. One of the main jobs of any hospital pharmacist, in addition to dispensing medicine, is to make sure the medicines will not be harmful to patients.

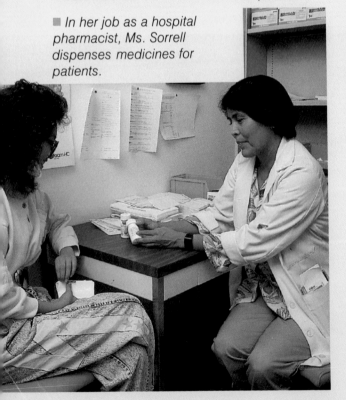

■ *In her job as a hospital pharmacist, Ms. Sorrell dispenses medicines for patients.*

How can you make sure that the medicines are safe for the patients?

All hospitals keep detailed charts about their patients. These charts include information about the medicines they are taking and about those to which they may have an allergy. Before I give out any medicine, I read the chart about the particular patient. My responsibility is to make sure the medicine I supply will not interfere with other medicines the patient may be taking. I also must be sure that the medicine will not cause an allergic reaction or harm the patient in any other way.

How do you get the medicines ready for the patients?

I fill the prescription orders given by the hospital physicians. Then I prepare the medicines for the nursing staff to deliver to the patients. The nurses use a cart with little drawers. Each drawer is assigned to a certain patient. A pharmacy technician under the supervision of a pharmacist puts the correct dosage of the right medicine into each drawer. If a patient is to receive a certain medicine four times a day, for example, then four doses of that medicine are put into the drawer. Each dose is individually packaged.

Do you give instructions about the medicines to the nurses?

Whenever a prescription is ordered for a patient, I give the nursing staff information about the medicine. I tell them how the patient might react to the medicine and what the side effects are. This information helps the nurses guard the patient's health.

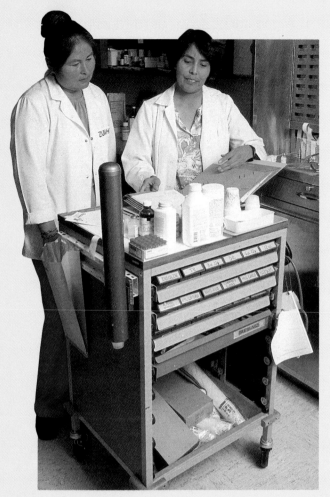

■ *A hospital pharmacist informs the nursing staff about a medicine's possible side effects.*

Do you have any contact with patients?

I have contact with people who are patients at the hospital's outpatient clinic. An *outpatient* is a person who receives medical treatment at the hospital but does not need to stay there. Each outpatient, like each inpatient, has a chart. I work from an outpatient's chart just as if the person were a patient in the hospital. When an outpatient hands me a prescription, I consult the chart and check for possible problems he or she might have with the medicine. If I foresee a problem, I call the person's physician.

What do you tell people about medicines?

I tell everyone how important it is for them to read the instructions on medicine labels. They must understand how their medicines should be taken. Some medicines need to be taken with food; others do not. It is very important to know how much medicine to take and how often to take it. If a medicine is to be taken four times a day and the label does not state how much time should pass between doses, the patient should ask the pharmacist for more information.

Why is it important for a person to take a medicine for as long as the label directs?

Sometimes after a person takes a medicine for a few days, he or she feels better. However, some of the microbes that caused the health problem may still be present in the person's body. As soon as the person stops taking the medicine, the problem can start again. That is why it is important to finish taking a medicine according to the instructions given on the label or by the pharmacist.

Learn more about the safe use of medicines and about people who work as pharmacists. Interview a hospital pharmacist. Or write for information to the American Pharmaceutical Association, 2215 Constitution Avenue, N.W., Washington, DC 20037.

Main Ideas

- A drug that is used for the purpose of preventing or treating health problems is called a medicine.

- Prescription medicines can be ordered only by a physician or other authorized prescriber.

- OTC medicines are those medicines that do not require a prescription and are considered safe if used responsibly and according to directions.

- Once a new medicine is developed, it must undergo tests of its safety and effectiveness.

- Medicines can cause unwanted reactions if they are taken in a manner or for a purpose other than that intended.

- Medicines must be taken according to all directions if they are to be used safely.

Key Words

Write the numbers 1 to 14 in your health notebook or on a separate sheet of paper. After each number, copy the sentence and fill in the missing term. Page numbers in ( ) tell you where to look in the chapter if you need help.

drug (220)
medicine (220)
prescription (220)
antibiotic (221)
anesthetic (221)
analgesic (222)
OTC medicines (222)
decongestants (222)

antihistamines (223)
intravenous (228)
intramuscular (228)
side effects (228)
overdose (228)
dosage (233)

1. A general ___?___, used during major surgery, makes the patient unconscious.

2. Because they are injected directly into the circulatory system, ___?___ medicines work very quickly.

3. A drug that is used for the purpose of preventing or treating health problems is called a ___?___ .

4. Pain can be relieved with an ___?___ .

5. ___?___ are medicines that do not require a prescription.

6. ___?___ injections must first pass through muscle tissue before they can be absorbed by the circulatory system and take effect.

7. The ___?___ is information about the amount of a medicine to take at one time and how often to take the medicine in order to gain the proper effects.

8. An ___?___ of a medicine is an unusually large amount that can cause a person to become very ill or die.

9. A ___?___ is any substance, other than food and water; that causes a change in a person's body.

10. A ___?___ medicine can be used only on the order of a physician or other authorized prescriber.

11. A person with a cold can use ___?___ to relieve a stuffy nose.

12. ___?___ are unwanted reactions to medicines.

13. A bacterial infection is often treated with an ___?___ .

14. The effects of an allergy can be relieved with ___?___ .

Remembering What You Learned

Page numbers in ( ) tell you where to look in the chapter if you need help.

1. What is the difference between a medicine and a drug? (220)

2. What is the difference between a prescription medicine and an OTC medicine? (220–222)

3. Why does an intravenous injection take effect faster than an intramuscular injection? (228)

4. What things might cause a medicine to change? (231–232)

5. Why should you treat OTC medicines as carefully as you treat prescription medicines? (232–234)

6. Why should you ask your pharmacist whether there are any foods or drinks you cannot have while you are taking a certain medicine? (233)

7. What are the eight guidelines that you should follow for taking medicines safely and responsibly? (233–234)

8. Why should you avoid taking more than one medicine at a time? (234)

Thinking About What You Learned

1. You cannot get to sleep. You remember that the antihistamine prescribed for your allergies last summer made you sleepy. You are considering taking some of the antihistamine. Explain why you should or should not take the medicine.

2. Why is it important to follow exactly the directions for taking any medicine?

3. A friend had a sore throat and was given a prescription for an antibiotic. After he had taken three doses of the medicine, the sore throat went away, so he stopped taking the medicine. Two days later, he had a sore throat again. Explain what happened.

Writing About What You Learned

1. Interview five people about the way they use prescription medicines. Find out how many have ever used another person's prescription, how many have ever used an old prescription for a new illness, and how many have ever taken a larger-than-directed dose of a medicine. Write a report about their attitudes toward the use of prescription medicines.

2. Write a short story about a boy with indigestion. His father has given him a dose of an antacid and has left for work. The boy is still uncomfortable, and his mother wants him to take another dose. The story should not have an ending; it should invite discussion of the most responsible course of action for the boy.

Applying What You Learned

ART

Create two posters that warn people about the dangers of using medicines incorrectly.

SOCIAL STUDIES

Investigate the effects of the incorrect use of medicine on a person's ability to perform his or her job. Write a short report on your findings and present it to the class.

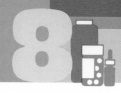

Modified True or False

Write the numbers 1 to 15 in your health notebook or on a separate sheet of paper. After each number, write *true* or *false* to describe the sentence. If the sentence is false, also write a term that replaces the underlined term and makes the sentence true.

1. A drug that is used to cure an illness or to reduce pain or other symptoms is a <u>medicine</u>.
2. A <u>parent</u> can write a prescription.
3. A medicine that acts on your nervous system and causes you to become unconscious is a <u>local</u> anesthetic.
4. If you wanted to relieve the stuffiness of a cold, you might take a <u>decongestant</u>.
5. Allergic symptoms in the body are caused by <u>histamines</u>.
6. Most medicines must enter the <u>respiratory</u> system before they can have an effect.
7. <u>Intravenous</u> injections go directly into the circulatory system.
8. Hair loss is an example of a <u>side effect</u> of a medicine.
9. The amount of medicine to be taken at one time and how often it is to be taken are called the <u>overdose</u>.
10. A medicine that kills bacteria is an <u>analgesic</u>.
11. <u>Aspirin</u> is an analgesic.
12. Companies must get approval from the <u>FDA</u> before they can offer medicines for distribution in the United States.
13. The <u>strength</u> of medicine can change over time.
14. <u>Medicines</u> change the way your body works.
15. A decongestant is a <u>drug</u>.

Short Answer

Write the numbers 16 to 23 on your paper. Write a complete sentence to answer each question.

16. Give two examples of situations in which anesthesia might be used.
17. Why should you take a medicine for the entire time described on the label?
18. When is a drug not a medicine?
19. What is an allergic reaction?
20. Why should you not take medicines together unless instructed to by your physician?
21. Why should you always store medicine in its original container?
22. What is the danger of taking a medicine to treat a condition not listed on the label?
23. How can medicine change?

Essay

Write the numbers 24 and 25 on your paper. Write paragraphs with complete sentences to answer each question.

24. Summarize the guidelines all people should follow when taking medicines.
25. Why is it better to deal with small discomforts through proper diet and exercise rather than by taking OTC medicines?

ACTIVITIES FOR HOME OR SCHOOL

Projects to Do

1. Work with several classmates to create a bulletin board that will illustrate rules for the safe and responsible use of prescription and OTC medicines.

2. Make a collage of advertisements for OTC medicines. For each advertisement, write the name of the magazine or newspaper in which it was found, the date of the publication, and your impression of the advertisement. Describe how the ad is trying to influence people. Write a report on medicine advertising, telling whether you think it plays a negative or positive role.

3. Select an illness for which you might take an OTC medicine. Go to a pharmacy, and make a list of all the medicines that might be used to treat the illness. For each medicine, list the brand name, ingredients, symptoms it is supposed to treat, side effects it might cause, and any warnings that are given. Make a wall chart of your findings.

■ *Collect advertisements for OTC medicines from magazines.*

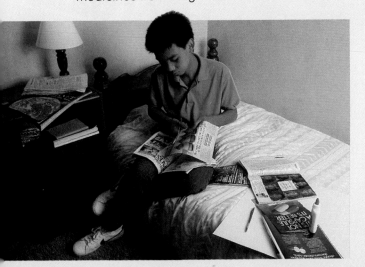

Information to Find

1. The Food and Drug Administration is constantly investigating new medicines. Select a serious illness, such as heart disease, cancer, or high blood pressure, and write to the FDA for information on current testing of new medicines to treat the illness. (FDA, National Office of Consumer Affairs, 5600 Fishers Lane, Rockville, MD 20857.)

2. Many physicians try to help people feel better without the use of medicines whenever possible. Interview a physician or pharmacist about treatments that do not involve medicines.

3. Sometimes prescription medicines are available in different strengths as OTC medicines. Interview a pharmacist to find out which OTC medicines fall into this category. Ask him or her why the FDA approves the sale of these medicines over the counter. Present a report to your class.

Books to Read

Here are some books you can look for in your school library or the public library to find more information about medicines and their safe use.

Graedon, Joe, and Teresa Graedon. *The People's Pharmacy, Totally New and Revised*. St. Martin's.

Levy, Stephen J. *Managing the Drugs in Your Life: A Personal and Family Guide to the Responsible Use of Drugs, Alcohol, and Medicine*. McGraw-Hill.

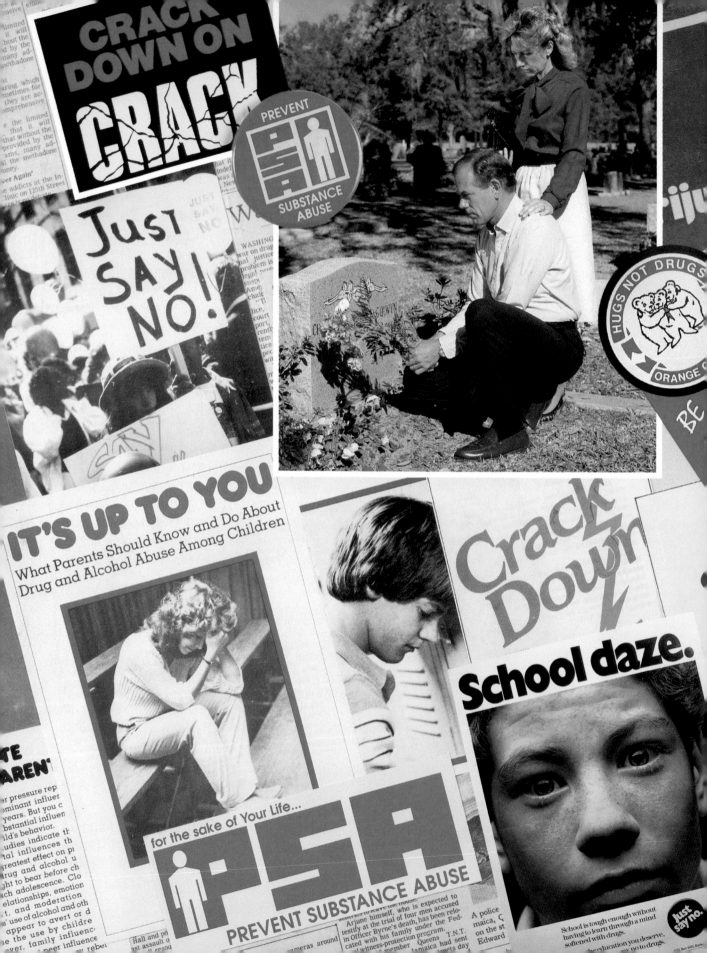

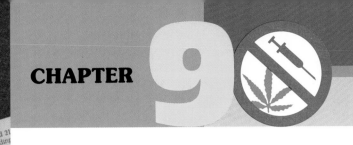

CHAPTER 9

DANGERS OF ILLEGAL DRUGS

People who use illegal drugs are drug abusers. They give many different reasons for abusing drugs. No matter what reasons they give, their actions are irresponsible and are harmful not only to themselves but also to the people around them. Using illegal drugs can result in loss of life and property, and it destroys relationships with other people.

The decision you make not to use illegal drugs can be one of the smartest decisions you will ever make. More and more young people are learning how to resist curiosity and the pressures to use illegal drugs. Their skills for refusing illegal drugs also can help build self-esteem.

GETTING READY TO LEARN

Key Questions

- Why is it important to know the dangers of illegal drugs?
- What risks do illegal drugs pose to a person's life and health?
- Why is it important to know how you feel about the use of illegal drugs?
- How can you refuse an offer of illegal drugs?

Main Chapter Sections

1 The Effects of Using Illegal Drugs
2 Stimulants, Depressants, and Narcotics
3 Hallucinogens, Cannabis Products, and Inhalants
4 Refusing Illegal Drugs

1 The Effects of Using Illegal Drugs

Friday, 9:00 P.M.—Michael arrives at a friend's house for a party.

Friday, 9:30 P.M.—Several people at the party bring out a white powdery drug and spread it on a mirror. They begin inhaling the drug into their noses through thin straws.

Friday, 9:45 P.M.—Michael decides to try the drug and inhales a small amount.

Friday, 9:55 P.M.—Michael passes out, his heart begins to beat irregularly, and his breathing is uneven. People at the party leave him in a bedroom to recover on his own. They assume he will be all right if he "sleeps it off." They are wrong.

Saturday, 11:00 A.M.—Michael is pronounced dead in the emergency room.

Tuesday, 10:00 A.M.—Michael is buried.

Illegal drugs are dangerous and unpredictable. The effects of illegal drugs on a person's body cannot always be predicted. When a person takes an illegal drug, he or she takes a dangerous risk. There is always a danger because the person cannot be certain of how strong the drug is.

■ *A person using illegal drugs is gambling with his or her life. Michael gambled only once — and lost his life.*

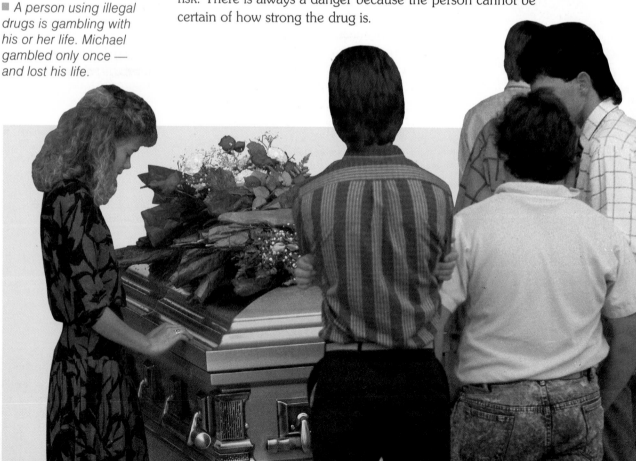

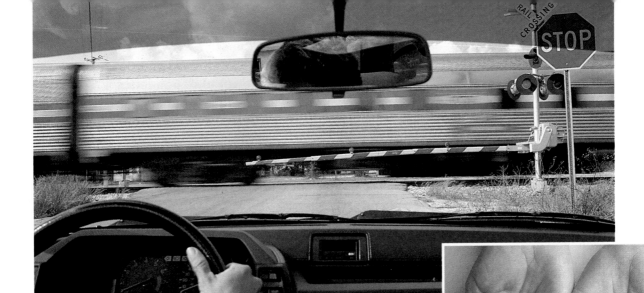

What Are the Immediate Effects of Using Illegal Drugs?

Illegal drugs have a wide variety of harmful effects on the human body. Some of these effects are easy to see in just seconds after a person takes a drug. Other effects may not show up for several hours.

Depending upon the drug that is taken, different effects may be experienced. The person may feel more alert or more relaxed. Heart rate and breathing may change. With some drugs, the parts of the brain that control the senses are chemically changed, affecting the way the person thinks and behaves. The exact effect of a drug depends upon the person's own body chemistry. This means that each person reacts differently to any drug.

Some drugs can cause a person to do things that are dangerous. The drug abuser may be physically injured or may injure another person. For this reason, the use of illegal drugs cannot be considered harmful only to the drug abuser.

■ Some drugs may not kill a person directly. Instead, they may cause a person to do things that are dangerous.

What Are the Long-term Effects of Using Illegal Drugs?

Although any use of an illegal drug is dangerous, long-term abuse of such a drug can cause a buildup of effects. For example, using a certain drug repeatedly will lead to tolerance. **Tolerance** is a state in which the person no longer feels the desired effect from the same amount of the drug. He or she will have to keep taking larger amounts in order to feel the desired effect.

tolerance (TAHL uh ruhns), a state in which a person no longer feels the same effect from the same amount of a drug.

245

emotional dependence
(ih MOH shuhn uhl • dih PEHN duhns), a state in which a person feels uncomfortable if he or she is not experiencing the effects of a drug.

physical dependence
(FIHZ ih kuhl • dih PEHN duhns), a state in which a person's body becomes accustomed to the presence of a drug and cannot function normally without it.

withdrawal (wihth DRAWL), stopping the use of a drug that has produced a physical and emotional dependence; usually produces painful reactions.

At this point, the drug abuser has formed an emotional dependence on the drug. **Emotional dependence** is a state in which a drug abuser feels uncomfortable if he or she does not keep experiencing the effects of the drug.

If the drug abuser continues using the drug, he or she risks forming a physical dependence. **Physical dependence** is a state in which the body becomes used to a drug and cannot function normally without it. The person needs the drug to feel all right.

Once a person has a physical dependence on a drug, the person will suffer painful reactions to its absence if he or she stops taking it. This condition is called **withdrawal.** The symptoms and seriousness of withdrawal vary with the kind of drug being used. Withdrawal from some drugs can lead to violent illness, convulsions, and even death. For this reason, a drug abuser who is physically dependent on a drug must go through withdrawal only with the help of a physician or other health-care worker.

If drug abuse lasts for many months or years, many of the person's organs and body systems will be seriously damaged. As tolerance grows, the drug abuser will need larger and larger amounts of the drug. Sometimes the person may take such a large amount of the drug that he or she will experience an overdose. An overdose of any drug can cause serious reactions in the body. The person may become unconscious, stop breathing, and die.

Who Is Affected by the Use of Illegal Drugs?

Using illegal drugs is selfish and inconsiderate. Yet many drug abusers believe they are not hurting anyone but themselves. In fact, illegal drugs affect many people in addition to the drug abuser. Families, friends, co-workers, classmates, neighbors, and society in general are all affected by a person's use of illegal drugs.

Family and Social Problems. People who abuse drugs often blame their problems on poor relationships with family members and friends. But a person who is using illegal drugs has little time to improve or maintain relationships with other people. The use of illegal drugs makes relationships worse by adding new problems. The person is often abusing drugs to escape reality.

If a drug abuser is emotionally and physically dependent on a drug, most of his or her time is probably spent on trying to get and use the drug. Most drug abusers deny their dependence

246

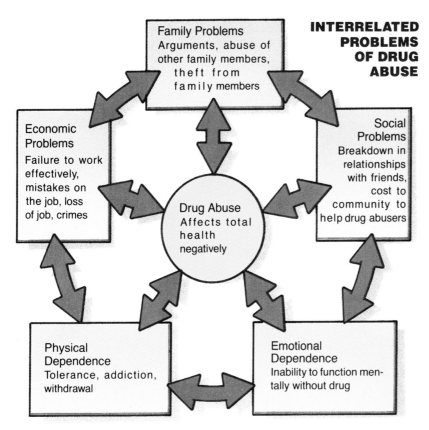

INTERRELATED PROBLEMS OF DRUG ABUSE

Family Problems
Arguments, abuse of other family members, theft from family members

Economic Problems
Failure to work effectively, mistakes on the job, loss of job, crimes

Drug Abuse
Affects total health negatively

Social Problems
Breakdown in relationships with friends, cost to community to help drug abusers

Physical Dependence
Tolerance, addiction, withdrawal

Emotional Dependence
Inability to function mentally without drug

■ *Some people blame family problems for leading them to drug abuse and dependence. Dependence causes more problems, which usually increase drug abuse.*

because they believe they are in control of their drug use. But failure to see that there is a problem can have serious consequences. The longer the time before the drug abuser receives professional help, the harder the withdrawal will be.

Economic Problems.   A drug abuser is almost always worried about getting money. Illegal drugs are very costly. As tolerance increases, the person must get larger and larger amounts of a drug. Many drugs cost more than $300 for a day's supply.

■ *Many drug users steal the money they need to buy drugs. These people often get arrested.*

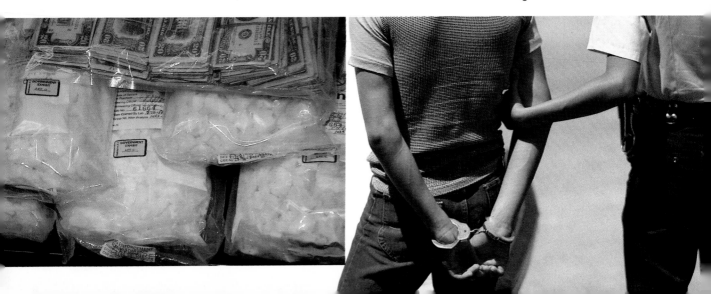

A person with a $300-a-day habit, which is not uncommon, will spend $109,500 a year on drugs. That is enough money to pay cash for a house in many parts of the United States.

Often, a drug abuser will get money by stealing from family members and friends. When this source of money runs out, the drug abuser will steal from other people and from businesses. Some drug abusers will do almost anything to get money for drugs.

STOP **REVIEW**
SECTION 1

REMEMBER?

1. What are some of the immediate effects of using illegal drugs?
2. What are some of the long-term effects of using illegal drugs?
3. How does one person's use of illegal drugs affect many other people?

THINK!

4. What are some of the consequences of being "mixed up with drugs"?
5. How is it that of two people who take the same amount of the same drug, one overdoses and the other does not?

Thinking About Your Health

Analyzing Your Attitudes About Drugs

Written below are seven unfinished sentences about the use of illegal drugs. On a separate sheet of paper, complete each sentence. This paper will not be handed in and does not have to be shared with anyone.

- People use illegal drugs because . . .
- I can say no to illegal drugs because . . .
- My parents feel that illegal drugs . . .
- My friends feel that illegal drugs . . .
- I feel that illegal drugs . . .
- A drug dealer . . .
- The drug laws . . .

Analyze each sentence to understand the kind of pressure that influenced the way you completed it. Did the pressure come from personal feelings, family values, the beliefs of friends, or society in general? Explain how these pressures work together to help you say no to the use of illegal drugs.

2 Stimulants, Depressants, and Narcotics

Different drugs affect a person's body in different ways. Some cause body systems to speed up. Others cause body systems to slow down. Still other drugs keep the brain from sensing pain. If certain drugs are properly prescribed by a physician and used properly, they can have great medical benefit. However, if drugs are used improperly, they can cause great harm and even death.

What Are Stimulants?

The young man's heart is pounding at 160 beats per minute, and his blood pressure has gone from a normal 120 over 60 to 160 over 110. Everything is exciting. He has energy that he never felt before. Suddenly, his feelings change. Now he is anxious, irritable, and exhausted. He finds everything annoying, his head is pounding, and all he wants to do is sleep. This person has experienced the changing effects of a stimulant. **Stimulants** are drugs that speed up the working of the nervous system, which in turn speeds up other body systems.

Not all stimulants affect the nervous system as strongly as just described, and not all stimulants are illegal. Stimulants are sometimes prescribed to treat certain illnesses. Stimulants that are prescribed are safe as long as they are used as they were intended to be used.

stimulants (STIHM yuh luhnts), drugs that speed up the functioning of the nervous system.

■ *Stimulants speed up heartbeat and breathing rates.*

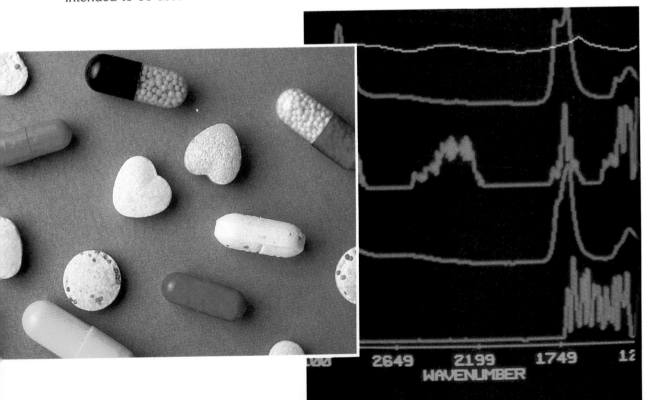

2649   2199   1749   12
WAVENUMBER

Stimulants in Foods and Tobacco. Certain stimulants are often used without the need for a prescription. Coffee, tea, and cola drinks, for example, all have the natural stimulant *caffeine*. Chocolate also has caffeine. Products with caffeine can be dangerous if they are abused. Use of caffeine can increase heart rate, change heart rhythm, and raise blood pressure. Caffeine can also cause headaches, nervousness, sleeplessness, diarrhea, and loss of concentration.

■ *Many common products contain small amounts of natural stimulants. Coffee, tea, cola drinks, and chocolate contain caffeine. Tobacco products contain nicotine.*

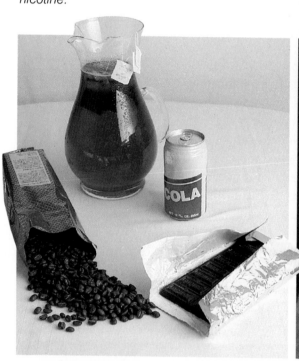

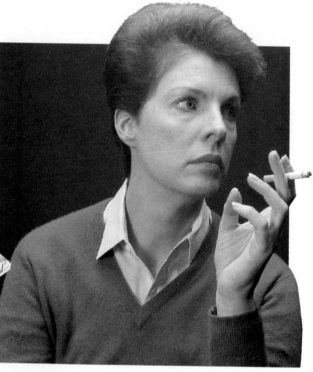

A second common stimulant is *nicotine*. Nicotine is found in all tobacco products. It causes the same effects as other stimulants. The United States surgeon general has stated that the use of products with nicotine can cause **addiction** to, or severe physical and emotional dependence on, that drug.

Most stimulants are far more powerful than caffeine and nicotine. Some of these stimulants have legal uses, but they are often used illegally.

addiction (uh DIHK shuhn), a severe physical and emotional dependence on a drug.

Amphetamines. The *amphetamines* form a group of very powerful stimulants. Physicians sometimes prescribe low dosages of amphetamines to fight drowsiness, relieve depression, or reduce appetite. Amphetamines are also prescribed to improve concentration in children who have attention disorders. Before prescribing these drugs or any other stimulants, however,

250

physicians try non-drug methods to relieve the patient's problems. Only after all other methods have failed will a physician prescribe amphetamines. When obtained illegally, amphetamines are usually taken too often and in amounts that are too large. This often leads to addiction.

Some of the signs of amphetamine abuse are enlarged pupils of the eyes, trembling, nervousness, sleeplessness, and diarrhea. If amphetamine abuse lasts for a long time, it can cause uncontrollable violent behavior and death.

Cocaine. Cocaine does have a few specific medical uses. For example, it is used as an anesthetic in certain kinds of nose surgery. People who use cocaine illegally inject, swallow, or sniff it. Repeated sniffing of cocaine destroys the nasal lining and septum—the cartilage down the center of the nose. When the cartilage is destroyed, the nose collapses.

Cocaine gives a person a burst of energy, excitement, and great happiness for a short time. As the drug's effects wear off, the person becomes very depressed. As a result, the person who uses cocaine often takes repeated doses of the drug to relieve the depression. This leads to cocaine addiction.

Long-term use of cocaine causes behavior changes. The person becomes very suspicious and fearful of people. The person may also believe that he or she has special mental powers and great physical strength. Feeling this way, the person becomes a danger to himself or herself and to others.

■ *Cocaine is made from the leaves of the coca plant, top, and is usually a white powder, lower right. Cocaine users can call a hotline to get help, lower left.*

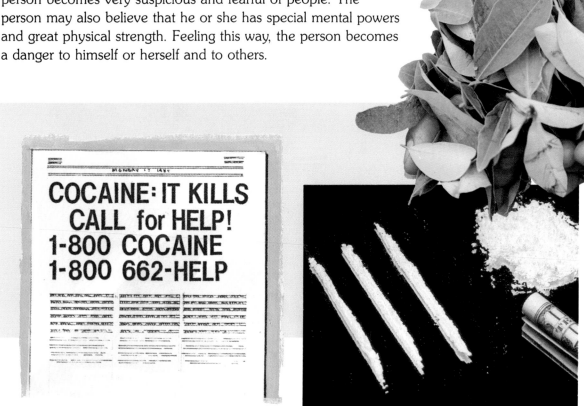

COCAINE: IT KILLS
CALL for HELP!
1-800 COCAINE
1-800 662-HELP

Cocaine is an especially serious threat to an unborn child. Research has shown that even one dose of cocaine taken during a pregnancy can cause lifetime damage to a baby. During the first three months, cocaine can damage developing organs. "Cocaine babies" are more likely to die before birth or become victims of sudden infant death syndrome (SIDS) than babies of mothers who do not use cocaine. Often, babies born to mothers who used cocaine have nervous-system problems that make them very irritable.

Crack Cocaine.   A very powerful and dangerous form of cocaine is called *crack*. This form of cocaine is made by chemically changing the drug to make a hard, waxy-looking chunk of material that can be broken into small pieces.

The small pieces are smoked, and the intense effect of the drug is felt almost immediately. The effect, however, lasts for only a short time, and then the person slips into a deep depression. In order to relieve the depression, the person may take more of the drug. He or she quickly forms a strong addiction to crack.

Like other stimulants, crack changes the heart rate and heart rhythm. Crack is such a powerful and concentrated form of cocaine that a small amount can cause heart failure and death.

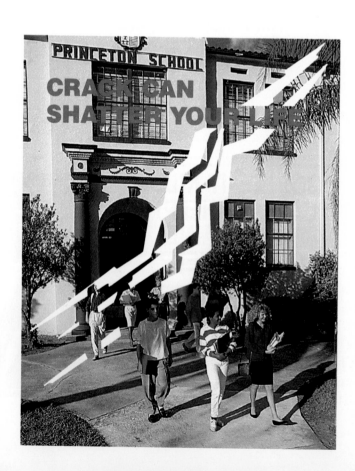

What Are Depressants?

Depressants are drugs that slow down the working of the nervous system. When this happens, all other body systems are slowed as well. Some depressants are prescribed by physicians to treat certain illnesses. These depressants are safe as long as they are used with proper medical supervision. However, depressants that are used illegally can be deadly.

Depressants are very dangerous when they are used with other drugs. For example, sleeping pills and alcohol are both depressants. When taken together, they can lead to unconsciousness and even death.

depressants (dih PREHS uhnts), drugs that slow down the functioning of the nervous system.

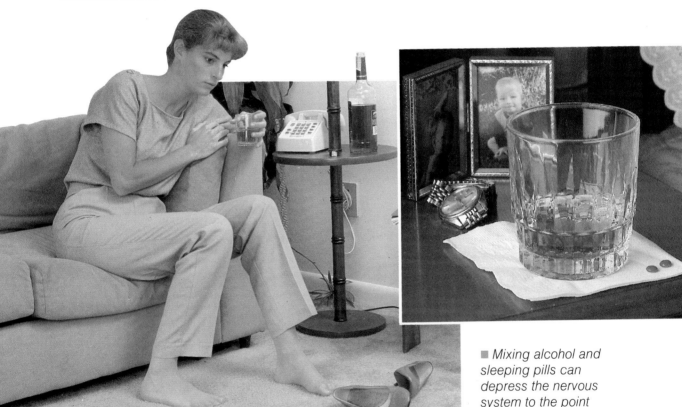

■ Mixing alcohol and sleeping pills can depress the nervous system to the point where breathing and the heartbeat stop.

Physicians may prescribe *barbiturates* to relieve anxiety and help a person sleep. Barbiturates may also be prescribed as long-term treatment for controlling seizures. However, barbiturates that are obtained illegally are most often used in amounts much larger than the dose needed for medical reasons. As a result, people abusing these drugs will experience an effect much like severe intoxication. If barbiturates are taken for a long time, they can cause sleeplessness, hallucinations, depression, emotional instability, and addiction.

253

What Are Narcotics?

For thousands of years, people have looked for ways to prevent or stop pain. Of all the things tried, the most effective has been the use of narcotics. **Narcotics** are drugs that reduce the brain's ability to recognize pain. Although the way narcotics work is not fully understood, scientists think narcotics cause the release of certain chemicals in the central nervous system that block the sensation of pain. Many prescription medicines that are used to relieve pain contain narcotics.

Opium. Until the early 1800s, physicians thought opium was the most effective drug for relieving pain. Opium comes from the unripe seeds of a certain kind of poppy plant. As well as relieving pain, opium was used to stop coughing, relieve diarrhea, ease nervousness, and cause drowsiness. Physicians in the 1800s discovered, however, that people who used opium very quickly became addicted to it.

When first used, opium causes a feeling of great calm. Troubles seem unimportant, and the person lives in an unreal world of contentment. With continued use, these calming effects are replaced by dreams and daydreams that can be very unpleasant. By this time, however, the person is emotionally and physically dependent upon the drug. Unfortunately, the user cannot stop taking it without the help of a physician.

■ *Opium is made from the sticky sap of the seed pods of certain poppies.*

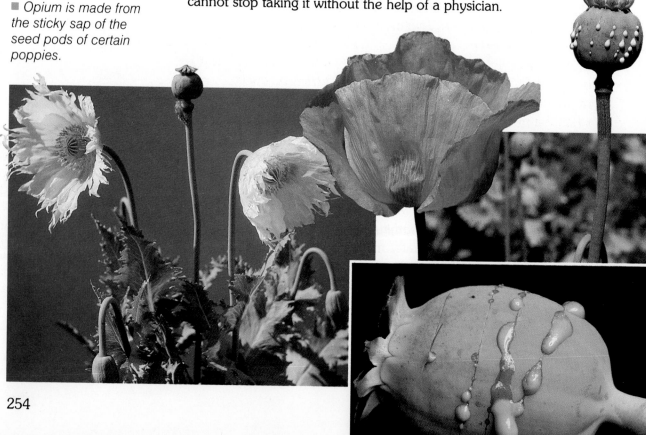

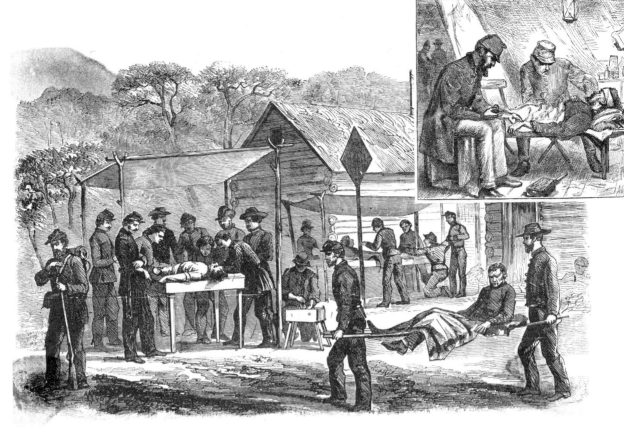

■ *Morphine was used during the Civil War to reduce the pain of wounds and surgery. As a result, many soldiers became addicted.*

Morphine.   Some other narcotics are made from opium. As a group, these are known as **opiates.** An opiate, such as *morphine,* comes from chemical changes made to opium. In the United States, federal laws prohibit the use of morphine unless it is prescribed by a physician. When taken in small amounts, morphine blocks pain and leaves the mind fairly clear. But even when the prescribed dosage is very small, morphine use can cause addiction.

Used illegally in larger amounts, morphine clouds the mind and makes the person feel very lazy. It may also depress the respiratory system, interfere with heart rhythm, and cause vomiting. Long-term use will lead to physical addiction, and the user will not be able to stop using the drug without professional help.

Heroin.   The most dangerous of all the opiates is *heroin.* Heroin is made from morphine but is far more powerful and addictive. Heroin cannot be used legally in the United States, even by prescription. Since the drug cannot be obtained legally, heroin users can never be sure of its purity or strength. A heroin user is always in danger of death from an overdose.

opiates (OH pee uhts), drugs that are made from opium; cause dullness and inaction.

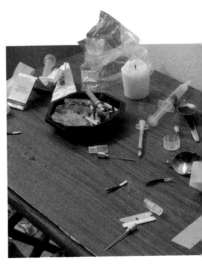

■ *By sharing needles, many heroin users spread diseases such as hepatitis B and AIDS.*

255

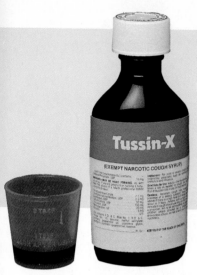

■ *A prescription medicine with codeine in it needs to be used wisely.*

Heroin addicts also face other dangers linked to their use of drugs. Heroin is mostly injected directly into a vein. Most people who use heroin are not careful about using sterile needles for these injections. Addicts often share needles. Because of this, heroin addicts risk getting diseases such as blood poisoning, hepatitis B, and AIDS.

Codeine.   One of the more common opiates is *codeine*, which is made in laboratories. Codeine is used in some prescription medicines to relieve pain or reduce coughs. However, physicians are very careful about prescribing any medicine with codeine because of the chance of addiction.

Methadone.   Another narcotic made in laboratories is *methadone*. However, methadone is not an opiate. This drug is made of chemicals. Although first used as a painkiller, methadone is now used to help cure heroin addiction. The use of methadone helps heroin addicts slowly get over their need for opiates. Methadone can be obtained only by prescription and must be taken under direct medical supervision. Methadone is also addictive.

MYTH AND FACT

Myth: A person cannot overdose the first time he or she uses a drug.

Fact: The first time a person uses a drug, he or she has no tolerance at all, so there is a good chance of over-dosing on the drug.

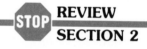 **REVIEW**

SECTION 2

REMEMBER?

1. How do stimulants and depressants differ in the way they affect the nervous system?
2. What are some narcotics that are used as painkillers?
3. What special dangers do heroin users face from their use of this illegal drug?

THINK!

4. Why is it so difficult to stop using cocaine?
5. Why are physicians hesitant to prescribe amphetamines to help a person lose weight?

Health Close-up

Drug Use and Pregnancy

The use of any drugs, legal and illegal, either before or during pregnancy, can cause serious problems in an embryo or fetus. A woman's general health before pregnancy is an important factor in the health of her child. During pregnancy, the blood supplies of the mother and fetus are closely connected. The fetus receives nutrients and oxygen through the circulatory system of the mother. Any substance that is present in the mother's bloodstream will also be present in the bloodstream of the fetus.

Even nonprescription drugs, such as caffeine and aspirin, can affect the health of a fetus. Excessive caffeine has been linked to an increased risk of miscarriage. If a woman uses too much aspirin during pregnancy, bleeding may occur in the fetus.

Antibiotics should also be taken with care during pregnancy. Some antibiotics can cause the fetus to have bone deformities and stained teeth.

Taking drugs illegally before or during pregnancy is the most serious problem because the woman is taking the drug without the knowledge of her physician. Taking illegal drugs causes serious problems for the fetus, in three main ways:

1. Use of illegal drugs before pregnancy can have a lasting effect on either parent's chromosomes. Any changes in the chromosomes will be passed on to the child. The problems that develop will depend on the chromosomes damaged by the drugs.
2. Use of illegal drugs during the early stages of pregnancy can cause damage to developing body parts and systems of the fetus.
3. Use of illegal drugs during the late stages of pregnancy can cause poor physical or mental development.

After birth, the baby may face another problem if the mother used an illegal, addictive drug during the pregnancy. Like the mother, the fetus would have become dependent on the illegal drug. The newborn goes through withdrawal. The effect of this withdrawal can be very serious, especially if the drug used by the pregnant woman was cocaine, a barbiturate, or an opiate.

Thinking Beyond

1. If a child is born physically dependent on an illegal drug, what drug effects might that child experience?
2. How might a woman's use of illegal drugs during pregnancy affect the future of her child?

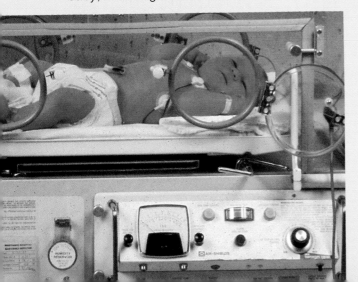

■ Drug use during pregnancy can cause serious problems for a newborn baby, including addiction.

3 Hallucinogens, Cannabis Products, and Inhalants

Some drugs cause changes in the way the drug abuser's brain senses the world. Other drugs can have the effects of both stimulants and depressants. In addition, certain substances that are not drugs can cause dangerous effects like those of drugs.

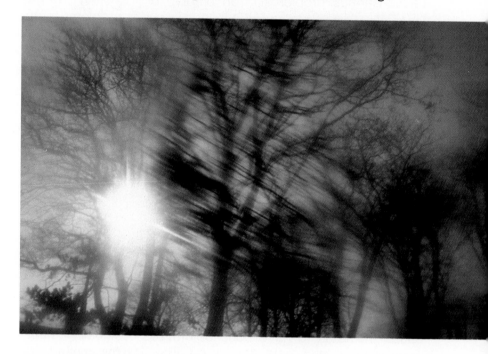

■ *Hallucinogens change the way a person perceives his or her surroundings.*

What Are Hallucinogens?

Some drugs are able to change the way a person perceives the surroundings. Drugs that affect a person's perceptions are called **hallucinogens.** Hallucinogens cause the abuser to experience sights and sounds that seem real but are really only in his or her mind. Colors may seem brighter. Visual images may seem distorted, and things that cannot move by themselves may seem to move.

hallucinogens (huh LOOS uhn uh juhnz), drugs that affect the way a person senses the world.

People who use hallucinogens often have rapid mood changes. One minute, they may feel joy, and the next minute, terror. Sometimes, these rapid mood changes lead to self-destructive behavior. There are several kinds of hallucinogens, but they all change the way the person experiences time, space, and reality.

LSD. The most powerful known hallucinogen is LSD. *LSD* stands for *l*ysergic acid *d*iethylamide. A dose of LSD the size of a grain of sand can have a dangerous effect that lasts for hours.

This illegal drug has caused the death of many people who had terrifying visions while using it. In trying to escape such visions, a person may physically harm himself or herself or die in an accident. LSD also causes depression, brain damage, and birth defects.

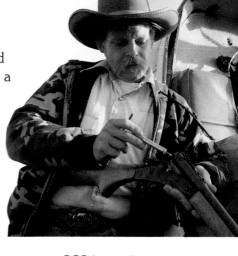

PCP. Another very dangerous hallucinogen is *PCP*. PCP is the drug phencyclidine. This drug is used chiefly as an animal tranquilizer. When used by people, PCP has the unusual quality of causing both depressant and stimulant effects. The effects are different from one person to another. A small amount of the drug may cause an effect similar to intoxication by alcohol. The drug may also cause violent rage, convulsions, memory loss, and even death.

■ *PCP is used as a tranquilizer for some large animals. PCP is too dangerous to be used legally by humans.*

Mescaline and Psilocybin. Unlike LSD and PCP, which are made in laboratories, *mescaline* and *psilocybin* are natural hallucinogens. Mescaline is made from the peyote cactus, and psilocybin comes from a certain kind of mushroom. Both of these drugs are illegal and can cause mood changes that range from joy to terror. There is no way of knowing which effect will occur at any given time.

What Are Cannabis Products?

cannabis (KAN uh buhs), the hemp plant, from which marijuana and hashish are made.

Probably the most often used illegal drugs are cannabis products. Marijuana and hashish are drugs that come from the **cannabis,** or hemp, plant. *Marijuana* is the dried leaves and flowers of the plant. *Hashish* comes from a liquid made by the plant.

Tetrahydrocannabinol (THC) is the active chemical found in cannabis. In small amounts, THC acts first as a stimulant and then as a depressant. In large amounts, THC's effects are

■ *The peyote cactus, left, and the hemp plant, right, contain chemicals that may be abused for their effects on the body.*

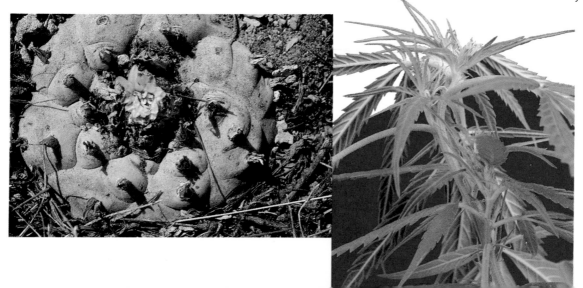

similar to those of hallucinogens. To a person who has taken marijuana or hashish, time may seem to pass very quickly or very slowly. Distances and sizes of objects may appear to be twisted out of shape. People who use marijuana risk harm to themselves because they are not aware of hazards in their environment. Marijuana often makes people feel lazy and unconcerned about what is happening around them. Long-term use of cannabis products can cause loss of memory and lack of motivation. It can also interfere with the person's ability to think.

DRUG ABUSE AND ITS EFFECTS

KINDS OF DRUGS

	Drugs	Possible Immediate Effects	Possible Long-Term Effects/Overdose
Stimulants	Amphetamine Cocaine Crack	increased alertness, increased heart rate and blood pressure, loss of appetite, sleeplessness, dry mouth, irritability, talkativeness, muscle twitching, extreme nervousness, chest pain, anorexia, marked psychological dependence	agitation, increase in body temperature, tremors, delusions, violent behavior, hallucinations, delirium, convulsions, death
Depressants	Alcohol Tranquilizers Barbiturates	slurred speech, flushing, headache, slowed heart rate and breathing, increased reaction time, drunken behavior, impaired coordination, confusion, narrow attention span, faulty judgment, poor memory, nausea, vomiting, respiratory depression, delirium	shallow breathing, cold and clammy skin, dilated pupils, weak and rapid pulse, anxiety and depression, emotional instability, respiratory depression, coma, death
Narcotics	Codeine Morphine Heroin Opium Methadone	drowsiness, watery eyes, constricted pupils, itching, breathing difficulties, nausea, vomiting	slow and shallow breathing, flushing, clammy skin, decreased body temperature, spasticity, hypotension, increased chance of hepatitis, convulsions, coma, death
Hallucinogens	LSD PCP Mescaline Psilocybin	lack of coordination, poor perception of time and distance, anxiety, withdrawn state, panic states, extreme apprehensiveness, hallucinations	persistent psychotic effects, flashbacks, permanent brain damage, death
Cannabis	Marijuana Hashish	disoriented behavior, laziness, poor concentration, increased appetite, distortion of spatial perception, difficulty with depth perception, altered sense of timing, lowered testosterone levels, increased heart rate, panic attack	fatigue, paranoia, lung damage, pulmonary system damage, reproductive cell damage, decrease in growth hormones, hallucinations, psychosis, brain damage, cancer
Inhalants	Paint thinner Model glue Gasoline Correction fluid Freon Aerosol spray	sneezing, coughing, nosebleeds, fatigue, lack of coordination, loss of appetite, headaches, disorientation, confusion, memory loss, nausea, decreased heart and respiratory rates, involuntary passing of urine and feces	bronchial irritation; decreased respirations; drunkenness; stupor; pulmonary congestion and edema; violent behavior; hallucinations; dyspnea; ketosis; hepatitis; permanent damage to brain, kidneys, liver, and bone marrow; death

What Are Inhalants?

There are other chemicals that can be just as dangerous as any drug. Chemicals that form vapors that are inhaled are called **inhalants.**

There are several kinds of inhalants. Freon and aerosol sprays are inhalants that are gases. The most common inhalants are *solvents.* Solvents are liquids that give off fumes. Substances such as paint thinner, model glue, gasoline, and correction fluid are solvents. They all cause serious, druglike effects if their fumes are inhaled. If a person inhales the vapors given off by these chemicals, he or she will experience tingling, dizziness, loss of coordination, and slurring of speech. Continued use will cause permanent damage to the brain, lungs, heart, and other organs. Since the vapors can paralyze the respiratory system, death by suffocation can occur.

inhalants (ihn HAY luhnts), chemicals that have druglike effects if their vapors are inhaled.

■ *Some household products contain chemicals that produce druglike effects if their vapors are inhaled. These vapors can cause permanent damage to the heart, lungs, and brain.*

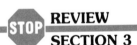

(STOP) **REVIEW**
SECTION 3

REMEMBER?

1. How do hallucinogens affect a person?
2. What are the cannabis products, and how do they affect a person?
3. Why are inhalants so dangerous?

THINK!

4. The effects of LSD often return months or years after the drug has last been used. Why is this particularly dangerous?
5. When you are painting or refinishing furniture, why is it necessary to make sure that fresh air circulates in the room?

4 Refusing Illegal Drugs

Most people do not use illegal drugs. They know that the only responsible decision about illegal drugs is to say no. These people know that the dangers of using illegal drugs are too great to risk. They know that any problems they have will not be solved through the use of these drugs but will, in fact, be made worse. What about people who do use illegal drugs? These people can still say no. However, they will need help in stopping their drug abuse. Then they, too, can say no to any future use of illegal drugs. Their self-esteem, lost through drug abuse, can be regained.

■ *Most people refuse to use illegal drugs.*

REAL-LIFE SKILL

Figuring the High Price of Drug Abuse

Assume that a person is spending $50 a day on an illegal drug. Determine how much money this person is spending on the drug per year. Then obtain catalogs from favorite stores and make a list of the items you could purchase with the yearly amount spent on the drug. Include the prices on the list. Share your results with the class.

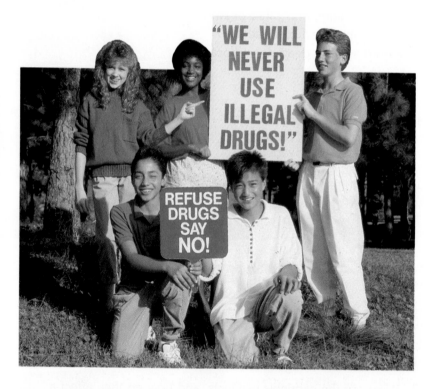

How Can a Person Who Uses Illegal Drugs Get Help?

Whatever their reasons may be, some people do use illegal drugs. Perhaps these people want to be accepted by a certain group. They may have problems they feel they just cannot handle by themselves. Some of these people may not know about the problems drugs can cause. No matter what has caused some people to start using illegal drugs, they need help to stop before they lose control of their lives.

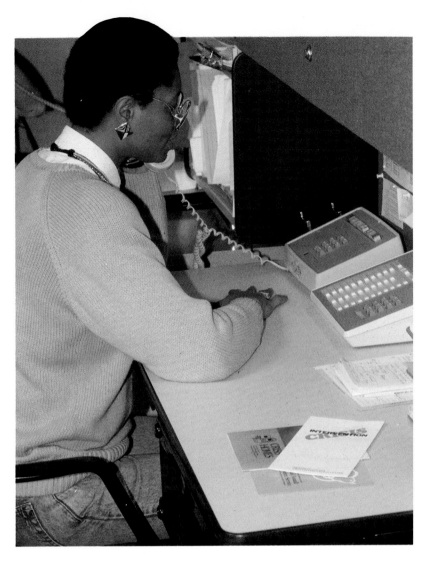

■ *A crisis intervention center provides help to people who have an emergency drug-related problem.*

Intervention and Treatment Centers.   People who use illegal drugs often do not seek help until they are in immediate danger. A person who has overdosed is in danger; so is a person who has mixed different drugs or who is having a severe reaction to a drug.

All these people need help quickly. Hospital emergency rooms have the staff and equipment to give the help that is needed. Also ready for such situations are *crisis intervention centers*. Both emergency rooms and crisis intervention centers have the trained workers and life-support equipment needed to help a drug abuser who is having trouble breathing or whose heartbeat is weak.

When the immediate danger to a patient has passed, he or she is usually sent to a *drug treatment center* for detoxification. **Detoxification** is a process in which a person receives medical care while the body rids itself of a drug. Detoxification is most often carried out over a long time.

detoxification (dee tahk suh fuh KAY shuhn), a process in which a drug user receives medical care while he or she stops using a drug.

263

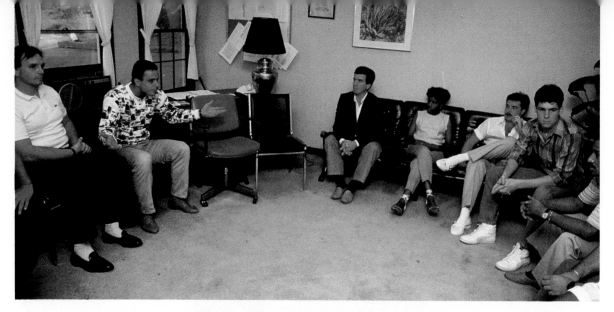

■ *Support groups provide help for people using or even thinking about using drugs.*

Counseling and Therapy Programs. If a person is using illegal drugs, the time to seek help is before he or she is in immediate danger. Help should be sought when a person is thinking about using illegal drugs. Parents and other trusted adults can give advice and help, but other sources of help may be needed. If a person needs advice, he or she can contact any of the following sources.

WHERE TO GO FOR HELP IN REFUSING ILLEGAL DRUGS

Yellow pages	Look in the telephone directory under the heading "Drug Abuse and Addiction Information and Treatment," or under "Counseling."
Hotlines	Most communities have toll-free hotlines that will provide information on counseling. Cocaine users, for example, can call a national 24-hour toll-free number (1-800-COCAINE).
Local hospitals	Hospitals can provide information on local counseling services. Call an emergency room or a hospital information number.
Religious organizations	If these organizations do not provide counseling, staff can direct a person to the proper counseling services.
School guidance counselors	Many school districts provide counseling, or referrals to counselors and support groups, for drug-related problems.

Why Do Most People Never Use Illegal Drugs?

Most young people never use drugs because they want to be in control of their lives. They enjoy their families, friends, school, hobbies, sports, and other interests too much to use drugs. They know that using drugs will interfere with their goals. Most young people see that illegal drugs can cause serious harm to their health. They do not take drugs because of the risk of harming their physical, intellectual, emotional, and social health. They know that taking drugs can damage a person's self-esteem.

■ *Most people do not use drugs, because they want to remain in control of their own lives.*

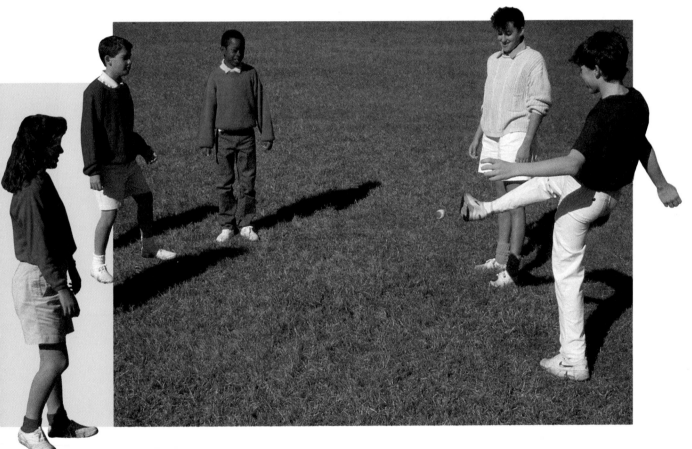

Most young people know that taking illegal drugs is against the law. You have read articles and seen television reports about people caught buying, selling, and abusing drugs. These people face criminal charges that will likely be with them the rest of their lives. Some abusers go to prison or pay fines or both. A criminal record may keep a person from getting a job that he or she wants.

Many young people know about saving money and spending it wisely. Young people who are concerned about this are not going to spend money on drugs. They know that drugs are expensive.

Drug abusers spend money on drugs and then have nothing to show for it. It takes a lot of money to keep buying more and more illegal drugs. Often drug abusers commit crimes to support their dependencies.

Everyone faces problems, some simple to handle and others more difficult. Through examples set by parents and teachers, many young people learn how to handle problems in positive ways. Abusing drugs does not help solve problems. A person

FEDERAL DRUG PENALTIES FOR BUYING AND SELLING MARIJUANA

Quantity	Description	First Offense	Second Offense
1,000 kg or more	Marijuana Mixture containing detectable quantity*	Not less than 10 years, not more than life. If death or serious injury, not less than 20 years, not more than life. Fine not more than $4 million individual, $10 million other than individual.	Not less than 20 years, not more than life. If death or serious injury, not less than life. Fine not more than $8 million individual, $20 million other than individual.
100 kg to 1,000 kg	Marijuana Mixture containing detectable quantity*	Not less than 5 years, not more than 40 years. If death or serious injury, not less than 20 years, not more than life. Fine not more than $2 million individual, $5 million other than individual.	Not less than 10 years, not more than life. If death or serious injury, not less than life. Fine not more than $4 million individual, $10 million other than individual.
50 to 100 kg	Marijuana	Not more than 20 years. If death or serious injury, not less than 20 years, not more than life. Fine $1 million individual, $5 million other than individual.	Not more than 30 years. If death or serious injury, life. Fine $2 million individual, $10 million other than individual.
10 to 100 kg	Hashish		
1 to 100 kg	Hashish Oil		
100 or more plants	Marijuana		
Less than 50 kg	Marijuana	Not more than 5 years. Fine not more than $250,000, $1 million other than individual.	Not more than 10 years. Fine $500,000 individual, $2 million other than individual.
Less than 10 kg	Hashish		
Less than 1 kg	Hashish Oil		

Source: United States Department of Justice, Drug Enforcement Administration, Narcotics Penalties & Enforcement Act of 1986
*Includes hashish and hash oil

266

who abuses drugs may be escaping from a problem and cannot think about positive ways to solve it.

Knowing these facts can prepare you to deal with someone who offers you illegal drugs. No one should pressure you to cause harm to yourself. If you are asked or pressured to take drugs, you can refuse. This is your right. You can walk away from the person making the offer. You may already have a response for refusing drugs. If your response works, keep using it and share it with your friends.

There are specific government regulations and penalties concerning all harmful and illegal drugs. For specific information about these penalties, you can write to the Department of Justice, Drug Enforcement Administration, Washington, DC 20537, or to the appropriate agency in your state.

STOP REVIEW SECTION 4

REMEMBER?

1. How is a crisis intervention center different from a drug treatment center?
2. What are some ways in which a person can get help if he or she is using illegal drugs?

THINK!

3. What are some things you can do to help a friend decide not to use illegal drugs?
4. Why must detoxification usually be combined with counseling and therapy?

Making Wellness Choices

Walter came running up to Janine. He was out of breath and excited. Walter and Janine had been friends since elementary school, and now they had gone to a few dances together. Everybody knew they really liked each other.

"There's going to be a big party at that new kid's house tomorrow night," said Walter. "Everybody has been invited. How about it—do you want to go?"

Janine had to think for a moment. She could not remember who Walter was talking about. Then she remembered. The day before, she had seen that boy giving pills to another student and taking money. She was worried about going to a party where someone might be selling or using drugs.

? What should Janine do? Explain your wellness choice.

267

People in Health

An Interview with a Drug Abuse Counselor

Osceola Wesley helps people with drug problems. He is a counselor at a drug abuse clinic in Coatesville, Pennsylvania.

What is a drug abuse counselor?

A drug abuse counselor is someone who helps people who have drug problems. When people with drug problems go to a drug abuse clinic, they meet with the counselors. The counselors decide what kind of treatment program is best for each person. Drug counselors may talk with people individually, or they may work with small groups.

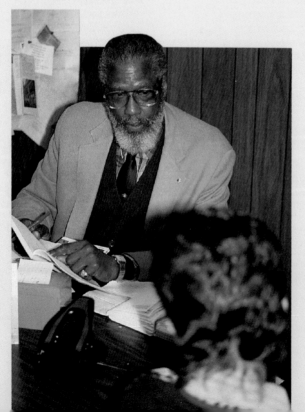
■ *A drug abuse counselor helps people who have drug problems.*

What do you actually do?

I begin by talking over the problem with the individual. I also talk about the person's family life, since we are really dealing with more than just the individual. The whole family is affected when someone has a drug abuse problem.

Do you give safe drugs or medicines to people to help them stop using illegal drugs?

Counselors at this clinic use no drugs or medicines to help people. This is a drug-free program.

Do people volunteer to go to your clinic?

Some come voluntarily. Many are sent to the clinic by their schools or their employers. A lot of people are sent to the clinic by the courts.

How did you become a drug abuse counselor?

I was recovering from my own drug addiction. I had been a heroin addict for many years and had been in jail twice. I entered a drug rehabilitation hospital. The day I entered the hospital, I went off drugs. That was 16 years ago, and I have not had any drugs since. I found I could help other drug abusers because I understood their problems.

What do you tell people about drugs?

I tell them my own story—how I was all messed up. I tell them that I lost half of my stomach because of all that drinking and taking drugs. Taking drugs is abuse—abuse of oneself.

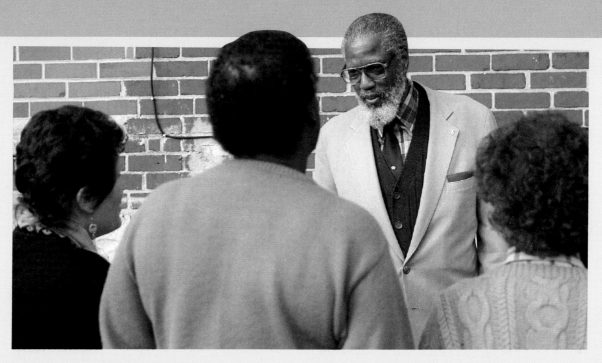

■ *Mr. Wesley and other counselors work with drug abusers and their families.*

Besides the physical damage, do drug abusers face other kinds of problems?

Drug abusers lose their normal feelings for others. Drugs chill emotions. That is the only way drug abusers can live with their guilt for abusing themselves and others. There is another problem. Once a person is a drug abuser, that person is always a slave to drugs. That means that even after a person becomes drug free, the danger of returning to drugs stays forever.

How do you treat teenagers at the clinic?

There is a counselor in this clinic who works especially with teenagers and their families. She goes into junior high schools each day. She also has group sessions here at the clinic. These young people must attend our program for at least 30 days. Their family members come in, and counselors work with them, too. A student cannot return to school until a urine test shows that he or she is drug free.

What are the best and worst parts of your work?

The best part of my job is the hardest part—working with the tough cases. I am given the hardest cases because I was one myself once. I let these people know that I was a loser and helped myself, and that if I could do it, then anyone can do it. What is really hard for me is watching someone self-destruct and knowing that I could help prevent it.

Learn more about drug abuse counselors. Interview a counselor. Or write the National Association of Alcoholism and Drug Abuse Counselors, 3717 Columbia Pike, Suite 300, Arlington, VA 22204.

269

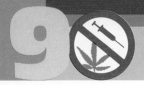

Main Ideas

- Drugs have a wide variety of effects on the human body.

- Drugs can cause a person to injure himself or herself or another person.

- Emotional dependence occurs when a person feels uncomfortable if he or she does not continue experiencing the effects of a drug.

- Physical dependence occurs when a person's body becomes accustomed to the presence of a drug and cannot function without it.

- Families, friends, neighbors, co-workers, classmates, and society in general are all affected by a person's use of illegal drugs.

- Solving problems without using illegal drugs builds self-esteem.

- The only responsible decision about illegal drugs is to refuse them.

Key Words

Write the numbers 1 to 13 in your health notebook or on a separate sheet of paper. After each number, copy the sentence and fill in the missing term. Page numbers in ( ) tell you where to look in the chapter if you need help.

tolerance (245)
emotional depen-
   dence (246)
physical depen-
   dence (246)
withdrawal (246)
stimulants (249)
addiction (250)

depressants (253)
narcotics (254)
opiates (255)
hallucinogens (258)
cannabis (259)
inhalants (261)
detoxification (263)

1. A person with an ___?___ on a drug feels uncomfortable if he or she does not continue to experience the effects of the drug.

2. As a person's ___?___ increases, he or she increases the dose of a drug to continue to feel its original effect.

3. Drugs called ___?___ are made from opium.

4. The body of a person with a ___?___ on a drug has become accustomed to the presence of the drug and cannot function normally without it.

5. An ___?___ is a severe physical dependence.

6. ___?___ of a drug on which a person is physically dependent will result in painful physical reactions.

7. ___?___ are drugs that work by speeding up the functioning of the nervous system.

8. Drugs such as marijuana and hashish come from the ___?___ plant.

9. ___?___ are drugs that slow down the functioning of the nervous system.

10. Drugs that reduce the brain's ability to recognize feelings of pain are ___?___ .

11. Drugs called ___?___ affect a person's perceptions.

12. During ___?___, a person receives expert medical care while the drug is completely eliminated from the body.

13. Spray paints, shellac, paint thinner, and gasoline, which are ___?___, have druglike effects if their vapors are inhaled.

Remembering What You Learned

Page numbers in ( ) tell you where to look in the chapter if you need help.

1. Why do the effects of a drug differ from person to person? (245)

2. What effect does tolerance to a drug have on a person? (245)

3. How are physical dependence and withdrawal symptoms related to each other? (246)

4. Why is an overdose often the direct result of tolerance? (246)

5. What are some stimulants, and how do they affect a person? (249–252)

6. Why is crack such a dangerous drug? (252)

7. What are some depressants, and how do they affect a person? (253)

8. From what substance are many narcotics made? (254)

9. What are some of the dangers of heroin use? (255–256)

10. Where can a person go for help if he or she is using an illegal drug? (262–264)

Thinking About What You Learned

1. Rita is emotionally dependent on a certain drug. Why is it not likely that she will stop using the drug before she becomes physically dependent?

2. How might a legal prescription medicine become an illegal drug?

3. How are the family, social, and economic problems of illegal drug users related?

4. Why is cocaine said to have an "up-and-down" effect?

5. Why do hallucinogens often cause self-destructive behavior?

Writing About What You Learned

1. Contact a local hospital, and arrange an interview with an emergency room physician or other health worker. Conduct an interview that concentrates on the treatments that are used for patients suffering from overdoses. Prepare a report, and present it to the class.

2. Write a short story about a group of friends who are being pressured to experiment with illegal drugs. Describe how each of the friends deals with the problem and makes a positive health decision.

Applying What You Learned

ART

Create a set of advertising posters warning about the dangers of using illegal drugs. Place the posters in your classroom or in other places around your school.

LANGUAGE ARTS

With some of your classmates, prepare and present a debate on the subject of current laws against both the sale and the use of drugs. Are they too strict or not strict enough?

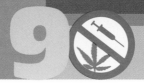

Modified True or False

Write the numbers 1 to 15 in your health notebook or on a separate sheet of paper. After each number, write *true* or *false* to describe the sentence. If the sentence is false, also write a term that replaces the underlined term and makes the sentence true.

1. If a drug user no longer feels the desired effect from the same amount of a drug, he or she has developed <u>tolerance</u>.
2. <u>Emotional</u> dependence occurs when the body cannot function normally without a drug.
3. <u>Stimulants</u> are drugs that speed up the functioning of the nervous system.
4. <u>Heroin</u> is a legal drug.
5. <u>Amphetamines</u> speed up the nervous system.
6. Sniffing <u>cocaine</u> can damage the nasal septum.
7. <u>Depressants</u> are drugs that reduce the brain's ability to recognize pain.
8. <u>Heroin</u> is produced from morphine.
9. Codeine is an <u>opiate</u>.
10. Methadone is used to treat <u>LSD</u> addiction.
11. <u>Mescaline</u> is used chiefly as an animal tranquilizer.
12. <u>Psilocybin</u> is a natural hallucinogen.
13. THC is the active chemical in <u>barbiturates</u>.
14. A <u>solvent</u> is one kind of inhalant.
15. To rid the body of an addictive drug, a person must go through <u>detoxification</u>.

Short Answer

Write the numbers 16 to 23 on your paper. Write a complete sentence to answer each question.

16. Where can a person get help if he or she is using drugs?
17. Why do some people never try drugs?
18. Why can taking cocaine be described as "a death-defying gamble"?
19. What are the dangers faced by a person who uses heroin?
20. What are some social and emotional problems of drug abusers?
21. How is drug abuse an economic problem?
22. How are the effects of stimulants like a "vicious circle"?
23. What are some of the medical uses of barbiturates?

Essay

Write the numbers 24 and 25 on your paper. Write paragraphs with complete sentences to answer each question.

24. Compare and contrast stimulants and depressants.
25. Summarize what you would say to someone who asked whether he or she should try drugs. Be sure to give specific reasons.

Projects to Do

1. Work with a team of classmates to create a bulletin board display that will illustrate the various short-term and long-term effects of using illegal drugs.

2. Work with your classmates to create a scrapbook of drug-related articles cut from newspapers and magazines. Each person should select an article and write a short summary of it. Attach each article to a left-hand page and its summary to the facing, right-hand page. Make the scrapbook available in your classroom

■ *Create a display about the short-term and long-term effects of drug abuse on a person's body.*

3. Arrange for a law-enforcement officer to come to your class and speak about local and state drug laws.

Information to Find

1. Drug treatment centers are found throughout the United States. Write to or call the center nearest you to obtain information on current methods of treating the use of illegal drugs. Share the information with your class in an oral report.

2. The United States Drug Enforcement Administration (DEA) can provide statistics on the use of specific illegal drugs. Select a particular drug you wish to research, and write to the DEA for information. Prepare a report, and present it to your class.

3. Write to your state legislature for information regarding proposed new drug enforcement laws. Make the information available to your class.

Books to Read

Here are some books you can look for in your school library or the public library to find more information about illegal drugs and drug dependence.

Berger, Gilda. *Addiction: Its Causes, Problems, and Treatment.* Franklin Watts.

Hyde, Margaret O. *Mind Drugs.* McGraw-Hill.

Madison, Arnold. *Drugs and You.* Messner.

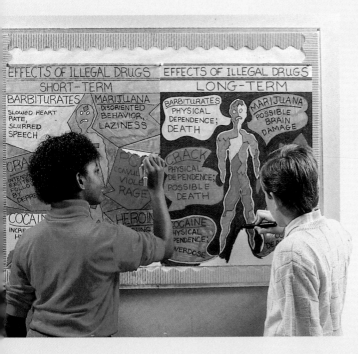

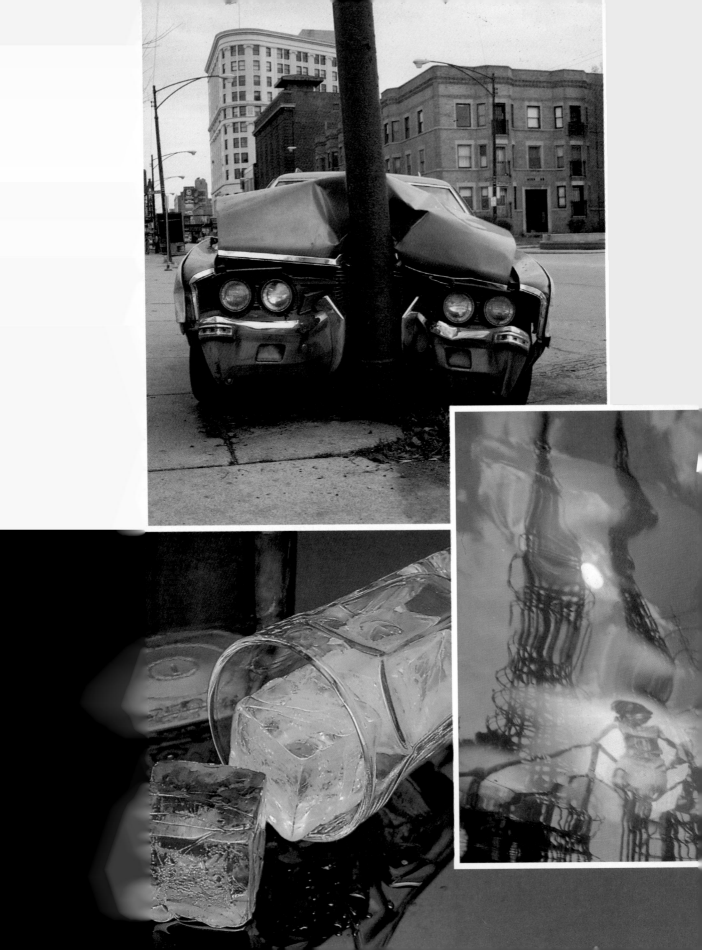

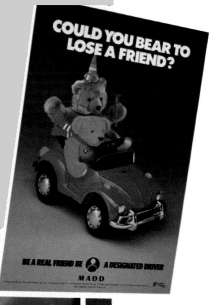

COULD YOU BEAR TO LOSE A FRIEND?

BE A REAL FRIEND BE A DESIGNATED DRIVER
MADD

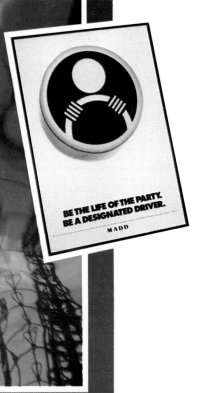

BE THE LIFE OF THE PARTY.
BE A DESIGNATED DRIVER.
MADD

ALCOHOL AND DRINKING

The use of alcohol can be traced all the way back to the Stone Age. In fact, some scientists believe that people began growing grain not to make bread, but to make alcohol.

The effects of this drug can threaten physical health and relationships with others. Nearly 60 percent of all deaths involving motor vehicles in the United States can be connected to alcohol abuse. Crime, illness, and family problems can also be directly tied to the abuse of alcohol. Yet many people do not take the effects of alcohol seriously.

Knowing about the effects of alcohol can help you make a responsible decision not to drink it during your teenage years. The information may also help you understand family members or friends who have alcohol-related problems.

GETTING READY TO LEARN

Key Questions

- Why is it important to learn about the effects of alcohol?
- Why is it important to know how you feel about the use of alcohol?
- How can a person refuse an offer of alcohol?

Main Chapter Sections

1 About Alcohol
2 Physical Effects of Alcohol
3 Social and Emotional Effects of Alcohol Abuse
4 Making Decisions About Alcohol Use

1 About Alcohol

What do you think of when you hear the word *alcohol*? Beer? Wine? Liquor? Would you think of antifreeze, fuel, stains, or dyes? Alcohol can be found in all of these things, as well as in hundreds of other products.

What Are the Different Kinds of Alcohol?

There are several different kinds of alcohol. Some are poisonous. One of these is *methyl alcohol.* It is made from wood materials and is found in paints and wood-finishing products. Another poisonous kind is *isopropyl alcohol,* also known as rubbing alcohol. Isopropyl alcohol is used to disinfect medical equipment and to kill microbes on the skin before medical workers give injections.

The kind of alcohol found in alcoholic beverages is *ethanol.* It is made from grains, fruits, and certain other substances that contain sugar. A chemical process known as **fermentation** changes the sugar into ethanol. Ethanol is a drug that is classified as a depressant.

fermentation
distillation
proof

fermentation (fuhr muhn TAY shuhn), a chemical process in which sugar molecules are broken down and alcohol is produced.

■ *There are several kinds of alcohol, and they have different uses. The alcohol that is consumed in beverages is ethanol.*

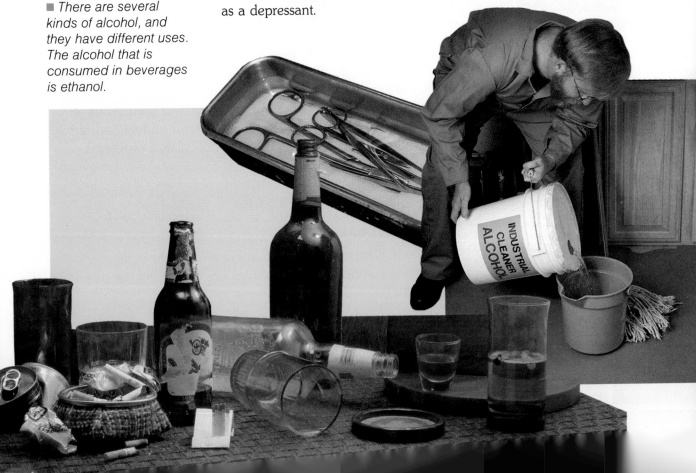

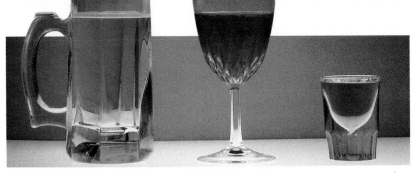

■ *A glass of beer, a small glass of wine, and a shot of liquor all contain about the same amount of alcohol.*

Liquors, which have more alcohol than beer or wine, are made through distillation. **Distillation** is a process in which an alcoholic liquid is boiled and then condensed from its vapor to liquid form again. The condensed, or distilled, liquid has a higher percentage of alcohol because some of the water was lost in the process.

distillation (dihs tuh LAY shuhn), a process in which a liquid is boiled and then its vapor is condensed to a concentrated liquid.

What Is Proof?

Each kind of alcoholic beverage, such as beer, wine, or liquor, has a different amount of ethanol. The amount of ethanol in liquor is given as a number with the word **proof.** The percentage of ethanol in liquor is always equal to one-half of the proof. For example, if a liquor is 100-proof, it is 50 percent ethanol. If it is 80-proof, it is 40 percent ethanol.

The amount of ethanol in wine or beer is stated in percentages. Wines have between 12 and 14 percent ethanol. Beer has between 2 and 6 percent ethanol. For alcoholic beverages made in the United States, a bottle of beer, a glass of wine, and a shot of 80-proof liquor each have about the same amount of ethanol.

proof, a term used to express the amount of alcohol present in a liquor.

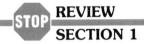 **REVIEW**
SECTION 1

REMEMBER?

1. What are some different kinds of alcohol, and how are they different from one another?

2. How is distillation used to increase the percentage of alcohol in an alcoholic beverage?

THINK!

3. Which has a greater amount of alcohol—a drink that is 85-proof or one that has 45 percent alcohol? Explain your answer.

4. Denatured alcohol is ethanol that has had methyl alcohol added to it. Why would it be dangerous, even fatal, to drink denatured alcohol?

2 Physical Effects of Alcohol

KEY WORDS

intoxicated
hangover
alcoholism

Imagine a group of scientists studying the effects of vinegar on the human body. After thousands of experiments, the results of the study cannot be denied by anyone. The continuous use of vinegar in large amounts will cause brain damage, heart disease, diseases of the liver and kidneys, emotional and physical dependence, and death at an early age. As a result, lawmakers pass laws making it illegal for anyone under the age of 21 to purchase or use vinegar, and physicians strongly recommend that adults limit their use of it.

What would you think about a teenager who continued to use vinegar? What would you think about an adult who continued to use large amounts of vinegar? Now substitute the word *alcohol* for the word *vinegar*. Ask yourself why some people keep using large amounts of alcohol when they know how their health will be affected. Are these people making responsible decisions?

What Are the Immediate Effects of Using Alcohol?

When a person drinks an alcoholic beverage, the alcohol is very quickly absorbed through the wall of the stomach. It enters the circulatory system. Once the alcohol is in the circulatory system, it is quickly carried to every part of the person's body.

The first part of the body affected by alcohol is the brain. Alcohol is a depressant drug. It slows nerve activity in the parts of the brain that control how a person feels and acts. As a person drinks more alcohol, more parts of the brain are affected and reflexes are slowed. The person's vision may blur. He or she may lose control over muscles and have trouble talking and walking. Alcohol also may irritate the stomach and small intestine.

The ways in which alcohol affects a person depend on how much of it is circulating in the blood. The amount of alcohol in the blood is called *blood alcohol concentration,* or BAC. The BAC is often expressed as the percentage of alcohol in the blood.

BAC is affected by the following:

- how much the person drinks
- how fast the person drinks
- the physical condition of the person

Body size and weight also influence BAC. A large person has more body mass and blood than a small person. Young people most often have smaller bodies than do adults. They can feel

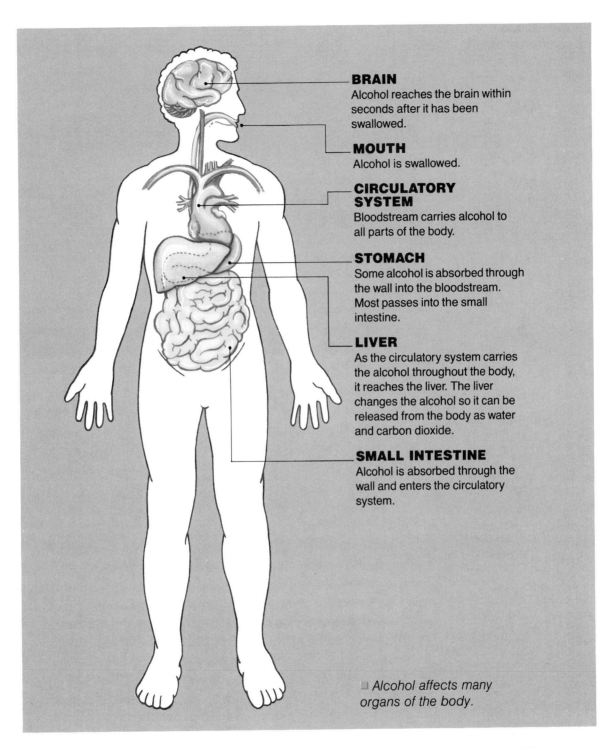

BRAIN
Alcohol reaches the brain within seconds after it has been swallowed.

MOUTH
Alcohol is swallowed.

CIRCULATORY SYSTEM
Bloodstream carries alcohol to all parts of the body.

STOMACH
Some alcohol is absorbed through the wall into the bloodstream. Most passes into the small intestine.

LIVER
As the circulatory system carries the alcohol throughout the body, it reaches the liver. The liver changes the alcohol so it can be released from the body as water and carbon dioxide.

SMALL INTESTINE
Alcohol is absorbed through the wall and enters the circulatory system.

▢ *Alcohol affects many organs of the body.*

rapid and severe changes by drinking even a small amount of alcohol.

When a person's BAC reaches a level that causes him or her to lose control over mental or physical abilities, the person is **intoxicated.** If BAC becomes high enough to cause the person

intoxicated (ihn TAHK suh kayt uhd), a condition in which a person lacks control over mental or physical abilities as a result of high BAC.

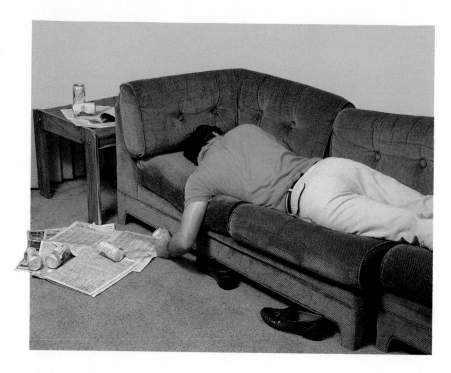

■ *A person who drinks too much alcohol may become intoxicated and pass out.*

hangover, the illness a person feels as the body rids itself of alcohol.

to be intoxicated, he or she will be likely to get a hangover later. A **hangover** is the illness the person feels as the body rids itself of alcohol. The symptoms of this illness can be nausea, vomiting, physical weakness, headache, rapid heart rate, nervousness, and inability to concentrate. A hangover is relieved only by time, as the body recovers from the effects of the alcohol.

What Are the Long-term Effects of Abusing Alcohol?

When people abuse alcohol for many months or years, they face many serious problems. These long-term effects of alcohol abuse are serious threats to a person's wellness. Problem drinking can become alcoholism. **Alcoholism** is the emotional and physical dependence on alcohol. A person who is dependent on alcohol is called an *alcoholic*. Alcoholics more often have a poor self-concept and often have lost confidence in their abilities.

alcoholism (AL kuh haw lihz uhm), the emotional and physical dependence on alcohol.

There is debate as to what causes alcoholism. Two chief causes are accepted. Some research has shown that a tendency for alcoholism may be inherited. Other research seems to show that alcoholism comes from a person's early development in a family or certain culture group. Some researchers feel that the causes may be factors of both heredity and environment.

As with any other drug, people who have a physical dependence on alcohol will experience withdrawal symptoms if they cannot get it. The withdrawal symptoms may be an inability to sleep, nervousness, rapid heart rate, and high blood pressure.

EFFECTS OF INCREASING BLOOD ALCOHOL LEVELS

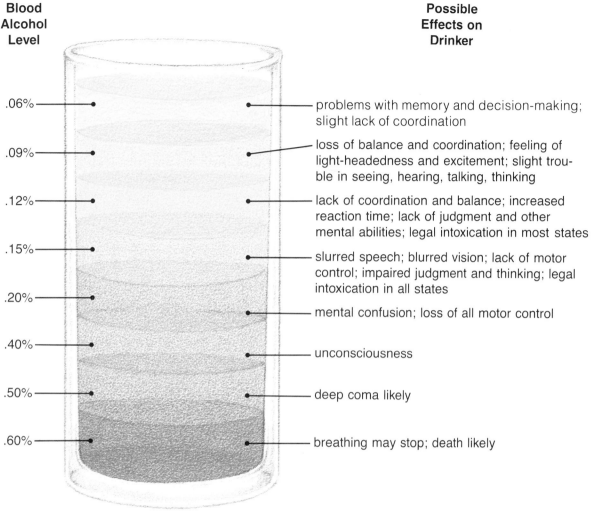

Blood Alcohol Level	Possible Effects on Drinker
.06%	problems with memory and decision-making; slight lack of coordination
.09%	loss of balance and coordination; feeling of light-headedness and excitement; slight trouble in seeing, hearing, talking, thinking
.12%	lack of coordination and balance; increased reaction time; lack of judgment and other mental abilities; legal intoxication in most states
.15%	slurred speech; blurred vision; lack of motor control; impaired judgment and thinking; legal intoxication in all states
.20%	mental confusion; loss of all motor control
.40%	unconsciousness
.50%	deep coma likely
.60%	breathing may stop; death likely

Source: National Highway Traffic Safety Administration

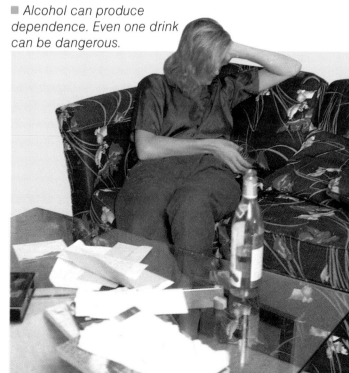

■ *Alcohol can produce dependence. Even one drink can be dangerous.*

Withdrawal can cause a person to feel confused and to see things that are not there. In some cases, very sudden withdrawal can cause death.

Along with alcoholism, there are many other health problems that can be directly related to long-term alcohol abuse. These problems affect different parts of the body.

Liver Damage.   When a person drinks alcohol, the liver must break it down and remove it from the body. If large amounts of alcohol pass through the liver over many years, damage in the form of scar tissue occurs. Then the liver is not able to function properly. This damage to the liver leads to a disease called *cirrhosis*. Cirrhosis is the leading cause of death among alcoholics.

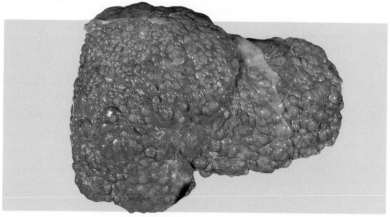

■ *Years of drinking large amounts of alcohol can cause cirrhosis, a liver disease.*

Cancer.   The heavy, repeated use of alcohol over many years can damage the lining of the stomach and of the mouth. This damage can lead to stomach cancer or mouth cancer or both. Women who use alcohol may also have a greater risk of getting breast cancer than women who do not use alcohol.

Brain and Heart Damage.   Long-term alcohol abuse can damage brain cells. This damage can cause loss of memory, trembling hands, and jerky movements of the head. If a person not only abuses alcohol but also smokes cigarettes, the alcohol increases the risk of getting heart disease.

■ *The cells of a healthy brain, left, can be damaged, right, by long-term alcohol abuse.*

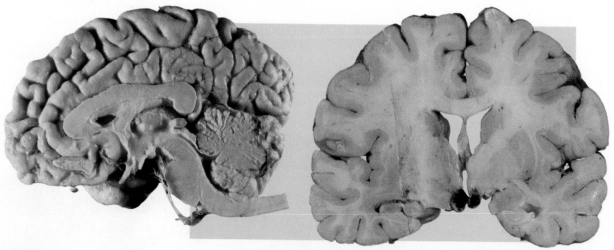

Fetal Alcohol Syndrome.   Women who drink alcohol during pregnancy may give birth to babies with *fetal alcohol syndrome*. These babies have physical and mental problems because the alcohol their mothers drank interfered with their development. This syndrome is totally preventable if pregnant women do not drink alcohol.

Malnutrition.   Alcoholics sometimes have no desire to eat. Many have malnutrition and vitamin-B deficiency. The alcohol may also irritate the digestive system so much that food cannot be absorbed properly.

STOP **REVIEW**
SECTION 2

REMEMBER?

1. List four factors that can influence the effect of alcohol on a person.
2. What are some of the immediate effects of alcohol abuse?
3. Describe four serious health problems that come from long-term alcohol abuse.

THINK!

4. If a person has a close relative who is an alcoholic, why might it be a good idea for that person not to drink alcohol?
5. Why is operating a motor vehicle after drinking alcohol an example of a negative risk-taking behavior?

Making Wellness Choices

On a very cold day in November, Bob and Jennifer went to a football game at the high school. They were both wearing heavy winter coats and were wrapped in blankets. But they were still very cold. In a short time, their hands and feet felt numb. About then, a man in front of them turned around and offered Bob a bottle of brandy. The man told Bob that the brandy would make them warmer. Bob held the bottle and looked at Jennifer as if to ask what they should do.

 What should Jennifer do? Explain your wellness choice.

3 Social and Emotional Effects of Alcohol Abuse

Dan is worried about his older sister. Over the past few months, he has noticed that she is not home very often. When she is home, she is either fighting with everyone or staying away from everyone. Her grades have dropped, and last week she was fired from her part-time job for always being late. Dan has also noticed that she seems confused and he often smells alcohol on her breath. He has become very anxious about her.

What Problems Does Alcohol Abuse Cause for Other People?

A person who abuses alcohol is hurting not only himself or herself. People who abuse alcohol may eventually have problems in their relationships with family members, friends, and people with whom they work. In many cases, alcohol abuse has caused the breakup of families and the loss of friendships.

School-related and work-related problems can often be tied to alcohol abuse. A person who abuses alcohol does not function

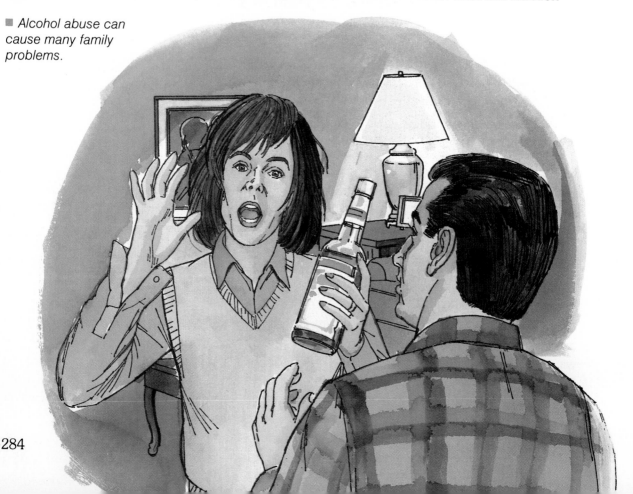

■ Alcohol abuse can cause many family problems.

284

efficiently and often misses school or work. When the person does go to school or work, he or she is often late. A person who abuses alcohol is likely to drop out of school or lose a job.

The problems of alcohol abuse extend to family members. Family members have to deal with the person who is abusing alcohol. Children in such families are sometimes physically or emotionally abused. Often these children are not given the attention or love that all people need. They do not have high self-esteem or the opportunity to express their feelings or satisfy their needs.

What Are Some Alcohol-Related Community Problems?

One of the biggest, yet most preventable, safety problems in the United States is that of people drinking alcoholic beverages and driving. Nearly 60 percent of all motor vehicle accidents involve a driver who has been drinking alcohol. In fact, the most common cause of death among teenagers is motor vehicle accidents involving alcohol. Many teenagers who have motor vehicle accidents have been drinking and driving, or riding with a driver who has been drinking.

Every year, alcohol abuse causes the loss of billions of dollars in the United States. The loss includes property damage from crimes and accidents as well as income lost due to family breakups and unemployment. Billions of dollars more are spent each year to pay for medical treatments, hospital costs, and police work relating to alcohol abuse.

Because of these social and economic problems, states set a legal minimum age at which a person may buy or drink alcohol. Some communities choose not to allow the sale of any alcoholic beverages to adults within city or county limits.

■ *A person suspected of driving while intoxicated is often given a breath test to determine his or her fitness to drive.*

How Can Alcohol-Related Problems Be Prevented and Treated?

Most communities have clinics, counseling services, and support groups to help people who abuse alcohol and people who are affected by abusers. Ask your principal or counselor to have someone from one of these groups talk to classes about alcoholism. Ask the visitor to leave posters with phone numbers students can call if they need to talk.

285

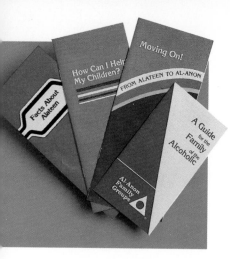

■ *Several organizations provide help for alcoholics and their families and friends.*

Alcoholics Anonymous.   Formed in 1935, Alcoholics Anonymous (AA) has chapters in most communities. AA holds regular meetings that are open to anyone with a present or past drinking problem. At these meetings, alcoholics help one another by talking about why they abused alcohol, how AA is helping them, and what they can do to help themselves.

Al-Anon.   Al-Anon is a part of Alcoholics Anonymous. It helps the families and friends of alcoholics. Al-Anon holds meetings to help these people learn to handle problems that occur in relationships with alcoholics.

Alateen.   Formed in 1957, Alateen helps the teenage children of alcoholics. At the meetings, teenagers help one another deal with their parents' drinking problems. Alateen helps young people realize that they did not cause their parents' alcoholism. Alateen also helps them accept the fact that they cannot control or cure their parents' problems.

Children of Alcoholics.   Formed in the early 1980s, this organization helps people who have grown up in homes with alcoholics. The group most often counsels adults. However, in some communities, Children of Alcoholics has meetings for children and teenagers who are still living at home.

Student Assistance Program.   This program was formed to identify and help students who are abusing alcohol. Schools that sponsor this program require these students to receive counseling, instead of expelling them from school for drinking. The program requires that family members receive counseling.

REAL-LIFE
SKILL

Gathering Information

You may want to learn how you can join a SADD program. Contact SADD at P.O. Box 800, Marlboro, MA 01752, 508-481-3568 for more information.

Students Against Driving Drunk (SADD).   In 1985, SADD started a special program for junior high school and middle school students. This program, which is called "I'm Special Because I'm Me," is also known as Students Against Doing Drugs. It gives information about harmful substances to parents and teenagers.

Parents and teenagers sign a contract with each other to learn as much as possible about the effects of harmful substances. The contract states that a teenager will discuss concerns about peer pressure with his or her parents. The teenager will also seek advice and guidance from his or her parents if faced with a situation in which harmful substances are being used.

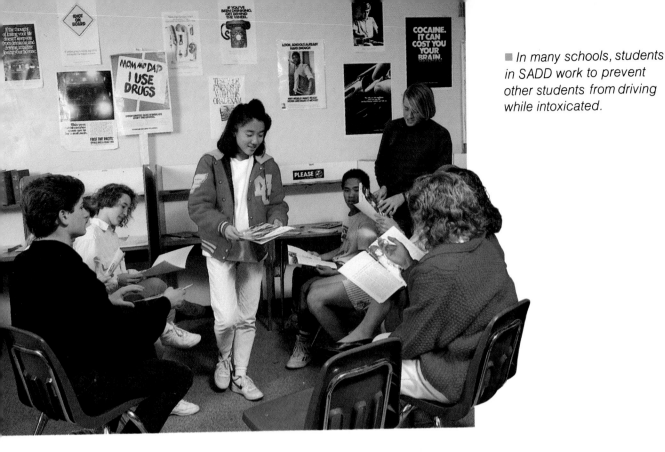

■ In many schools, students in SADD work to prevent other students from driving while intoxicated.

In turn, parents agree to be available for advice and communication. If your school does not have a chapter of SADD, you may want to start one with the help of a parent or other adults.

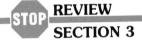 **REVIEW**
SECTION 3

REMEMBER?

1. What are two effects that alcohol abuse can have on a person and his or her family?
2. How does Alcoholics Anonymous help alcoholics?
3. How does a Student Assistance Program help stop alcohol abuse in schools?

THINK!

4. How could people have a chance to prevent as many as 60 percent of all motor-vehicle accidents?
5. What kinds of treatment are available in your community for people with drinking problems?

287

Health Close-up

Driving Under the Influence of Alcohol

To reduce driving under the influence of alcohol, the United States Congress voted to give extra highway-safety funds to states that passed strict drinking-and-driving laws. Many states passed such laws, which included tough penalties. After the laws went into effect, the number of highway accidents involving alcohol declined a lot.

However, strict enforcement of the new laws did not continue. The number of highway accidents involving alcohol increased again. As public awareness of the problem grew, groups such as Mothers Against Drunk Driving (MADD) and Remove Intoxicated Drivers (RID) were formed. These groups have pressured government officials for strict enforcement of laws and for even tougher ones.

Stiff penalties in the laws have stopped many people from driving when they have been drinking, and highway accidents have decreased. Because the laws have been successful, lawmakers have favored them.

In the future, new technologies will help law-enforcement authorities keep drinking drivers off the roads. One device in cars will sense alcohol on the breath of the driver and lock the ignition. Computers in restaurants and bars will determine whether a customer is intoxicated; then he or she could be prevented from driving.

Thinking Beyond

1. How might groups such as MADD and RID help educate people about the dangers of alcohol abuse?
2. How would a law against driving with an open container of an alcoholic beverage help prevent intoxicated driving?

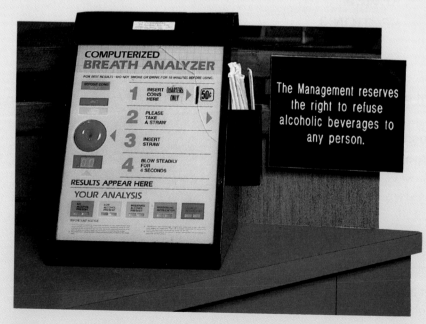

■ Places that serve alcohol must be careful not to sell drinks to intoxicated persons.

4 Making Decisions About Alcohol Use

You make many decisions every day. Most of the decisions you make are responsible and made after careful thought. However, if you are like most people, some of your decisions may not have been carefully thought out. Your actions may not have been as responsible as they could have been.

Many of the decisions you make are not critical ones. If you decide to wear a shirt that does not go with your slacks, you may just look a little odd. However, in certain other cases, your life and the lives of others can depend upon your making the right decision. Decisions about the use of alcohol are critical ones.

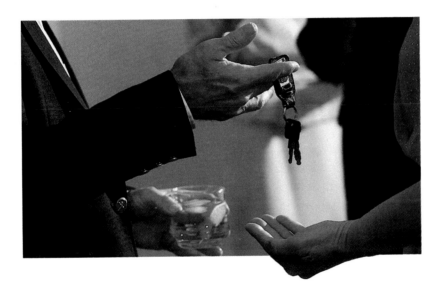

■ *If a person has been drinking, deciding not to drive shows responsibility.*

What Are Some Steps Toward Responsible Decision Making?

You know that it is dangerous to ride in a car driven by anyone who has been drinking alcohol. How would you handle the situation if a close relative who had been drinking offered you a ride? This situation requires that you make a responsible decision. The following five steps can be helpful:

1. Realize that a problem exists and that a decision is required.
2. Decide what choices can be made to solve the problem. You can choose to ride, or you can choose not to ride.
3. Consider all the positive and negative results, or consequences, of each choice. If you ride with your relative, you are putting yourself in a dangerous situation.

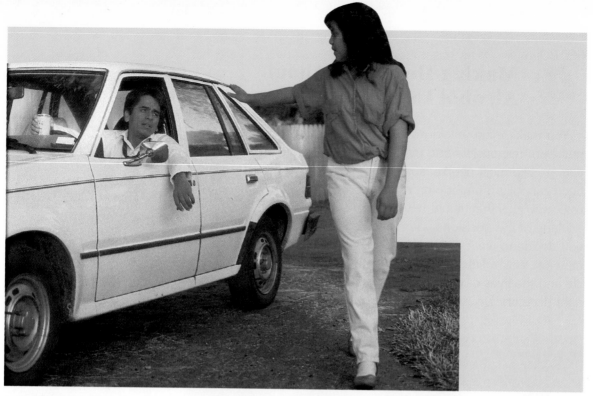

■ *Deciding not to get a ride from someone who has been drinking shows you are responsible for your own health and well-being.*

If you choose not to ride, your relative may be angry with you. Also, you may have to walk if you cannot find another ride.

4. Choose what you will do, and take action. What would be your responsible decision?

5. Evaluate your decision. Discuss your decision with a parent or another trusted adult.

How Can You Refuse Alcohol?

Have you ever found yourself in a situation where you did not want to do something because you knew it was not right? Perhaps someone was trying to influence you to do it. There are several ways you can handle this kind of pressure. Knowing what you can do before you are faced with the problem can help you say no.

- If someone wants you to do something that you do not want to do, you can say "No" or "No, thank you." You can be polite, but convincing.
- If you find that the pressure continues after you have said "No," you can respond by saying you have something else to do. You might even ask the person pressuring you how he or she would feel about being pressured to do something.
- You can change the subject.

- You can walk away from the person who is pressuring you.

Making a responsible decision about alcohol use when you are being pressured can be very hard to do. However, carefully thinking about what might happen if you do not make a responsible decision will help you resist the pressure. People will respect you for taking charge of your own health.

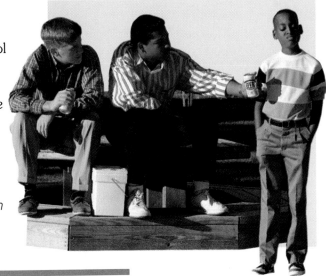

■ *If someone offers you something that will harm you, say no, and walk away.*

STOP REVIEW SECTION 4

REMEMBER?

1. List the five steps for making a responsible decision.
2. What are some actions you can take if you are pressured to drink alcohol?

THINK!

3. You are about to accept a ride with someone when you discover that he or she has been drinking. What would you do?
4. How can you help someone else make a responsible decision about alcohol use?

Thinking About Your Health

Can You Make a Responsible Decision?

At the top of a sheet of paper, write the title "I Can Make a Responsible Decision." On the left, write "Problem." Underneath, write two or three problems you would like to solve. On the right, use the five steps for problem solving to decide on a solution for each of your problems. Discuss your decisions with a parent or another trusted adult, and keep this paper in a safe place. You can check yourself from time to time.

291

People in Health

An Interview with a State Trooper

Marlene Carroll-Auerbach understands the dangers of drinking alcohol and driving. She is a state trooper with the Wisconsin State Patrol in Iowa County, Wisconsin.

What does a state trooper do?

A state trooper enforces state traffic laws. Most of the time, a state trooper is on the road doing just that. An important part of a state trooper's work is testing drivers suspected of DWI, OMVI, OWI, or DUI.

What do the abbreviations *DWI, OMVI, OWI,* and *DUI* mean?

They all refer to drunk driving. *DWI* stands for *driving while intoxicated; OMVI* stands for *operating a motor vehicle while intoxicated, OWI* stands for *operating while intoxicated;* and *DUI* stands for *driving under the influence.* Different states use different terms, but they all mean the same thing. Wisconsin uses the abbreviation *OWI.*

When do you test a driver for OWI?

I test a driver for OWI only after I have stopped him or her for breaking a traffic law. This might be driving through a red light or not using headlights at night. If, while I am talking to the driver, I suspect that he or she has been drinking, I give the tests. I might suspect drinking if I smell alcohol on the person's breath or if I see a bottle or can from an alcoholic beverage in the car.

What do you do when you suspect a driver has been drinking?

I have the driver get out of the car to do field tests. I keep detailed records of the results for my report, which goes to a judge.

What are some examples of field tests?

For one test, the driver stands on one leg, arms at his or her sides, and counts to 30. A person who is intoxicated will have trouble counting and standing. In another test, the

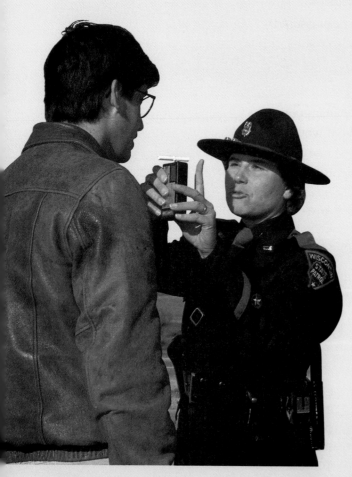

■ *State troopers stop and test persons suspected of driving while intoxicated.*

292

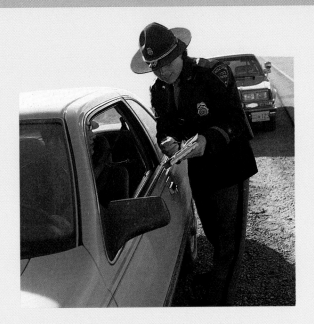

■ *Intoxicated motorists are subject to arrest in most states.*

person walks heel to toe for nine steps. At the end of the nine steps, he or she turns on one foot and walks back nine steps. Most people who are intoxicated cannot turn on one foot.

If people fail the field tests, do you arrest them?

After giving the person all the field tests, I often give him or her a breath test. The driver blows air into a tube. A connected meter shows how much alcohol is in the person's breath. If the breath test shows a high level of alcohol, I can arrest the person. I can also arrest a person whose breath test shows a low level of alcohol if he or she did poorly in the field tests.

What happens when you arrest a driver?

I put handcuffs on the person and put him or her into my car. I may search the driver's car for evidence of drinking. Then I take the person to the trooper station for another, more scientific breath test on a machine called the Intoxilizer 5000. This machine uses a computer and is very accurate.

Does the arrested driver go to jail?

Each state has its own laws about drunk driving and jail. In Wisconsin, if a person has been arrested for the first time, he or she may be allowed to go home with an adult relative or friend who has not been drinking. If there is no one who can take the driver home or if the person is from out of state, then even the first-time offender goes to jail. After 12 hours, the driver must take another breath test. He or she will not be released until the breath alcohol content is safe.

What if the driver is a teenager?

Each state has its own laws for under-age drinkers. In Wisconsin, drivers under the legal drinking age are not allowed to have any alcohol on their breath. They can be arrested even if they are not legally intoxicated. The law was written to show young people the serious consequences of drinking and driving.

Learn more about the work of state troopers in your state. Contact your state Highway Patrol office and interview a state trooper. Or write for information to the National Trooper's Coalition, 222 N. Verlinden Avenue, Lansing, MI 48915.

Main Ideas

- There are different kinds of alcohol.

- The rate at which alcohol is absorbed into the blood depends upon body size and weight, how much food is in the stomach, the physical condition of the person, how fast the person drinks, and how much the person drinks.

- When the alcohol level in the blood is high, a person loses control over mental and physical abilities.

- Abuse of alcohol over a long time causes health problems including malnutrition, liver disease, brain and heart damage, an increased risk of cancer, and fetal alcohol syndrome.

- A person with an alcohol-related problem can get help from community clinics and groups such as Alcoholics Anonymous, Alateen, Al-Anon, and Children of Alcoholics.

- There are steps a person can take to make good decisions. Following these steps can help you find ways to handle pressures on you to drink alcohol.

Key Words

Write the numbers 1 to 6 in your health notebook or on a separate sheet of paper. After each number, copy the sentence and fill in the missing term. Page numbers in ( ) tell you where to look in the chapter if you need help.

fermentation (276)   intoxicated (279)
distillation (277)   hangover (280)
proof (277)   alcoholism (280)

1. The number given as the ___?___ of a liquor is twice the percentage of alcohol in the liquor.

2. ___?___ is a chemical process in which sugar molecules are broken down and alcohol is produced.

3. A process called ___?___ increases alcohol content by boiling and condensing a liquid so that some water is lost.

4. A condition in which a person has a dependence on alcohol is ___?___ .

5. When a person's BAC causes a loss of control over mental and physical abilities, the person is ___?___ .

6. The illness a person feels as the body rids itself of alcohol is called a ___?___ .

Remembering What You Learned

Page numbers in ( ) tell you where to look in the chapter if you need help.

1. Explain the differences among isopropyl alcohol, methyl alcohol, and ethanol. (276)

2. Why are beer, wine, and liquor equally harmful? (277)

3. What factors can affect the blood alcohol concentration in a person's body? (278)

4. What are some of the immediate effects of drinking alcohol? (278)

5. How can you tell that a person has a hangover? (280)

6 What are two possible causes of alcoholism? (280)

7. What are some serious long-term effects of alcohol abuse? (280–283)

8. What are some emotional and social problems related to alcohol abuse? (284–285)

9. What are some sources of help for people who abuse alcohol? (285)

10. Where can family members and friends of those with alcohol problems go for help? (286)

11. List the five steps of the decision-making process. (289–290)

Thinking About What You Learned

1. Why is it dangerous for a person to become intoxicated?

2. If someone in a family abuses alcohol, how might other family members recognize the problem? What can they do about it?

3. How can student groups tackle the problem of alcohol abuse among their peers? In what ways might they be more effective than adults?

4. You have realized that your best friend has been missing a lot of school recently and that his grades have been slipping. On weekends, all he wants to do is go to parties with a group of young people who use alcohol. Describe what you think his problem is and how you could help.

5. Recently, four teenagers were killed in an automobile accident. When police investigated, they found empty beer bottles in the car. What can young people do to prevent accidents involving alcohol from happening to them?

Writing About What You Learned

1. You have been asked to give a speech to a younger class on how alcohol affects the body. Write a two-page speech on this topic. Include information on the different kinds of alcohol, the forms of alcoholic beverages, how alcohol affects a person, and the damage long-term alcohol abuse can cause to various parts of the body.

2. Write a story related to the use of alcohol, demonstrating the use of the five steps for making a responsible decision.

3. Make a list of things you might say to someone to stop him or her from pressuring you to drink alcohol.

Applying What You Learned

SOCIAL STUDIES

Research the figures on teenage alcohol abuse during the 1950s, 1960s, 1970s, and 1980s. Prepare a report on your findings, and present it to the class.

MATHEMATICS

Determine how much money is spent in one year by a person who drinks a case of 24 bottles of beer a week. Make a list of other items that a person might purchase with that money to make his or her life more enjoyable.

Modified True or False

Write the numbers 1 to 15 in your health notebook or on a separate sheet of paper. After each number, write *true* or *false* to describe the sentence. If the sentence is false, also write a term that replaces the underlined term and makes the sentence true.

1. Alcoholic beverages contain <u>methyl alcohol</u>.

2. <u>Distillation</u> is a process that changes sugar into ethanol.

3. Alcohol is a <u>depressant</u>.

4. Liquor contains <u>more</u> alcohol than beer.

5. Liquor that is 80-proof is <u>20</u> percent ethanol.

6. The first part of the body affected by alcohol is the <u>liver</u>.

7. <u>Alcoholism</u> is the emotional and <u>physical</u> dependence on alcohol.

8. Many alcoholics suffer from <u>malnutrition</u>.

9. One of the biggest problems related to alcohol abuse is <u>theft</u>.

10. <u>Al-Anon</u> is a group open to anyone with a drinking problem.

11. A person who has a high BAC is <u>intoxicated</u>.

12. Nausea, vomiting, and headache are symptoms of a <u>hangover</u>.

13. Alcohol is quickly absorbed through the <u>lungs</u>.

14. BAC is affected by how <u>fast</u> the person drinks.

15. Alcoholics usually have <u>positive</u> self-concepts.

Short Answer

Write the numbers 16 to 23 on your paper. Write a complete sentence to answer each question.

16. How does distillation affect the alcohol content of liquor?

17. What does the proof figure tell you about a liquor?

18. What are the short-term effects of drinking alcohol?

19. What are three things that affect BAC?

20. How is body size related to the effect of alcohol?

21. How does alcohol damage the liver?

22. How can a pregnant woman make sure her child will not be born with fetal alcohol syndrome?

23. How does an alcoholic's problem affect his or her family?

Essay

Write the numbers 24 and 25 on your paper. Write paragraphs with complete sentences to answer each question.

24. What are some of the organizations dedicated to dealing with alcohol problems? What does each organization do?

25. How can practicing the skills of responsible decision making help you say no to drugs more easily?

ACTIVITIES FOR HOME OR SCHOOL

Projects to Do

1. Collect advertisements for alcoholic beverages, and paste each on a sheet of paper. Below each advertisement, write a short paragraph that answers these questions: What are the people in the advertisement doing as they are drinking? How do they appear to feel? Do these activities and feelings really depend on the use of alcohol? How do you know this?

2. Make a poster about the dangers of alcohol abuse. On the poster, draw or paste pictures that show the effects that alcohol has on the body. Ask permission to display your poster at school or at home.

3. Work with a small group to write a short skit for younger students about how alcohol abuse harms people's health and safety. Ask your teacher to arrange for your group to visit one or more elementary classes and perform the skit.

■ *Help younger students learn about the effects of alcohol.*

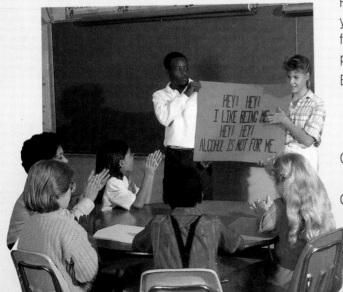

Information to Find

1. Telephone a local alcohol treatment clinic. Ask what programs it has for alcoholics and for families and children of alcoholics. Through your library or your community telephone book, find out what other groups offer help to alcoholics and their families. Prepare a written or an oral report describing the programs that are available.

2. Call your local AA group. Ask if it would be possible to interview a group member. Ask this person why he or she began drinking, how the person recognized the problem, and what treatment he or she has received. Invite the person to your class to speak.

3. Write to the National Clearinghouse for Alcohol Information, P.O. Box 2345, Rockville, MD 20847-2345. Ask for free information concerning teenage drinking and the teenage children of alcoholics.

Books to Read

Here are some books you can look for in your school library or the public library to find more information about alcohol and problems caused by alcohol.

Buxbaum, Ann, and Gilda Gussin. *Alcohol and Other Drugs: Using Skills to Make Tough Choices.* Management Sciences for Health.

Claypool, Jane. *Alcohol and You.* Franklin Watts.

Goodwin, Donald. *Alcoholism: The Facts.* Oxford University Press.

297

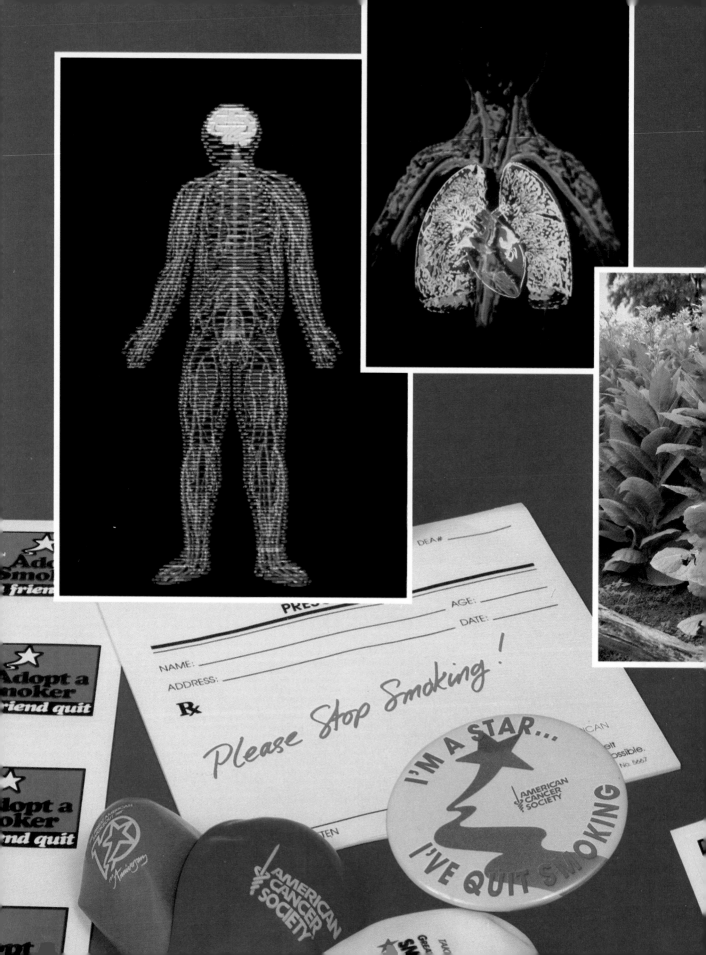

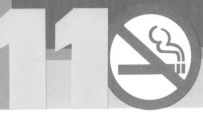

DANGERS OF TOBACCO USE

It is hard to believe that anyone would knowingly harm his or her own health. Yet every day, millions of people do just that. They use tobacco products despite overwhelming evidence that the use of these products can cause serious health problems.

Refusing harmful substances, such as tobacco, is an important skill. Unfortunately, it is not always an easy skill to learn or to apply. The pressure to use tobacco products or any other harmful substances can be extremely hard to resist. However, an understanding of the dangers can make refusing easier.

GETTING READY TO LEARN

Key Questions

- Why is it important to learn about the harmful effects of tobacco?
- Why is it important to know how you and your family feel about the use of tobacco?
- How can you resist the pressure to use tobacco?
- How can you take responsibility for your health regarding the use of tobacco?

Main Chapter Sections

1 About Smoking
2 Long-term Effects of Tobacco Use
3 Deciding Not to Use Tobacco

SECTION

1 About Smoking

KEY WORDS

tar
nicotine
carbon monoxide
ammonia
formaldehyde
arsenic
cyanide

When asked what three sentences of advice he would give to teenagers, a physician said, "Do not smoke. Do not smoke. Do not smoke."

Physicians have long believed that smoking cigarettes is harmful. In the last 30 years, studies have revealed the following facts about smoking:

- Cigarette smoking is a leading cause of lung cancer.
- There is a link between cigarette smoking and heart disease.
- Smokers with cancer or heart disease are more likely to die from these diseases than nonsmokers.
- Smokers suffer more chronic respiratory diseases and other health problems than nonsmokers.
- A pregnant woman who smokes can injure her fetus and cause her baby to be underweight at birth, a serious threat to survival.

■ *As surgeon general of the United States, C. Everett Koop was active in making people aware of the connection between cigarette smoking and health problems.*

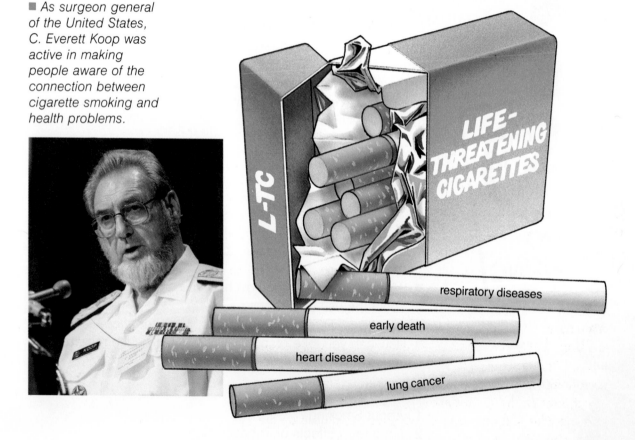

300

What Are the Harmful Substances in Tobacco Smoke?

More than 1,200 different substances have been found in tobacco smoke. Most of these substances are gases and particles of solid matter. Three of these substances are thought to be very harmful to health.

Tar. Tobacco contains tiny bits of solid matter that form **tar,** a sticky brown substance. You can see tar as a yellow-brown stain on the filters of burning cigarettes. Inside the body, tar causes problems. It builds up inside the respiratory system of smokers. It sticks to their bronchial tubes and lungs. It also sticks to their teeth. The teeth of people who smoke are often stained yellow from tar.

tar, a sticky brown substance that is produced when tobacco is burned.

■ Tar from cigarettes discolors teeth, builds up inside the respiratory system, and affects the heart and blood vessels. Another substance in cigarettes is nicotine, a highly addictive stimulant.

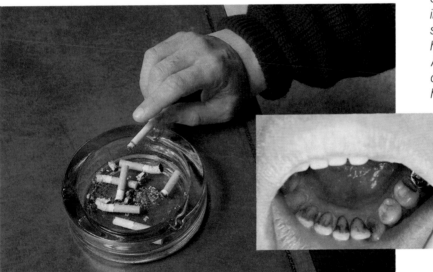

Tar is made up of several chemicals that can harm many parts of the body. Some of these chemicals affect the heart and blood vessels. Others damage lung tissue and other parts of the respiratory system. Some of the chemicals in tar are the primary causes of cancer in smokers.

Nicotine. Another substance in tobacco is nicotine. **Nicotine** is a drug that is classified as a stimulant. When tobacco smoke is inhaled, the nicotine in it causes all blood vessels in the body to narrow. Since the heart has to pump harder and faster to get blood through the narrow blood vessels, the smoker's blood pressure rises. Chronic high blood pressure, caused by the nicotine in tobacco smoke, can cause heart disease.

nicotine (NIHK uh teen), a drug that is classified as a stimulant.

When a person starts smoking, he or she quickly forms an emotional dependence on the nicotine. If the person continues to smoke, tolerance grows and addiction forms.

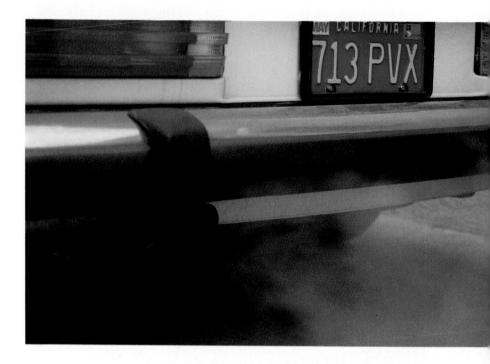

■ *Cigarette smoke contains carbon monoxide, the same poisonous gas found in automobile exhaust.*

carbon monoxide (KAHR buhn • muh NAHK syd), a poisonous gas that combines easily with red blood cells.

ammonia (uh MOH nyuh), a substance commonly used in household cleaners.

formaldehyde (fawr MAL duh hyd), a substance used as a disinfectant and as a preservative.

arsenic (AHRS nihk), a strong poison used in weed killers and insecticides.

cyanide (SY uh nyd), a deadly poison that causes severe respiratory problems.

Carbon Monoxide. Also present in cigarette smoke is carbon monoxide. **Carbon monoxide** is a poisonous gas that combines easily with red blood cells. When cigarette smoke enters the lungs, many of the red blood cells pick up carbon monoxide instead of oxygen. As a result, there is less oxygen available for use by the body's cells. To get enough oxygen, the person has to breathe harder. The heart also has to beat faster to pump enough oxygen to the body's cells. As a result, smokers often feel tired and out of breath.

Other Harmful Substances. Along with tar, nicotine, and carbon monoxide, tobacco smoke has a number of other harmful substances in it. Among these are ammonia, formaldehyde, arsenic, and cyanide. **Ammonia** is a substance commonly used in household cleaners. When tobacco smoke is inhaled, the ammonia in it irritates the nasal passages. **Formaldehyde** is a colorless poison that is used as a disinfectant and as a preservative. **Arsenic** is a strong poison that is used in weed killers and insecticides. **Cyanide** is a deadly poison that causes severe respiratory problems.

How Does Tobacco Smoke Affect Smokers?

You may think it takes years of smoking to cause changes in the health of a smoker. In fact, smoking even one cigarette has an effect on the body. Smoking one cigarette causes the heart rate to increase and the blood vessels to narrow. Because of this narrowing, the surface skin temperature drops, especially in the fingers and toes. The lining of the nose, mouth, and throat becomes irritated, and the smoker may experience a headache, dizziness, or an upset stomach.

Smoking cigarettes also affects a smoker's appearance. Smoking one cigarette causes bad breath and bloodshot eyes, and it makes clothes and hair smell of smoke. Smoking one cigarette makes a home stuffy and smelly. Cigarettes ashes make it look dirty.

Smoking can also create a fire hazard. If the smoker is not careful, he or she may burn holes in furniture and clothes or set fire to the home. Smoking in bed is a major cause of home fires.

■ *Smoking in a car can be especially unpleasant because of the small space. Smoking can be a fire hazard if someone falls asleep while smoking.*

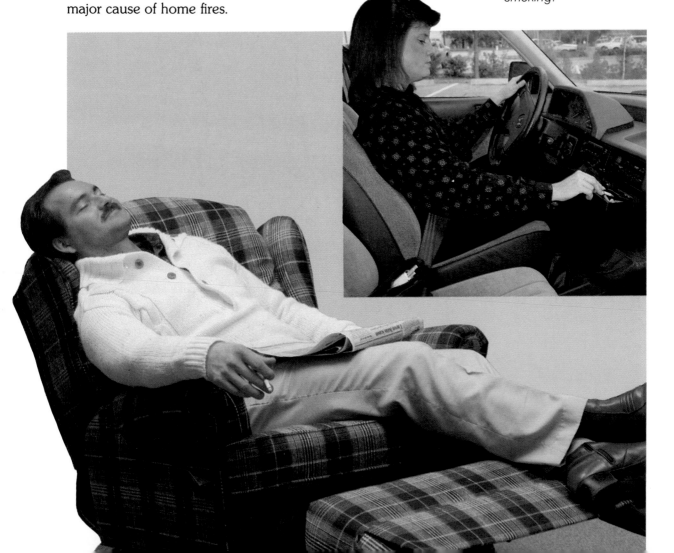

How Does Tobacco Smoke Affect Nonsmokers?

Researchers have discovered that the smoke from another person's cigarette, pipe, or cigar can threaten the health of nonsmokers. For example, this smoke can set off asthma attacks and can cause headaches, coughing, sneezing, and watery eyes. It can also add to the chance of a nonsmoker getting a respiratory illness.

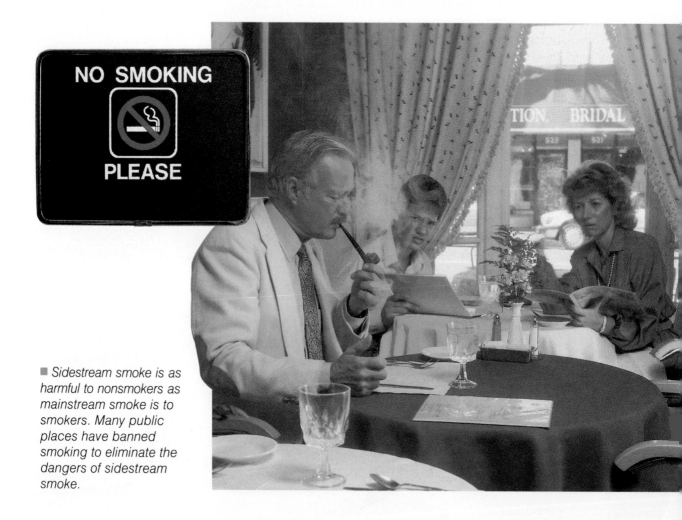

■ Sidestream smoke is as harmful to nonsmokers as mainstream smoke is to smokers. Many public places have banned smoking to eliminate the dangers of sidestream smoke.

Smoke from burning tobacco that goes directly into the air is called *sidestream smoke*. Studies show that sidestream smoke has five times as much carbon monoxide as the smoke inhaled by a smoker. It also contains a high percentage of other harmful substances. Smoke inhaled and exhaled by a smoker, which is called *mainstream smoke,* also can harm a nonsmoker. Mainstream smoke contains high levels of all the harmful substances inhaled by a smoker.

To protect nonsmokers from the dangers of tobacco smoke, many states and communities have passed laws to restrict smoking in public places. Restaurants, hotels, and airlines have set aside no-smoking areas or have banned smoking totally. Organizations of nonsmokers work to protect the rights of nonsmokers to breathe clean air.

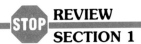

REVIEW
SECTION 1

REMEMBER?

1. What three substances in tobacco smoke are particularly harmful to a person's wellness?
2. What are four other substances that are found in tobacco smoke?
3. What are two ways in which tobacco smoke affects smokers and nonsmokers?

THINK!

4. Why do smokers experience withdrawal symptoms when they stop smoking?
5. Why would the tobacco industry want to say that smokers have a right to smoke wherever they choose?

Making Wellness Choices

Rick and Bob are at a campaign strategy meeting for the upcoming class elections. They are part of a committee that has been organized to support Devon in his campaign for class president. During the meeting, which is being held in a small room, two other members of the committee begin to smoke cigarettes. These two people seem to light one cigarette after another for about an hour. Soon the room is filled with a blue haze. Rick and Bob feel as if their eyes are filled with sand. Their throats are burning, and their chests ache.

 What should the boys do? Explain your wellness choice.

2 Long-term Effects of Tobacco Use

In the early 1960s, the surgeon general of the United States issued a report titled *Smoking and Health*. The report presented a great deal of information linking cigarette smoking with health problems such as lung cancer and heart disease. In 1964, the United States Congress passed a law requiring that all packages of cigarettes carry the following warning.

CAUTION: Cigarette Smoking May Be Hazardous to Your Health.

As a result of further studies, all cigarette packages must now carry one of the following warnings:

- Smoking Causes Lung Cancer, Heart Disease, Emphysema, and May Complicate Pregnancy.

- Quitting Smoking Now Greatly Reduces Serious Risks to Your Health.

- Smoking by Pregnant Women May Result in Fetal Injury, Premature Birth, and Low Birth Weight.

- Cigarette Smoke Contains Carbon Monoxide.

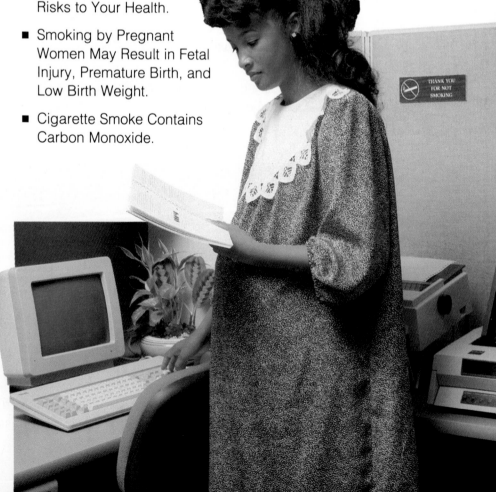

■ *Pregnant women need to avoid cigarette smoke. It can cause problems for unborn babies.*

Scientists have discovered that the dangers increase with each cigarette smoked. As tolerance increases, addiction develops, and the person smokes more cigarettes. People who smoke know that people die from diseases caused by smoking every year. However, they find quitting their habit very hard.

How Does Smoking Damage the Circulatory System?

Cigarette smoking has a harmful effect on the heart and blood vessels. Nicotine narrows the blood vessels and makes the heart beat faster and the blood pressure rise. Carbon monoxide reduces the supply of oxygen in the blood and makes the heart work harder to get oxygen to the body's cells. Over time, the heart can be permanently damaged.

Smoking can also cause other kinds of damage. When blood vessels leading to the heart muscle are narrowed, the heart itself may not get enough oxygen. As a result, smokers have a much greater risk of suffering heart attacks than do nonsmokers.

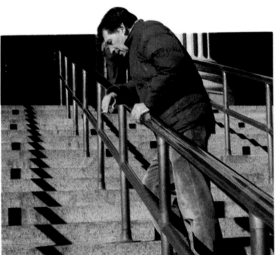

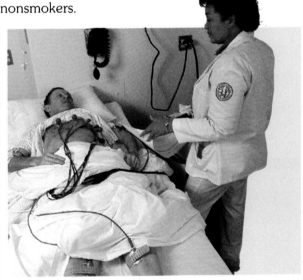

■ The carbon monoxide in cigarette smoke makes the heart work harder to supply body cells with oxygen, left. Smokers have a higher risk of suffering heart attacks than do nonsmokers, right.

Smoking can also increase the effects of other diseases of the circulatory system. One example is atherosclerosis, a disease in which cholesterol and fat deposits build up on the inner walls of arteries. Smoking narrows the arteries further, putting an even greater strain on the heart. Again, if the condition affects the blood vessels of the heart, a heart attack may result.

Smokers are also more likely to have blood clots form than are nonsmokers. If a blood clot forms in an artery leading to the heart, it may cause a fatal heart attack. If a clot forms in an artery leading to the brain, it may cause a stroke. Strokes can cause temporary or permanent paralysis and even death.

How Does Smoking Damage the Respiratory System?

Since tobacco smoke is inhaled, its greatest damage is to the respiratory system. Continued damage to the respiratory system often leads to chronic respiratory diseases.

One sign of disease is sometimes called *smoker's cough.* Smoker's cough is the result of damage done by certain chemicals in tar to the cilia in the bronchial tubes. When the cilia are damaged, they are no longer able to sweep harmful matter and mucus away from the lungs. These materials remain in the bronchial tubes and settle into the lungs due to gravity. The only way to move them out of the lungs and bronchial tubes is by frequent coughing.

Smoker's cough can irritate the bronchial tubes, making them raw and sensitive. The irritation causes the bronchial tubes to produce more mucus, which makes the coughing even worse. It may also cause the bronchial tubes to swell. Constant swelling and overproduction of mucus in the bronchial tubes, or chronic bronchitis, can last for many years. If smoking continues, the condition becomes worse. Chronic bronchitis makes breathing very difficult and can lead to more serious diseases by lowering a person's resistance.

■ *Smoking can lead to chronic coughs, right, from lung diseases such as emphysema, left.*

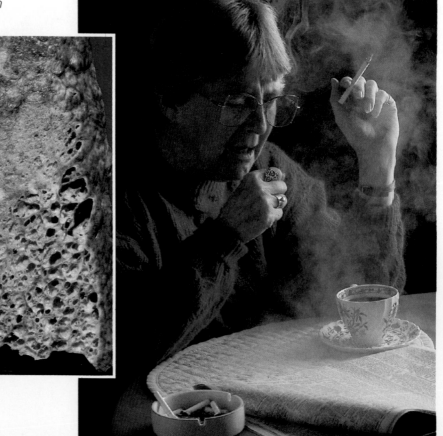

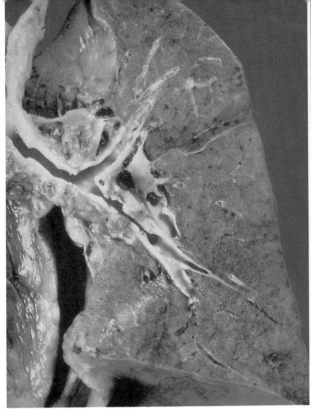
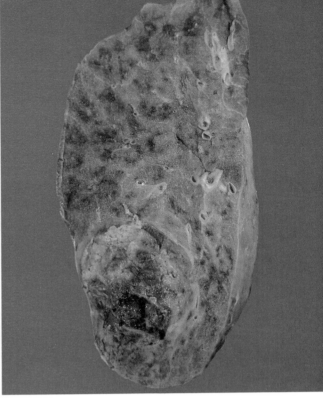

■ *The damage in a lung of a smoker, right, is easy to see when compared with a lung of a nonsmoker, left.*

One lung disease that is often caused by cigarette smoking is emphysema. Emphysema begins when mucus blocks the breathing tubes and traps air in the alveoli. The walls of the alveoli tear, scar tissue forms, and the tiny alveoli become large sacs. As a result, there are fewer surfaces in the lungs through which oxygen can pass into blood. Because people with emphysema have less oxygen in their bodies, they tire easily. Even mild physical activity may be difficult for them.

There is no cure for emphysema. Once the air sacs tear, they cannot be repaired. Although other factors, such as air pollution, can also cause emphysema, it is most often related to smoking cigarettes.

Cigarette smoking is also the major cause of lung cancer. Certain chemicals in tar may cause normal cells in the respiratory system to become cancer cells. Cancer cells multiply rapidly, crowd out normal cells, and destroy normal lung tissue. When lung tissue is destroyed, the body cannot get the oxygen it needs.

Cigarette smokers are many times more likely to develop lung cancer than are nonsmokers. The more cigarettes a person smokes each day, the greater his or her chance of developing lung cancer. People who begin smoking as teenagers are even more likely to develop lung cancer than are people who start smoking later in life.

MYTH AND FACT

Myth: Smoking a pipe or cigar instead of cigarettes reduces the risk of lung cancer.

Fact: People who have switched from cigarettes to pipes or cigars may continue to inhale the tobacco smoke from habit. The greater strength of this smoke actually increases the risk.

What Other Health Problems Are Caused by Smoking?

Cigarette smoking causes still other problems. Smokers are more likely than nonsmokers to get cancer of the mouth, larynx, and esophagus. Cancers of the bladder and kidneys are also more common among smokers than among nonsmokers.

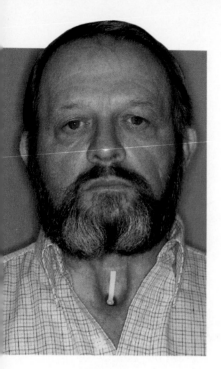

■ Cancer of the throat may result from cigarette smoking.

■ Cigarette smoking may cause several different kinds of cancer.

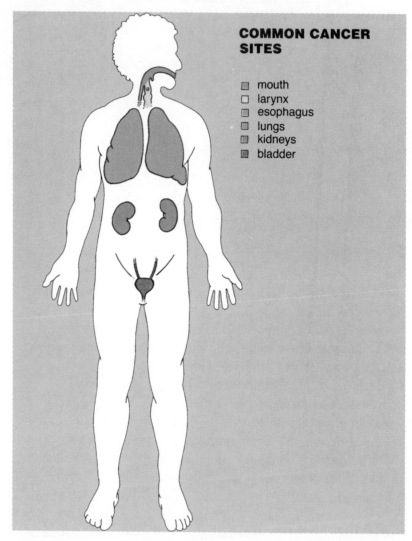

COMMON CANCER SITES

- ▨ mouth
- ▢ larynx
- ▨ esophagus
- ▨ lungs
- ▨ kidneys
- ▨ bladder

Studies show that a pregnant woman who smokes can harm the health and development of the embryo and fetus. Substances in the cigarette smoke are passed from the woman to the fetus. Because smoking causes blood vessels in the mother and fetus to narrow, the fetus may not get enough nutrients and oxygen to develop as it should. Children born to women who smoke tend to weigh less at birth than children of nonsmoking women. The smokers' children are also more likely to be born dead or to die soon after birth than nonsmokers' children.

What Are the Dangers of Using Smokeless Tobacco?

Not all tobacco is smoked. Some is used as smokeless tobacco. **Smokeless tobacco** is chewed, held in the mouth for a while, or sniffed. Some people have been misled into believing that smokeless tobacco is safe to use because smoke is not inhaled. There are, in fact, no safe tobacco products.

Smokeless tobacco is manufactured in the form of *chewing tobacco* or *snuff*. Some people use these forms by putting a small amount between the lower lip and gum or between the cheek and gum. Saliva mixes with the smokeless tobacco and the user must either swallow or spit out the juice. From the moistened smokeless tobacco, nicotine and other dangerous chemicals enter the blood through the tissues in the mouth.

Some people use snuff by sniffing it into their nostrils. When the tobacco enters the nose, it comes in contact with the moist tissues inside. The nicotine and other chemicals enter the circulatory system through these tissues.

smokeless tobacco
(SMOH kluhs • tuh BAK oh), tobacco that is chewed, held in the mouth for a while, or sniffed.

■ *Snuff and chewing tobacco are types of smokeless tobacco. They can discolor teeth and can cause sores in the mouth that become cancerous.*

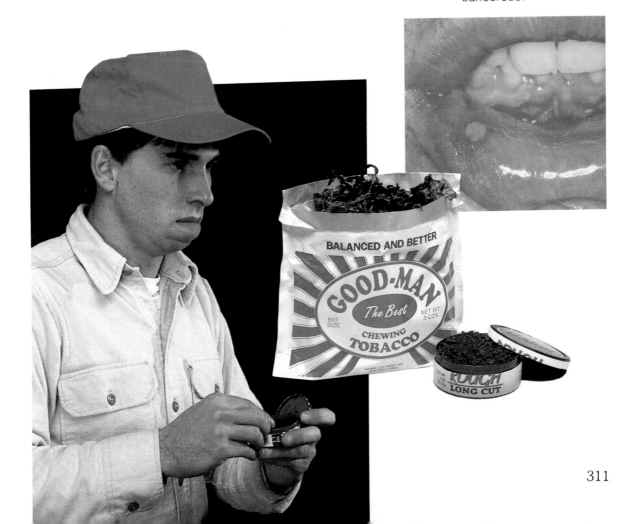

As with smoking tobacco, there are many hazards with the use of smokeless tobacco. The nicotine in smokeless tobacco has the same harmful effects as tobacco that is smoked. However, people who use smokeless tobacco also face other hazards.

People who use this kind of tobacco risk developing cancer of the gums, tongue, throat, and jaw. The tobacco juice often causes sores in the mouth, and people who swallow it may have problems with their digestive organs. Sniffing or chewing smokeless tobacco usually dulls the senses of smell and taste. The tobacco causes people to develop bad breath. It also has small amounts of sugar, which contributes to tooth decay, gum disease, and loss of teeth.

Because of the dangers of smokeless tobacco, tobacco companies are now required by law to print one of the following warnings on smokeless tobacco products:

- This Product May Cause Mouth Cancer.

- This Product May Cause Gum Disease and Tooth Loss.

- This Product Is Not a Safe Alternative to Cigarettes.

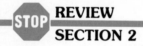

REVIEW

SECTION 2

REMEMBER?

1. What are the specific hazards of tobacco use that are mentioned on tobacco packages?

2. How does the use of tobacco affect the circulatory system?

3. In what ways does smoking affect the respiratory system?

THINK!

4. Why should smokeless tobacco not be considered less dangerous than tobacco that is smoked?

5. If a woman who smokes becomes pregnant, how can she protect the development of the fetus?

Health Close-up

Tobacco Advertising

What causes a person to begin using tobacco? One of the answers often given to that question is advertising. Newspapers, magazines, and billboards all provide manufacturers with the means of advertising their products. Some advertisements are for products that can help make your life easier or more enjoyable. Some of the things you see advertised, however, can be harmful, as is the case with tobacco products.

Although advertisements for tobacco products are banned from television and radio, manufacturers continue to use other advertising sources. Seldom can you go through a magazine or newspaper without finding at least one advertisement for a tobacco product. In addition, highways have many billboards advertising tobacco products.

How are these products portrayed? The advertisements usually show happy, healthy, young people using the tobacco products in exciting situations, so that tobacco use seems glamorous. The advertisements never show the disease and death that can come from tobacco use.

How people react to the advertisements is important. The manufacturers want to make money, so they use advertisements to convince people to buy their products. However, an understanding of the dangers of using tobacco can help you withstand the pressures of advertising. Notice that each tobacco advertisement contains one of the surgeon general's warnings. You have a responsibility to yourself to analyze these advertisements and withstand the pressures they try to exert on you.

■ *Tobacco advertising often shows exciting activities or beautiful scenery to make smoking look attractive.*

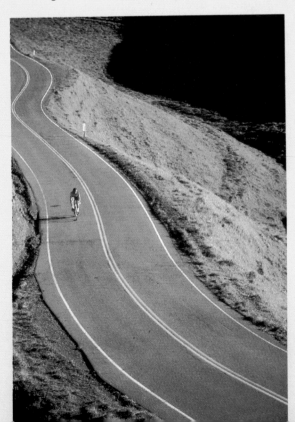

Thinking Beyond

1. Why, do you think, have advertisements for tobacco products been banned from television and radio?
2. What are some ways in which you might overcome pressures exerted on you by tobacco advertisements?

3 Deciding Not to Use Tobacco

The total number of people who use tobacco is declining in the United States, yet cigarette smoking among teenagers continues to increase. Most teenagers do not realize how quickly they can become dependent on nicotine. Drug dependence, they think, is something that happens to other people, not to them.

The physical dependence, or addiction, to nicotine is very hard to break. The longer a person uses tobacco, the harder it is to stop. Many people who try to stop using tobacco are able to succeed only with great difficulty. A decision not to start using tobacco is much easier to stick with than a decision to stop using tobacco.

Why Do Some People Start Using Tobacco?

Despite the fact that the dangers of tobacco use are well known, some people still begin to smoke or to use smokeless tobacco. In surveys, people give several reasons when they are asked why they started to use tobacco.

- They wanted to go along with friends who smoked.
- They wanted to look and feel more grown-up.
- Their parents or older brothers or sisters used tobacco.
- Advertisements had suggested that people who use tobacco were attractive and mature.
- They wanted to show their independence from those who had told them not to use tobacco.
- They felt they could always quit later.
- They wanted to satisfy their curiosity.

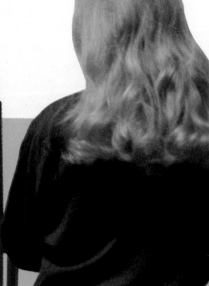

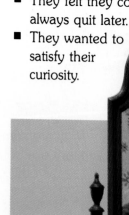

■ *Some people think they look attractive or more mature if they smoke.*

Considering the dangers involved in using tobacco and the difficulty of giving it up, what do you think of these reasons?

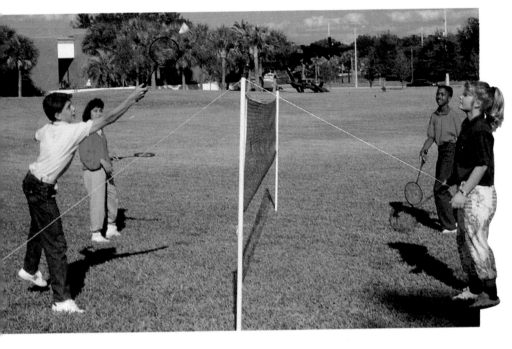

■ *Most people do not smoke. They know that staying away from harmful substances helps keep them healthy.*

Why Do Most People Decide Not to Use Tobacco?

There are actually fewer people smoking today than there were 10 or 20 years ago. Why have many people made the responsible decision not to use tobacco products? Just as people give many reasons for using tobacco, people also give many reasons for not using tobacco.

- They know that staying away from harmful substances helps them enjoy good health.
- They believe that they do not have to do what other people are doing. Instead, they make their own decisions.
- They believe that the use of tobacco makes them less attractive.
- They know that it is against the law for anyone under the age of 16 to purchase tobacco products in most places in the United States.
- They believe that smoking is a fire hazard.
- They believe that tobacco products are a waste of money.
- They believe that smoke, ashes, and cigarette butts bother other people.
- They believe that the use of tobacco will cause serious disease.
- They know that sidestream and mainstream smoke can be harmful to others.

315

How Can You Refuse an Offer to Use Tobacco?

You have a right and a responsibility to refuse to do anything that can harm you. By refusing to use tobacco, you make a responsible decision to stay healthy and safe. Your refusal may make the person offering the tobacco product uncomfortable or angry at first. However, your concern must be for your own health and well-being, not for the person's feelings.

When you are offered tobacco, there are several ways to refuse. These methods can be used to refuse any substance that presents a risk to your health and life.

- If someone asks you to try a cigarette, say, "No, thank you." If the person keeps asking you, say "No!" in a firm and convincing manner.
- Tell the person offering the tobacco that you have something else to do. You can tell the person you are going to visit friends, or play some sport, or work on a hobby. Then leave.
- Knowing the facts about tobacco can help you say no. If someone asks you to try a tobacco product, you can say, "No, thanks. Tobacco use causes too many problems."
- Another way to say no to tobacco is to change the subject. For example, if someone offers you tobacco or any other harmful substance, say, "No, thanks" and then suggest that the two of you do something else.
- Sometimes the pressure from peers to try tobacco can become strong. If, after all your efforts to refuse, the person continues to pressure you, the best thing to do is walk away.

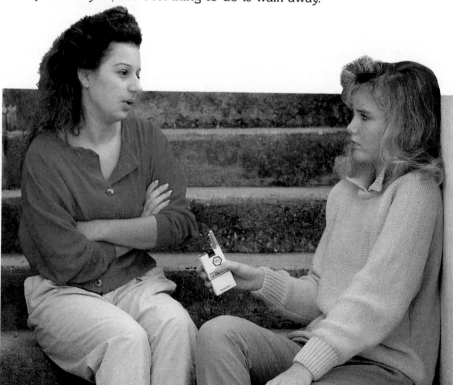

■ If someone offers you a cigarette, say no.

316

Refusing something that can harm you is a responsible health decision. You demonstrate your self-confidence, and you show responsibility for your own health. Knowing that you can follow through on your decision not to use tobacco can make you feel good about yourself. People will respect you for taking charge of your own health.

STOP REVIEW
SECTION 3

REMEMBER?

1. What are some reasons people give for using tobacco? How do you feel about these reasons?
2. What are some reasons people give for not using tobacco? How do you feel about these reasons?
3. How might you go about refusing to use tobacco?

THINK!

4. What kinds of pressure might cause a person to quit using tobacco?
5. How might someone turn the pressure to use tobacco against the person making the offer?

Thinking About Your Health

Are You Prepared to Say No to Smoking?

Listed below are five health effects of smoking.

- shortness of breath
- frequent coughing
- bad breath
- tiredness
- yellow-stained teeth and fingers from nicotine and tar

For each effect, think of a refusal statement that you could use when someone pressures you to smoke. For example, you might say, "No, thanks; I don't want to be short of breath when I get on the basketball court." Be creative. Write each refusal statement on an index card. Practice saying each statement until you feel comfortable enough to use it if necessary.

317

People in Health

An Interview with a Stop-Smoking Director

Victoria Holloway knows about the harmful effects of cigarette smoking. She is a stop-smoking director in Cincinnati, Ohio.

What does a stop-smoking director do?

A stop-smoking director helps people who want to stop smoking. The director conducts classes that help people understand why they smoke and how they can stop. He or she also educates both smokers and nonsmokers about the harmful effects of tobacco use.

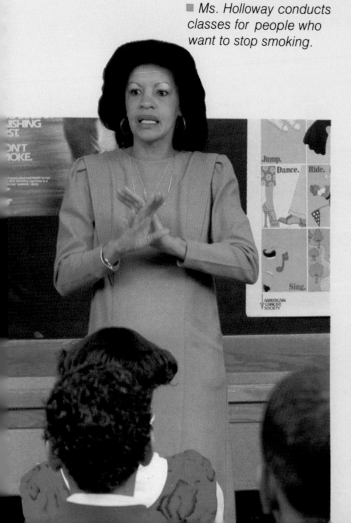

■ Ms. Holloway conducts classes for people who want to stop smoking.

Do you conduct programs for people of all ages?

I work with people of all ages. However, I am currently involved in a program for middle school students. It is a voluntary program that is conducted during school lunch hours. The program has eight sessions and lasts eight weeks.

What happens during a session?

Each smoker either chooses or is assigned a "buddy." A buddy is a nonsmoker who serves as a friend, offering encouragement and support to the smoker. The buddy and the smoker participate in activities together. This helps the smoker realize that activities do not have to include smoking. A smoker needs a buddy to replace the cigarette, which often has been treated as a friend. After the first session, I meet with the smokers and the buddies on different days and share the same information with both groups. This way both groups have similar knowledge about smoking.

What do you do during these sessions?

I help young people identify the reasons they smoke. Many of them smoke because they are around others who smoke and they want to gain the approval of their peers. Others smoke because they want to show their independence. After I help these young people identify the reasons they smoke, I ask them to write a list of positive qualities about themselves. When they have completed their lists, I remind them of the importance of self-esteem and that they can say no to cigarettes. I also discuss the dangerous effects of smoking.

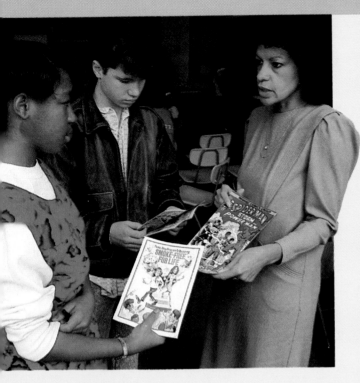

■ *Some pamphlets and magazines contain helpful messages about not smoking.*

What do you tell people in your programs who want to stop smoking?

First, I tell them that they must really want to stop smoking. It takes a lot of willpower to stay away from cigarettes. I also let them know that they will have to change their behavior in order to stop smoking. For example, instead of having a cigarette after a meal, they might go for a walk with their buddy or with a family member. Some people are able to smoke fewer and fewer cigarettes until they have completely quit smoking. Others find that quitting "cold turkey" works best for them. They stop all at once. I also tell people who are trying to stop smoking to chew sugarless gum or eat carrot sticks and to find activities to keep their hands and minds occupied. Different methods work for different people.

What happens at the end of the eight-week program?

We have a ceremony in which all the young people who participated receive a certificate. It is important for these young people to realize that others care about them and are proud of their efforts.

Is the stop-smoking program successful?

Yes. It is successful because it educates nonsmokers, smokers, and the buddies of smokers about the harmful effects of cigarette smoking. Not everyone who stops smoking is able to stay away from cigarettes. However, students who participate in the program learn how they can stop smoking if they choose to do so.

What tips do you like to share with young people about avoiding cigarette smoking?

I tell young people that it is never too late to stop smoking. It is important to keep trying and to have a good support system—a friend or relative that the smoker can call.

Learn more about people who help others stop smoking. Interview a stop-smoking director. Or write for information from your local American Cancer Society office or from the American Cancer Society, 1599 Clifton Road N.E., Atlanta, GA 30329.

Main Ideas

- More than 1,200 different substances have been identified in tobacco smoke.
- By law, all cigarette packages must now carry one of four health warnings.
- Nicotine narrows the blood vessels, raises the blood pressure, and makes the heart beat faster.
- Since tobacco smoke is inhaled, its greatest damage is to the respiratory system.
- The number of adult tobacco users is declining in the United States, yet the number of teenagers who use tobacco is increasing.
- By refusing to use tobacco, you are making a responsible decision to stay healthy and safe.

Key Words

Write the numbers 1 to 8 in your health notebook or on a separate sheet of paper. After each number, copy the sentence and fill in the missing term. Page numbers in ( ) tell you where to look in the chapter if you need help.

tar (301)
nicotine (301)
carbon monoxide (302)
ammonia (302)
formaldehyde (302)
arsenic (302)
cyanide (302)
smokeless tobacco (311)

1. A sticky brown substance called ___?___ is produced when tobacco is burned.

2. ___?___ is a drug in tobacco and is classified as a stimulant.

3. A poisonous gas that combines easily with red blood cells is ___?___.

4. One substance in tobacco smoke, called ___?___, is commonly used in many household cleaners.

5. Present in tobacco smoke, ___?___ is a substance used as a disinfectant and as a preservative.

6. Present in tobacco smoke, ___?___ is a strong poison used in weed killers.

7. A deadly poison called ___?___, which is found in tobacco smoke, causes severe respiratory problems for smokers.

8. Tobacco that is chewed, held in the mouth for a while, or sniffed is called ___?___.

Remembering What You Learned

Page numbers in ( ) tell you where to look in the chapter if you need help.

1. What substance in tobacco stains the teeth yellow? (301)

2. Name three substances in tobacco that are particularly harmful. (301–302)

3. How does smoking even one cigarette affect your body? (303)

4. How can smoking cigarettes be considered a fire hazard? (303)

5. What is the difference between mainstream and sidestream smoke? (304)

6. What are some ways in which tobacco smoke affects nonsmokers? (304–305)

7. Why have some states passed laws against smoking in public places? (305)

320

8. What are the warnings that must be placed on all packages of cigarettes? (306)

9. How does smoking damage the circulatory system? (307)

10. How does smoking damage the respiratory system? (308–309)

11. Why do people with emphysema have difficulty breathing? (309)

12. In what way does smoking during pregnancy harm the unborn baby? (310)

13. What are some of the dangers of smokeless tobacco? (311–312)

14. What are some reasons people start smoking? (314)

15. What are some things a person might say or do to refuse an invitation to use tobacco? (316)

Thinking About What You Learned

1. A person has decided to quit smoking "cold turkey." Why will this person probably have a difficult time quitting?

2. How can one family member's smoking affect the rest of the family?

3. Why is smoking a cigarette all the way to the filter more dangerous than smoking it only halfway?

4. Why should a person not smoke if he or she is taking a prescribed stimulant?

5. How would you refuse tobacco offered to you by an older family member who you like? It is sometimes more difficult to walk away from people you know well.

Writing About What You Learned

1. Contact your local chapter of the American Heart Association, the American Lung Association, and the American Cancer Society. Ask for up-to-date information on the incidence of smoking among teenagers. Ask about differences in the figures for girls and boys and for different cultural groups. Determine how the figures have changed in the last ten years. Prepare a report, and present it to the class.

2. Write an article for the school newspaper about methods of quitting smoking and ways of refusing to smoke.

Applying What You Learned

SOCIAL STUDIES

Research the history of tobacco use throughout the world. Include information about tobacco production as a business. Prepare a report, and present it to the class.

ART

Prepare a series of posters that detail ways of quitting smoking. With your principal's permission, display the posters around the school.

Modified True or False

Write the numbers 1 to 15 in your health notebook or on a separate sheet of paper. After each number, write *true* or *false* to describe the sentence. If the sentence is false, also write a term that replaces the underlined term and makes the sentence true.

1. Cigarette smoking is a leading cause of <u>lung cancer</u>.

2. Chemicals in <u>nicotine</u> are the primary causes of cancer in smokers.

3. <u>Tar</u> in tobacco smoke causes high blood pressure.

4. <u>Carbon monoxide</u> is present in tobacco smoke.

5. <u>Cyanide</u> is a poison found in tobacco smoke.

6. Smoking cigarettes causes your heart rate to <u>decrease</u>.

7. Smoke that comes from the end of a cigarette is called <u>sidestream smoke</u>.

8. Tar in tobacco smoke damages the <u>cilia</u> in the bronchial tubes.

9. People with <u>emphysema</u> have large amounts of scar tissue around their alveoli.

10. Children born to women who smoke usually weigh <u>more</u> at birth than children of nonsmoking women.

11. <u>Snuff</u> is a kind of smokeless tobacco.

12. <u>Ammonia</u> is a common household cleaner that is found in tobacco smoke.

13. If a person keeps pressuring you to smoke, you should <u>refuse</u> the offer.

14. There are <u>more</u> people smoking today than there were 20 years ago.

15. In most states, it is against the law for anyone under the age of <u>16</u> to buy tobacco products.

Short Answer

Write the numbers 16 to 23 on your paper. Write a complete sentence to answer each question.

16. What does being able to walk away from something that can harm you say about you?

17. What are three substances in tobacco smoke that are poisonous in other uses?

18. How does smoking reduce your ability to take in oxygen?

19. What are two immediate physical effects of smoking a cigarette?

20. How does smoking cigarettes affect the smoker's appearance?

21. How does tobacco smoke affect nonsmokers?

22. Why is sidestream smoke more harmful than mainstream smoke?

23. What are the long-term effects of tobacco use?

Essay

Write the numbers 24 and 25 on your paper. Write paragraphs with complete sentences to answer each question.

24. What are the effects of tobacco smoke on the respiratory system?

25. Explain how cigarette smoking affects not only the individual who smokes but also those around him or her.

ACTIVITIES FOR HOME OR SCHOOL

Projects to Do

1. Create a scrapbook of advertisements for tobacco products obtained from newspapers and magazines. Attach to each advertisement your analysis of how the advertisement encourages people to use tobacco.

2. Develop an antismoking campaign for your school. Organize the campaign with help from your teacher and classmates. Run the campaign for a week.

3. Some cigarette manufacturers claim that their filters remove most of the harmful substances in cigarette smoke. Collect cigarette advertisements that make this claim. From each advertisement, find the name and address of the cigarette manufacturer. Write the company and ask for factual information that proves each advertisement claim.

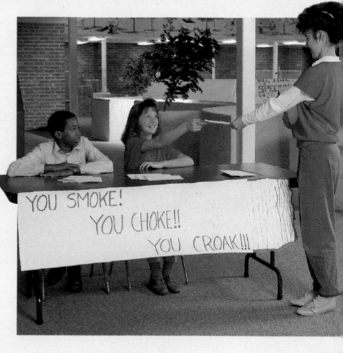

■ *Participate in an antismoking campaign at school.*

Information to Find

1. Write to your state legislature for information on state laws about tobacco use by teenagers. Make the information available to your class.

2. Contact some local companies, as well as the offices for your school district, and find out what their policies are on smoking within their buildings. Prepare a chart or table, and make it available to your class.

3. Find out what clinics and programs are available in your community for people who want to stop smoking. Compare the programs. Find out how many people have enrolled in each program and how many have stopped smoking. Then make a chart or graph that shows this information.

Books to Read

Here are some books you can look for in your school library or the public library to find more information about the dangers of tobacco use.

Casewit, Curtis W. *The Stop Smoking Book for Teens*. Messner.

Hyde, Margaret O. *Know About Smoking*. McGraw-Hill.

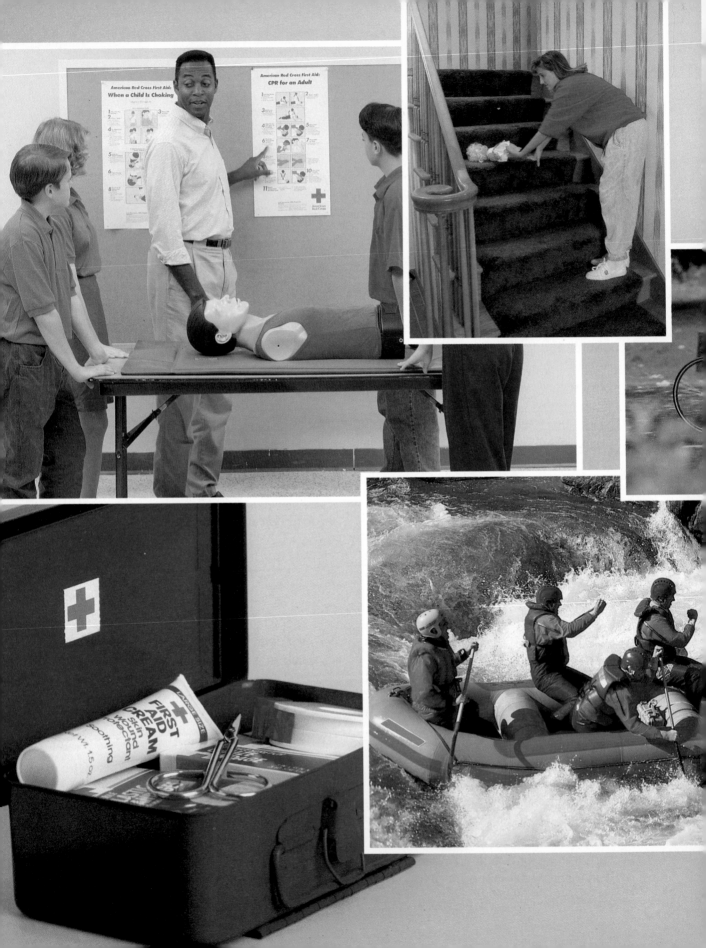

12

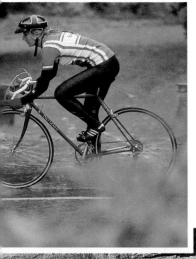

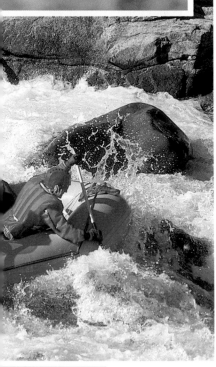

YOUR RESPONSIBILITY FOR SAFETY

Young people have more accidents than older people. More deaths among young people between the ages of 5 and 14 result from accidents than from all other causes of death combined. Twenty-five percent of all accidental deaths happen at home. You can prevent most accidents by following some basic safety rules and by being safety-minded.

When accidents do happen, however, you can help yourself or someone else who has been injured if you know basic emergency procedures. By using these procedures, you may even save a life.

GETTING READY TO LEARN

Key Questions

- Why is it important to learn about safety and first aid?
- Why is it important to know how you feel about keeping yourself and others safe?
- How can you learn to make choices that will help keep you safe?
- What can you do to become more responsible for your own safety?

Main Chapter Sections

1 Living Safely
2 First Aid for Life-Threatening Emergencies
3 Safety at Home

1 Living Safely

Every day, people make many decisions that affect their safety. Crossing a street, riding a bicycle, and using power tools require you to make choices about your actions. The consequences of being careless include property damage, personal injury, or even death. The results of being safety-conscious often go unnoticed. Nevertheless, your knowing how to be safe and being safety-conscious can prevent many accidents.

KEY WORDS

accident
hazards
emergency
first aid

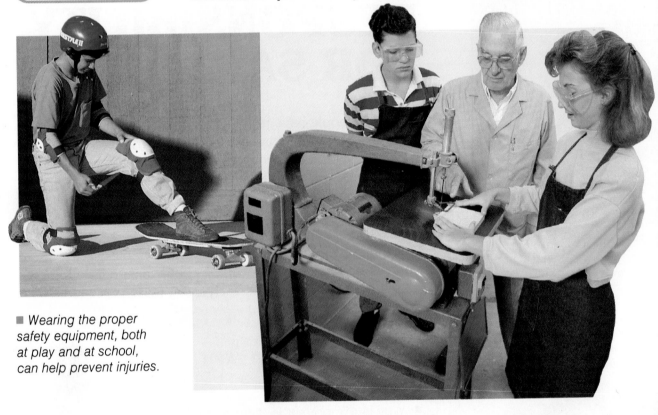

■ Wearing the proper safety equipment, both at play and at school, can help prevent injuries.

How Can You Prevent Accidents?

accident (AK suhd uhnt), a sudden, unplanned event that can cause a person harm.

An **accident** is a sudden, unplanned event that may cause a person harm. The harm may be choking, poisoning, a wound, or a burn. Many people believe that they have no control over accidents. Accidents, they think, "just happen." Yet people who study safety say that unsafe behavior is usually to blame. For a variety of reasons, many people do not think or act safely. If you do think and act safely, you can reduce your chances of having an accident. You can also develop an attitude of respect and responsibility for yourself and other living things around you.

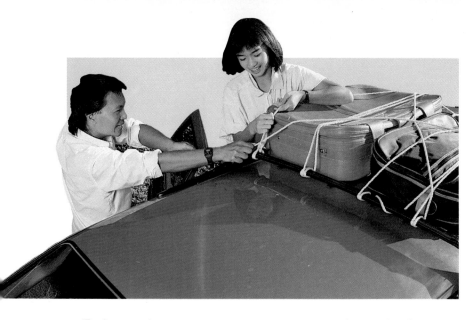

■ Unsafe behavior is the cause of most accidents. Thinking and acting safely can reduce the chance of having an accident.

To be a safety-conscious person, you must know the factors that contribute to being safe. You avoid accidents by

- understanding what you are doing.
- developing the skills to perform an activity in a safe manner.
- being aware of your physical and emotional condition.
- knowing the physical conditions in your environment that can lead to accidents.

Knowledge and Understanding.   Before a person can do something safely, he or she must understand important aspects of the activity. Before riding a moped, for example, a person needs to learn the motor vehicle laws for mopeds. He or she must know how to operate a moped and what protective gear to wear. The person also needs to know the dangers of riding a moped in traffic. The moped rider needs to understand that some drivers often ignore or cannot easily see mopeds.

■ Learning the motor vehicle laws and knowing how to operate a vehicle safely can help prevent accidents.

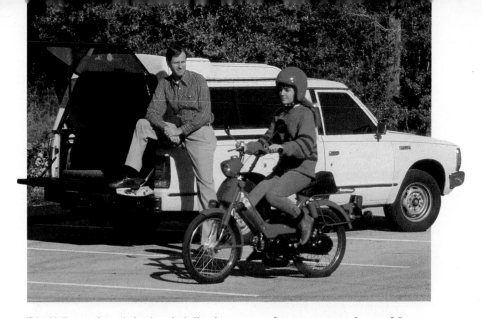

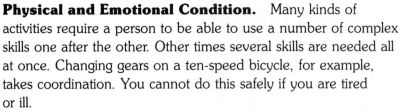
The skills for driving a motor vehicle need to be practiced away from traffic.

The time required to recognize a danger and take action is your reaction time.

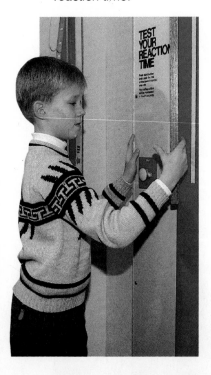

Skill Level. A lack of skill often contributes to accidents. Most moped accidents happen to persons who have been riding a moped for less than six months. Too often the beginning moped rider has not mastered steering, braking, and signaling skills. Learning the skills for using a moped begins with a moped rider education course and plenty of practice in a safe place, such as a vacant parking lot. An inexperienced rider is less likely to be injured in an empty parking lot than in a busy street.

Physical and Emotional Condition. Many kinds of activities require a person to be able to use a number of complex skills one after the other. Other times several skills are needed all at once. Changing gears on a ten-speed bicycle, for example, takes coordination. You cannot do this safely if you are tired or ill.

When you are tired or ill, your reaction time slows. *Reaction time* is the amount of time, usually given in seconds, required to recognize a danger and take action. A slow reaction time causes problems when you are riding a bicycle. You may not be able to react quickly enough to miss an obstacle on the road.

A person's performance can also be affected by emotions. For example, if you are angry, worried, showing off, or taking a dare, you might have trouble thinking about riding safely.

Conditions in the Environment. Knowing what to expect in your environment can help keep you and others safe. For example, it is essential to know the depth of a pool or lake before diving in. People who dive headfirst into shallow water can receive a permanent spinal injury. That is why the depth of the water is marked at community swimming pools. In unmarked areas, a good safety rule is: "First time? Feet first!"

In addition to any existing unsafe conditions in your environment, some other **hazards,** or possible dangers, may be added. For example, a gun stored with bullets in it is an unnecessary hazard. Even an unloaded gun left where an untrained person could find it is a hazard.

hazards (HAZ uhrdz), possible dangers.

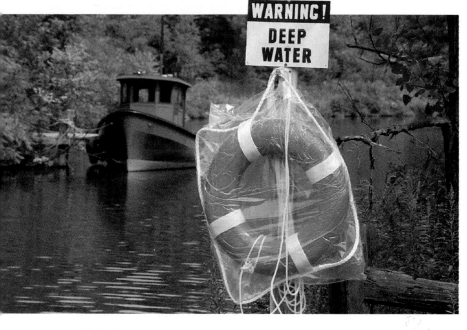

■ *Signs warn of dangerous conditions in the environment.*

Why Do Accidents Happen?

Being safe means more than just knowing the factors for accident prevention. You must also judge which conditions are safe and which are unsafe and then decide to act responsibly. Acting responsibly protects your safety and the safety of others. Not acting responsibly often leads to accidents.

People usually do not plan to act unsafely or irresponsibly. However, sometimes people are careless because they are thinking of other things, such as how fast they can finish what they are doing. Some people may also be overconfident of their knowledge and skill. Carelessness and overconfidence both lead to accidents.

Carelessness.   A major cause of accidents is carelessness. Forgetting to pick up toys, books, and other things from floors or stairs can result in people falling and being injured. Storing harmful substances where a child can find them and swallow them can cause the child serious harm. Failing to keep your bicycle in good repair can cause accidents, too. For example, a loose chain can slip off, causing a rider to fall. Failing to use seat belts in a car can result in serious injury if there is an accident.

329

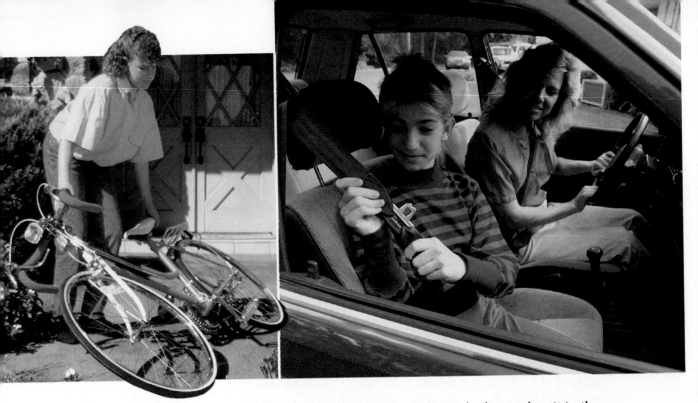

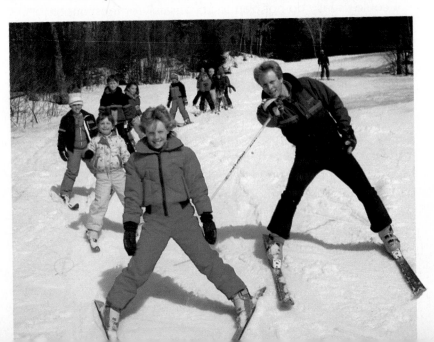

■ *Moving your bicycle from the sidewalk and always wearing a seat belt help prevent injuries.*

Some people mistakenly think that only those who sit in the front seat of a car need to wear seat belts. Car builders install seat belts in back seats, too, for the safety of back-seat passengers. Most states have laws requiring passengers to wear seat belts.

Overconfidence.   Many accidents are caused by people who know safety rules but choose to ignore them. Rather than try to act safely, they take unnecessary risks. Taking a dare to do something that is beyond your skill or that would require you to be in an unsafe place is taking an unnecessary risk. Young

■ *Learning proper skills from a trained instructor can help you stay safe.*

people learn skills better by taking controlled risks. This means challenging your skills while staying safely in control of the situation. In some cases, this is best done with the help of trained instructors. For example, a skating instructor knows what skating activities are safe for each student to attempt.

What Can You Do When an Accident Occurs?

Accidental injury and death can usually be avoided by being careful. Sometimes, however, no matter how careful you are, accidents happen. Often an accident creates a serious situation that requires immediate action. Such a situation is called an **emergency.** For example, choking can be an emergency. Without quick action, brain injury or even death can result. Any emergency, whether minor or major, can threaten a person's health.

The immediate care that is given to someone who has been injured or who suddenly becomes ill is called **first aid.** First aid can keep a person alive until trained medical help arrives. First aid can also protect an accident victim from further harm. You can learn first-aid procedures for many emergencies by taking a course given by the American Red Cross. Knowing first aid may help you save a life someday.

emergency (ih MUR juhn see), a serious situation that requires immediate action.

first aid, the immediate care that is given to someone who has been injured or who suddenly becomes ill.

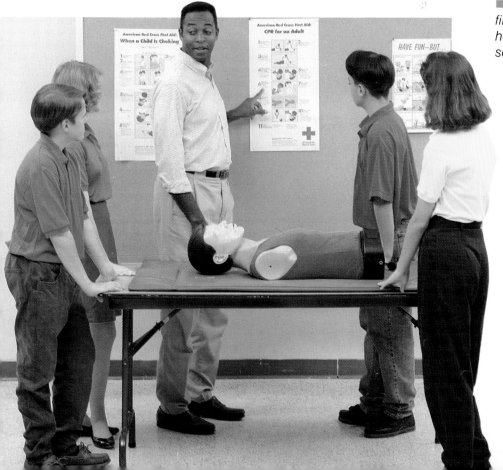

■ *Knowing certain first-aid procedures may help you save a life someday.*

A first-aid course can prepare you to handle many kinds of emergencies in case you are the first person to come upon an accident. Knowing first-aid procedures can help you feel good about yourself because you know you are able to help yourself and others. Before you learn first-aid procedures for specific injuries, however, you need to know some very basic steps that apply to most kinds of emergencies. These steps can lessen the chance of complications and even save a life. Remembering these steps in case of an emergency can help you feel confident about giving first aid.

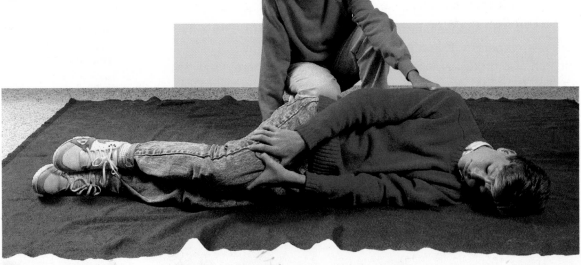

■ *If you are the first person at the scene of an accident, stay calm, check the scene and the victim, call for help, and care for the victim.*

Step 1: Check the scene and the victim.

First, stay calm so you will be able to think clearly. Make sure it is safe to approach the victim. If any dangers threaten—heavy traffic, a downed power line, fire, and so on—do not go near the victim. Stay at a safe distance and call 911 or your local emergency number immediately.

If it is safe to approach, check the victim to try to find out what is wrong. First, check to see if the victim is conscious. Sometimes that is obvious because the victim is talking, crying, or moving around. If the victim is lying still and does not respond to you, assume he or she is unconscious. Call for an ambulance at once.

Next, check to see if the victim is breathing, and then find out if he or she has a pulse. Check to see if the victim is bleeding heavily. If the victim is conscious and can talk, ask what happened and if he or she has pain or any other symptoms. Do not move a victim unless there is immediate danger, such as the possibility of a fire or an explosion.

Step 2: Call 911 or your local emergency number.

Certain conditions are life-threatening and require emergency first aid. These are choking, no breathing, unconsciousness, no pulse, severe bleeding, and poisoning.

*A*IRWAY
*B*REATHING
*C*IRCULATION

■ *Know the ABCs of first aid—Airway, Breathing, Circulation.*

Think of *ABC* when you look for life-threatening problems. *A* stands for *airway;* a person's airway is blocked if he or she is choking. *B* stands for *breathing;* a person who stops breathing for as little as four to six minutes may suffer brain damage. *C* stands for *circulation;* no pulse and severe bleeding are major circulatory emergencies. Poisoning can affect breathing by depressing brain stem activity. It can also affect circulation by speeding or slowing the heart or by changing the blood's chemistry.

If you discover any of these conditions, call 911 or your local emergency number at once. Local telephone books list emergency numbers on the inside front cover. If you are not sure which number to call, dial 0 (zero) for the operator. If a bystander is present, that person can make the call. If you are not sure whether the victim's life is threatened, call anyway. Emergency medical personnel would rather come and find no emergency than arrive too late.

■ *In an emergency, call 911 or 0 (zero) for help.*

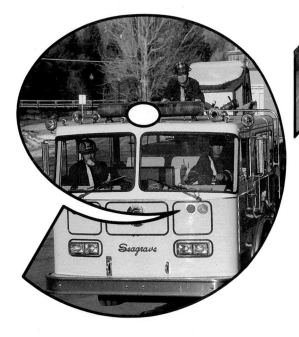
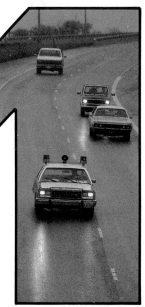
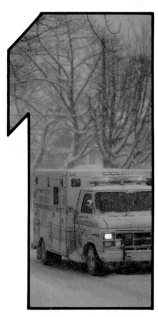

EMERGENCY TELEPHONE CALL FOR HELP

1. Tell *what* the emergency is—for example, a car accident, a fire in a house, a heart attack.
2. Tell *where* the emergency is. Give the address, or describe the location. Be sure to give complete directions for getting there, including the correct floor and room if you are in a building.
3. Give your complete name.
4. Give the telephone number from which you are calling.
5. If people have been injured, tell how many.
6. Describe each injury or illness as clearly as you can.
7. Do not hang up until the other person finishes the conversation. He or she may have questions to ask you. You may also get instructions about what to do until help arrives. If possible, write down the instructions.

Step 3: Care for the victim.

You may need to provide care after you have checked the scene and the victim. Always care for life-threatening emergencies first. Each life-threatening emergency calls for its own step-by-step first-aid procedures. Without immediate care, these emergencies can cause death.

When you have completed all the other steps, your responsibility is to keep the injured person calm and comfortable. Assure the person that medical help is on the way. Follow any instructions you have received from the emergency service.

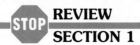

REVIEW
SECTION 1

REMEMBER?

1. What is the cause of most accidents?
2. List four factors that contribute to maintaining personal safety.
3. List three basic steps to follow in handling most emergencies.
4. Identify life-threatening situations that require emergency first aid.

THINK!

5. Why is it incorrect to say that accidents "just happen"?
6. How might a lack of skill while riding a bicycle be a threat to your safety?
7. Why is it important to stay calm during an emergency?

Health Close-up

Hazards While Cooking

Unsafe cooking practices are a common cause of fire in the home. Sometimes oil or bits of food on the cooking surface or in the oven catch fire. Oil can spatter out of a pan onto a burner. You can avoid fires at home by helping to keep your stove clean. Also, turn pot and pan handles to the center of the stove so that the pots and pans cannot be knocked over or pulled down by young children. Avoid placing the handles over other burners on the stove.

Microwave cooking also requires caution. Before you use a microwave oven, you should know how to use it properly. You also need to follow the special directions for microwave cooking.

Follow the rules of safety for outdoor cooking, too. When cooking with charcoal, use only proper lighting fluids. Never use other flammable liquids, such as gasoline. These explode and can spread fire. The improper use of fluids in starting outdoor charcoal fires causes many accidents. Never add charcoal-lighting fluid to hot coals. The fluid quickly turns to vapor and can explode. Lighting fluids are meant to be used 1 to 2 minutes before lighting the charcoal.

Charcoal is not safe for indoor cooking or heating. The burning charcoal releases a poisonous gas called carbon monoxide, which can be deadly in a closed place.

People can accidentally start serious fires with lighters and matches. Many fires are started because matches are thrown into wastepaper baskets after the matches are blown out but while the tips are still hot. Be sure that matches are cool before you throw them away. Keep all lighters, matches, and lighting fluids out of the reach of children.

■ *Be aware of possible hazards when preparing foods.*

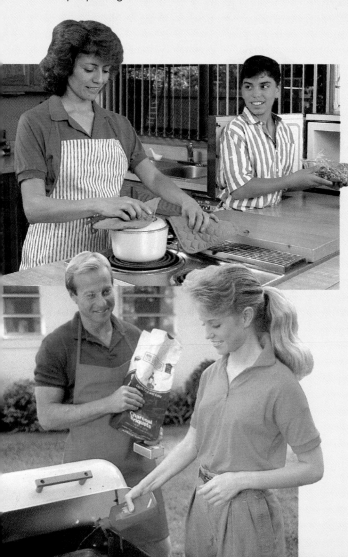

Thinking Beyond

1. Describe how the factors for accident prevention apply to cooking safety.
2. Make a list of safety rules to follow in your kitchen at home. Post your list in a place where it can easily be seen by those who use the kitchen.

2 First Aid for Life-Threatening Emergencies

Accidents that lead to choking, stopped breathing, no pulse, unconsciousness, and severe bleeding call for emergency first aid. Poisoning may cause a life-threatening condition. You can learn what emergency steps to take if one of these accidents happens. In many cases, the right kind of quick action will prevent more serious injuries or long-term health problems. Quick action may even save a life.

What Can You Do for Choking?

A person chokes when a piece of food or another object lodges in the trachea, or windpipe. People often choke on meat. This happens usually because a person takes too big a bite or does not chew the meat completely. Such choking can usually be prevented by cutting food into small pieces and chewing it well before swallowing. Choking can also be caused by laughing, running, or talking while chewing food.

■ *You need to be able to use and recognize the signal for choking.*

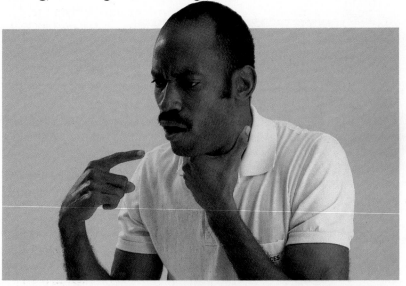

If you see a person choking, do not interfere if he or she is trying to cough out the object. Stay calm, and encourage the person to keep coughing. Do *not* slap the person on the back. This might cause the object to lodge deeper in the trachea.

If the person's trachea is completely blocked, he or she will not be able to speak, cough, or even breathe. When the trachea is blocked, air cannot enter the lungs. Often you can tell that a person's trachea is blocked because the person will grab at the

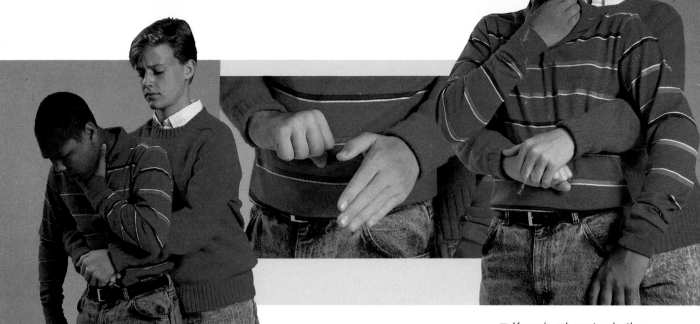

throat with one or both hands. This is a common reaction, and it is the international sign of choking. Ask, "Are you choking?" If the person nods yes, you must act quickly. Tell the person that you can help. The first-aid procedure to stop choking is called **abdominal thrusts.**

If you see someone grabbing at his or her throat, help the person stand up if he or she is sitting. Stay calm, and think of the steps for doing abdominal thrusts. Stand behind the victim, and put your arms around him or her but under the person's arms. Place the thumb side of one of your fists just above the person's navel and well below the lower tip of the breastbone. Grasp your fist with your other hand. Then, with a quick, hard, upward thrust, press your fist into the person's abdomen. Repeat this action until the object is forced out of the throat.

If you yourself should choke, you can perform abdominal thrusts alone. You can do this by leaning over the back of a hard chair. Put the back of the chair between your navel and breastbone. Press your body down quickly and forcefully on the back of the chair until the object is pushed out.

■ *Knowing how to do the abdominal thrust may help you save a life some day.*

abdominal thrusts (ab DAHM uhn uhl • THRUHSTS), the first-aid procedure to stop choking.

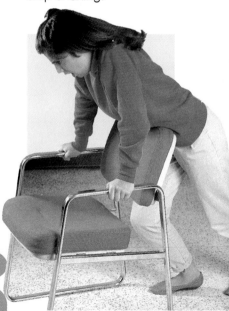

■ *If you are alone and choking, you can still perform abdominal thrusts.*

HOW TO HELP SOMEONE WHO IS CHOKING

1. Check to see if the person can speak, cough, or breathe.
2. Ask, "Are you choking?" If the person is choking, stand behind the person and put your arms around his or her waist.
3. Place a fist just above the person's navel, and hold the fist with your other hand.
4. Give several abdominal thrusts, pulling upward.
5. Repeat the thrusts until the object is dislodged.

What Can You Do for Stopped Breathing?

rescue breathing (REHS kyoo • BREETH ihng), an emergency procedure used when a person cannot breathe.

Rescue breathing is an emergency procedure used when a person appears to be unconscious and cannot breathe. It is a method of breathing air into the person's lungs. The actual procedure of rescue breathing begins after several steps of

RESCUE BREATHING

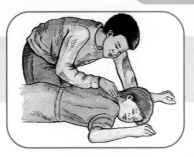

1. Tap the person and shout to see whether he or she responds.

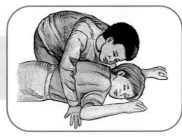

2. If the person does not react in any way, look, listen, and feel for breathing for about 5 seconds.

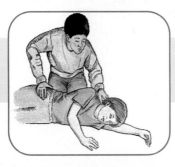

3. If the person is not breathing or you can't tell, roll the person onto his or her back, supporting the head and neck while you do so.

4. Tilt the person's head back and lift the chin. Recheck breathing.

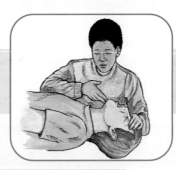

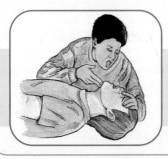

5. If the person is not breathing, keep the head tilted back and the chin lifted. Pinch the nose shut, using the thumb and index finger of your hand that is on the person's forehead.

preparation. The initial steps are very important if rescue breathing is to be done properly. The American Red Cross and American Heart Association provide classes for people ages 13 or older. Learning rescue breathing may help you save a life someday.

6. Blow air into the victim's mouth. Give two slow breaths. Blow in until the chest gently rises.

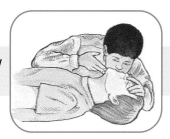

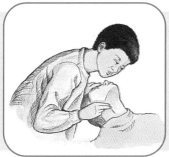

7. Check for a pulse. Put your fingers on the top of the person's neck just below the chin. Then slide your fingers into the grooves on the side of the neck. If the heart is beating, you will feel the pulse of the blood in one of the large blood vessels in the side of the neck. (If the victim does not have a pulse, you will need to give CPR.) Feel for the pulse for 5 to 10 seconds.

8. If the person has a pulse, give one slow breath about every 5 seconds. Do this for about 1 minute (12 breaths).

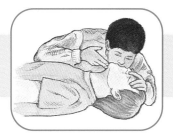

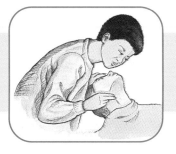

9. Recheck pulse and breathing about every minute. Continue breathing until the person starts to breathe on his or her own or until someone who has medical training arrives.

What Is CPR?

If a person's heart and breathing have stopped, *cardiopulmonary resuscitation* (CPR) can keep the person alive. CPR is an emergency procedure that combines rescue breathing and chest compressions. It works because a rescuer breathes air into a victim's lungs, getting oxygen into the blood. Then, with chest compressions, the rescuer causes the person's heart to move the blood throughout the body. For CPR to be successful, however, it must be combined with the proper medical care. CPR only keeps the cells of the victim's body from harm and possible death until more advanced medical help is given.

CPR

1. The victim needs to be flat on his or her back on a firm, level surface, like a floor. Kneel beside the victim between the head and the chest.

2. Lean over the chest. Place the heel of one hand just above the notch at the lower end of the breastbone. Place your other hand on top of the first hand.

3. Position your shoulders over your hands.

4. Press the chest down and then release. Push straight down, keeping your arms straight. Push the chest down about 2 inches. Let the chest all the way up before you push it down again. Compress the chest about 15 times in about 10 seconds. That is a little more than one compression per second.

5. Give 15 compressions, and then retilt the head and give 2 slow breaths.

6. Do 3 more sets of 15 compressions and 2 breaths.

7. Recheck the pulse and breathing for about 5 seconds.

8. Continue giving sets of 15 compressions and 2 breaths until the person begins to breath and has a pulse, or until an ambulance arrives.

What Can You Do for Severe Bleeding?

Things with sharp edges, such as knives or broken glass, can accidentally cut skin, tendons, muscles, and blood vessels. A cut artery in the neck, arm, or leg can result in heavy blood loss in a short time. Such a serious cut is a life-threatening emergency. Severe bleeding must be stopped immediately.

You can follow emergency procedures to stop severe bleeding. Keep the victim calm and lying down. Send for help if anyone is near. Fold a clean cloth and place it over the wound. To prevent infection, avoid touching the wound with your hand. Use the victim's hand to put pressure on the cloth over the wound. Keep applying firm pressure for five to ten minutes. Apply a bandage to help keep pressure on the wound.

You should not lift or remove the cloth. If you do, you may break up a clot that is beginning to form. If the cloth becomes soaked with blood, place another one over it and apply another bandage. Do *not* remove the soaked cloth. If the wound is on a hand, foot, leg, or arm, and you know there is no broken bone, raise the injured part higher than the heart. This will slow the flow of blood from the wound, since the heart will have to send the blood "uphill." When the bleeding stops, tie a bandage or another cloth around the same dressing to hold it in place. Then make sure the injured person receives trained medical help.

HOW TO STOP SEVERE BLEEDING

1. Keep the victim calm and lying down.
2. Call for trained medical help.
3. Fold a clean cloth to use as a dressing, and place it over the wound.
4. Have the victim keep firm pressure on the wound. Do not lift or remove the cloth. Apply a bandage over the cloth to help keep pressure on the wound.
5. If possible, raise the injured part above the person's heart.
6. When the bleeding stops, tie a bandage around the same dressing to hold it in place.

■ *A wound needs to be elevated and covered with a clean cloth to stop the bleeding.*

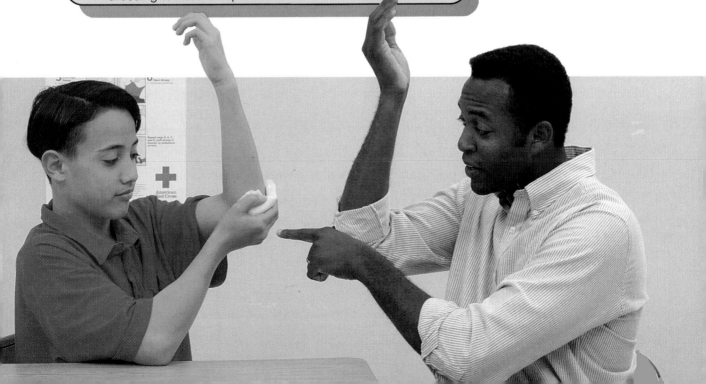

What Can You Do for Poisoning?

A **poison** is any substance that causes a chemical reaction in the body that results in injury, illness, or death. A poison may be in the form of a solid, a liquid, or a gas. A person who has swallowed a poisonous solid or liquid or has inhaled a poisonous gas needs immediate first aid. Poisoning may cause life-threatening conditions.

Follow these first-aid procedures to help a person who has been poisoned. First, keep calm and think about what you are doing. Second, try to determine what type of substance poisoned the person. Third, call for medical help. You can call the Poison Control Center in your community. If you do not know the number, dial 911 or 0 (zero). Do not give the person any fluid unless a worker at the Poison Control Center or another emergency service worker tells you to do so. Until help arrives, keep the victim as comfortable as possible.

MYTH
AND
FACT

Myth: You should make victims of poisoning drink soapsuds so they will vomit.

Fact: A burning poison, such as an acid or alkali, burns the esophagus when it is swallowed. It will burn the esophagus again if it is vomited. Do not give any liquid to a victim of poisoning unless instructed to do so by a rescue worker.

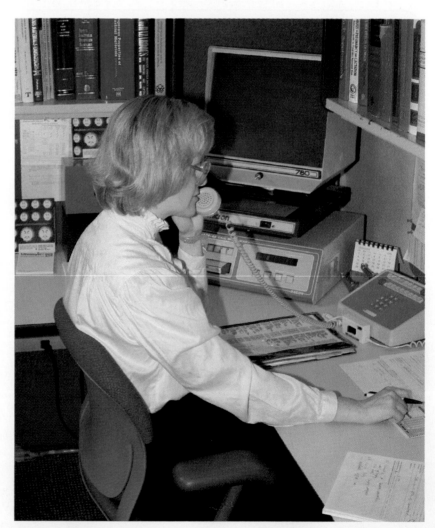

■ To help a person who has swallowed poison, call a Poison Control Center for information about first-aid procedures.

342

FIRST AID FOR POISONING

1. Stay calm and think about the steps for giving first aid.
2. Look for what caused the poisoning.
3. Call the Poison Control Center for help or dial 911 or 0 (zero).
4. Give a fluid only if the Poison Control Center tells you to do so.
5. Keep the victim calm until medical help arrives.

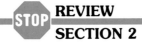

REVIEW
SECTION 2

REMEMBER?

1. How can you tell if a person is choking?
2. Why should you not remove a dressing that has been placed on a severe wound?
3. What service should you telephone if you find that someone has been poisoned?

THINK!

4. Suppose you do not know the first-aid procedure for a certain emergency and you are the only person to see a serious accident. How can you still act responsibly and be of help?
5. What are some responsible actions you can take to prevent poisoning in your home?

Making Wellness Choices

Brian and Joy are riding their bicycles near the park when they see a car hit a tree. The driver's door springs open, and they see a woman slumped over the steering wheel. No one else is in the car. No one else is nearby in the park. The woman is bleeding heavily from a wound on her arm. It also appears that her leg might be broken.

 What should Brian and Joy do? Explain your wellness choice.

343

SECTION

3   Safety at Home

Decisions about home safety can affect every member of your family. By developing safety habits at home, you can prevent common accidents and injuries, such as falls, burns, and electric shocks. If you also know emergency procedures, you can help the victims even if an accident should happen.

What Can You Do to Prevent Falls?

Falls cause about half of all injuries that happen in the home. Many falls can be prevented by practicing good safety habits. For example, by using a ladder instead of a chair to reach a high shelf, a person can avoid a fall. Ladders are made for safe climbing, but chairs are not. Keeping objects off the floor and the stairs can prevent falls. Wiping up spills from the floor and keeping electric-appliance cords off the floor can prevent falls, too.

Injuries Caused by Falls.   Falls can cause several different kinds of injuries. If you twist your ankle, the surrounding tissue may be damaged. This kind of injury is a sprain. A **sprain** is an injury in which the ligaments connecting the bones at a joint are stretched or torn. The tendons connecting the bones to the muscles may also be damaged.

KEY WORDS

sprain
strain
fracture
shock
electric shock

sprain (SPRAYN), an injury in which the ligaments connecting the bones at a joint are stretched or torn.

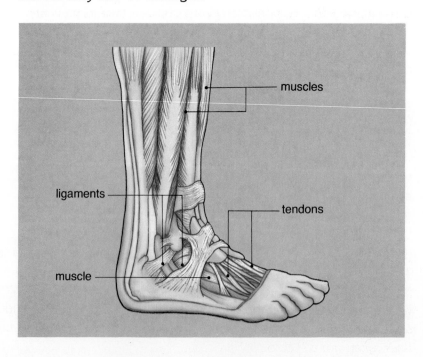

muscles

ligaments

tendons

muscle

■ *A strain results from stretched muscles or tendons. A sprain involves stretching or tearing of ligaments.*

344

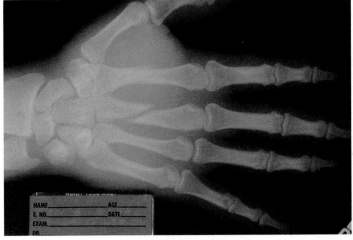
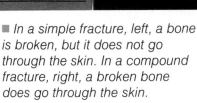
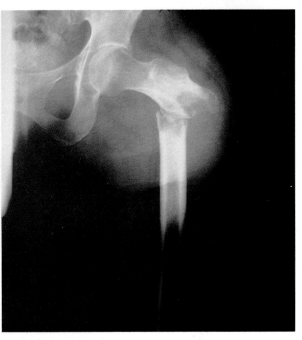

■ *In a simple fracture, left, a bone is broken, but it does not go through the skin. In a compound fracture, right, a broken bone does go through the skin.*

Falls sometimes cause strains. A **strain** is an injury in which a muscle or tendon is stretched or torn. It is sometimes difficult to tell a strain from a sprain.

Falls can also break bones. A break or crack in a bone is called a **fracture.** In a *simple,* or *closed, fracture,* the bone breaks or cracks but does not break the skin. A fracture in which the bone goes through the skin is called a *compound,* or *open, fracture.*

Emergency Procedure for Fractures.   A fracture is usually not life-threatening. However, the victim may develop signs of shock. **Shock** is a condition in which the circulatory system slows down and fails to provide a normal blood flow to the body. Shock may come from any injury. The signs of shock are pale and clammy skin, weakness, weak pulse, and rapid, irregular breathing. Keep the person lying down and elevate the legs to keep blood flow to the vital organs such as the lungs, heart, and brain. An unconscious person who is in shock should be kept lying on his or her side. This position allows saliva to drain from the mouth, preventing a blocked airway. Keep the person warm by placing blankets or extra clothing over and under the person. You must prevent the person from being chilled, but be sure the person does not get too warm. Then call for help.

Certain signs may indicate a broken bone. The person may be in pain, and the injured part may swell. An arm or leg may be bent in an unnatural way. You may see changes in skin color around the injured area. With a compound fracture, you will see the broken bone stick out of the skin.

strain (STRAYN), an injury in which a muscle or tendon is stretched or torn.

fracture (FRAK chuhr), a break or crack in a bone.

shock (SHAHK), a condition in which the circulatory system slows down and fails to provide a normal blood flow.

345

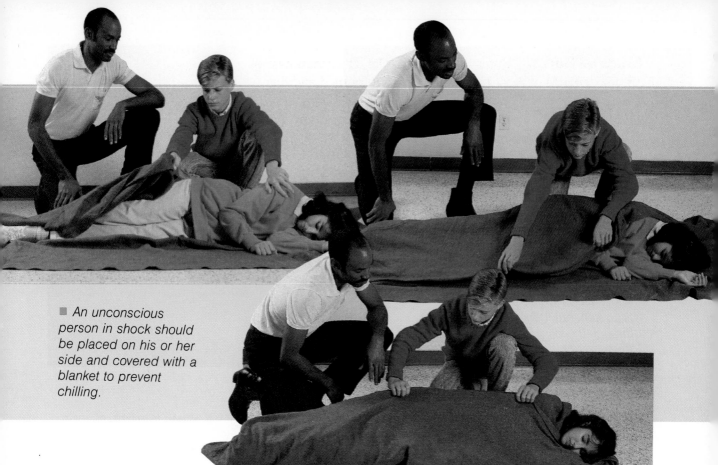

■ An unconscious person in shock should be placed on his or her side and covered with a blanket to prevent chilling.

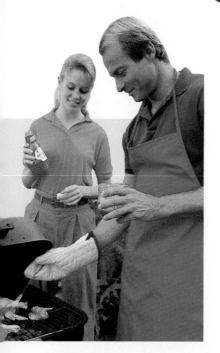

■ To avoid burns, pay close attention when working near open fires or hot surfaces.

If you are not sure whether a bone is broken, you should assume that it is. Do not try to straighten the broken bone or push it back into place. Moving the bone or the injured part of the body can cause even more damage to blood vessels, tissues, and nerves. This can also happen if the victim tries to use the injured part in any way. All fractures or suspected fractures should be checked and treated by a physician.

What Can You Do for Burns?

Burns are the third leading cause of accidental death in the United States. Nearly 2 million people are burned each year. More than 200,000 of them require hospital care, and about 6,000 of them die. Common causes of burns are boiling liquids, heaters, matches, cigarettes, fireworks, and home fires.

To avoid burns, always pay attention to what you are doing when you work near any source of heat. When cooking, do not wear loose-fitting clothing that could touch a flame or brush against a burner or hot stove. Be sure to read and follow directions on the labels of any chemicals that may cause a fire. The word *flammable* on a label means the chemical catches fire easily and burns quickly.

Kinds of Burns. Burns damage the skin. The seriousness of a burn depends on how much skin surface is burned and how deep the burn goes. The depth of a burn is described with the word *degree.* The least serious burns are *first-degree burns,* also called *superficial burns.* They damage only the outer layer of the skin. The skin's surface turns red. There is usually some swelling and some stinging pain. Most sunburns are first-degree burns.

Second-degree burns, also called *partial-thickness burns,* damage skin tissue more deeply. The skin turns red and blisters. Because water from the damaged tissue rises to the surface, the skin may be wet. Second-degree burns are very painful. The skin may be swollen for several days because fluid rushes out of the body cells in the area of the burn.

The most serious burns are *third-degree burns,* also called *full-thickness burns.* This kind of burn damages several layers of skin. The skin may be very white, or it may be charred gray. Third-degree burns often are less painful than second-degree burns because the nerves in the skin are destroyed.

■ *All burns need immediate first aid. A second- or third-degree burn needs to be treated by a physician.*

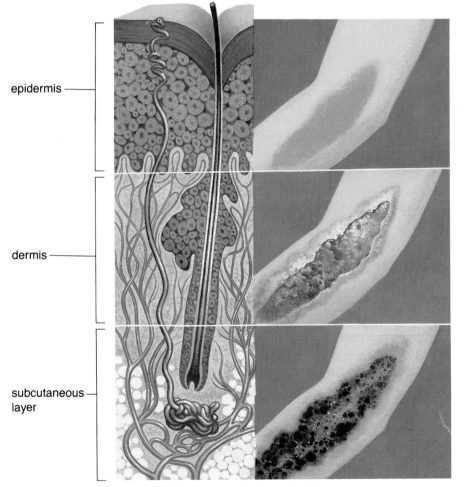

epidermis

dermis

subcutaneous layer

First-Degree Burn
Damage to the epidermis

Second-Degree Burn
Damage to the epidermis and dermis

Third-Degree Burn
Damage to the epidermis, dermis, and subcutaneous layer

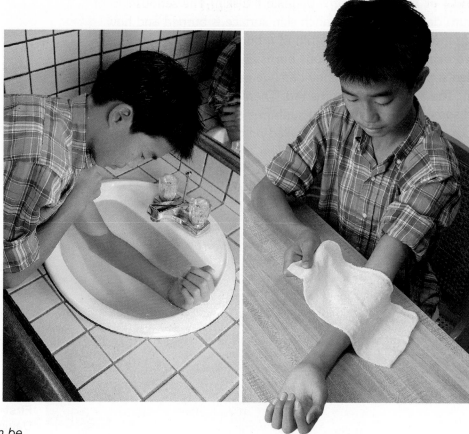

■ *Minor burns can be treated with cold water or a cold, wet cloth.*

First Aid for Serious Burns.   You can treat a burn by first removing the person from whatever is causing the burn. Then cool the burned area with large amounts of cool water for ten minutes or until the pain goes away. Cover the burned area loosely with dry sterile dressings, which help prevent infection. Do not use ice on second-degree or third-degree burns because it can cause the body to lose too much heat. Raise severely burned areas above the level of the heart, if possible.

Large second-degree and most third-degree burns are life-threatening and need immediate care. If you are faced with such an emergency, call for medical help as soon as possible. Do not try to remove any pieces of burned clothing stuck to the skin. This could cause further skin damage. Do not break any blisters on the skin. Do not use creams, lotions, butter, or grease of any kind on the burned area. Many people with serious burns go into shock, so treat the person for shock if necessary.

Third-degree burns can disrupt the way the whole body functions. A person may go into shock because the circulatory system is sending blood to the burned areas and not enough is reaching the vital organs. In some cases, shock can be more dangerous than the burn itself.

What Can You Do for Electric Shock?

Another common cause of home accidents is the unsafe use of electric appliances and tools. This carelessness often results in an electric shock. An **electric shock** is a painful, or even fatal, jolt, caused by direct contact with an electric current. A mild shock feels like a sharp, tingling stab and may cause a burn. A severe shock can cause death by stopping a person's heart and lungs. Bad wiring, faulty appliances and tools, and poor safety habits are the usual causes of electric shocks.

Causes and Prevention of Electric Shock. You can get an electric shock by touching a frayed electric cord. Children often suffer a shock when they stick something into an electrical outlet. To prevent such shocks, keep electric appliances and their cords in good repair, and place covers over unused outlets.

Electricity passes through water. People risk getting an electric shock if they use an appliance when they are wet or when they are standing on a wet surface. Using electric personal-care appliances near water in a bathroom is very risky. Even small appliances such as curling irons and radios can cause electric shocks. For the same reason, never operate an electric garden tool in the rain or when the grass is wet.

electric shock (ih LEHK trihk • SHAHK), a painful, or fatal, jolt caused by direct contact with an electric current.

■ A frayed wire, inset, can give a person a severe electric shock. Never touch a person who is receiving an electric shock. Follow the procedure shown in the picture.

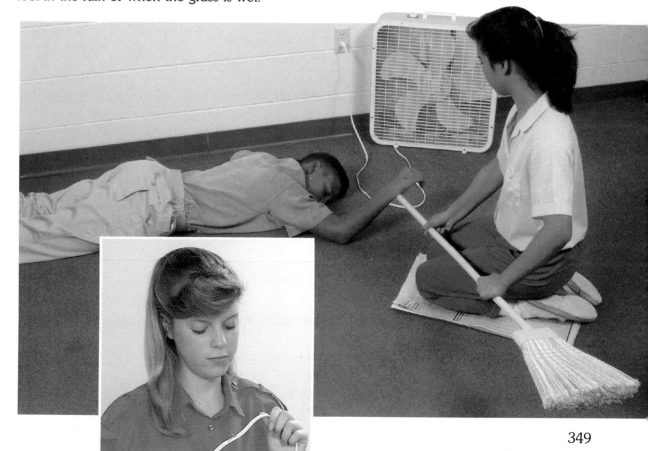

Emergency Procedure for Electric Shock. The first step to take for a serious electric shock is to make sure the power is off before you approach the victim. You can stop an electric current by turning off the main switch or circuit breaker for the building. At home, you should know where the fuse box or circuit-breaker box is located. Do not touch a victim who is still in contact with the electricity. If you do, you can get an electric shock yourself. If you are outside and a downed power line is involved, call the power company first. Never touch a low-hanging or downed power line.

If you do not know how to stop the electric current, carefully separate the victim from the source of electricity. If the injured person is touching an electric appliance, pull the plug from the wall using a newspaper or another form of insulation. Be sure your hands are dry and that you are standing on a dry surface.

Once the victim has been separated from the source of the electricity, call for emergency medical help. Check to see if he or she is conscious and breathing. To restore breathing, start the rescue breathing procedure. Treat the victim for shock.

■ *In case of an emergency, you need to know where the main electric switch for your home is located.*

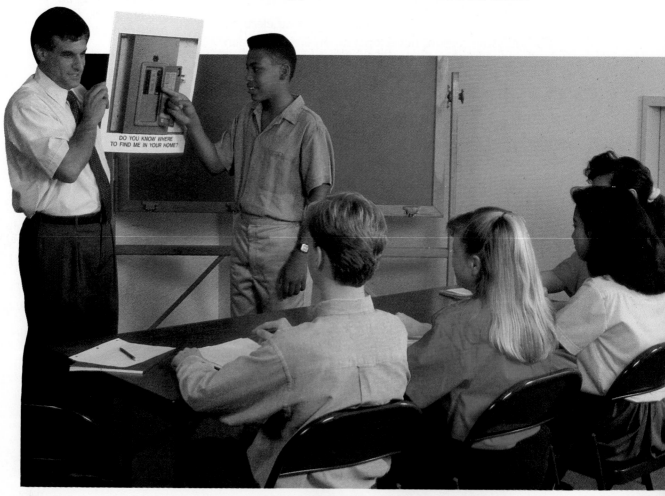

REMEMBER?

1. What are two signs that may indicate that a person has a broken bone?

2. What are the differences between second-degree burns and third-degree burns?

3. How should you treat a victim for shock?

4. What is a safe way to remove an accident victim from the source of an electric shock?

5. What is the difference between a strain and a sprain? How are they alike?

THINK!

6. Why is it still necessary to know emergency procedures if you always follow safety rules?

7. Suppose you are helping two injured people at the same time. One person has a large, bleeding wound, and the other has a second-degree burn. Which person would you treat first? Why?

Thinking About Your Health

What Is Your Safety Attitude?

On a sheet of paper, list three specific accident prevention actions that you have read about in this chapter. Next to each action, tell whether you are willing to carry it out. Some possible answers are "I'll try it," "I'll think about it," and "I won't try it." How would you describe your attitude about safety? Honestly evaluate how willing you are to take steps to prevent accidents.

Select one action that can prevent an accident. Try it. How did you make yourself and others safe because of your action?

People in Health

An Interview with a Building Inspector

Dave Hattrick knows about the importance of building safety. He is chief building inspector for the city of Boise, Idaho.

What does a building inspector do?

I make sure that buildings being constructed will be safe for people to live and work in. The buildings I inspect range from small sheds to huge shopping malls. I check many different things. For example, I check the foundation of a new building to make sure it is strong enough to support that building. I also check to see that the construction materials being used are the correct ones and the right sizes. When buildings are finished, I make sure they are safe in case of fire. I check to see if there are enough smoke detectors and exits. I make sure that doors open and close properly and that there are enough windows of the proper size.

Why do you have to check exits and exit routes in buildings?

In case of a fire, people have to be able to get out of a building quickly. For example, if there is a fire in a school, all students and adults must be able to get out of the classrooms and through the hallways as quickly as possible to leave the building safely. To allow this to happen, the building has to be designed and built properly. The exit doors must be in good working order so that they open easily to the outside. The hallways should be wide enough to hold many people at once.

How do safety requirements for houses and public buildings differ?

Public buildings must have at least two exits. They must also have lighted exit signs to mark the way out during an emergency. Houses are only required to have one exit door per room, though there should be two exits from the house itself. In houses, however, one window of each bedroom must be positioned so it can be used as an exit in an emergency. All new houses must have smoke detectors.

More public buildings are required to have sprinkler systems now than in the past. Smoke detectors need to be in all buildings. They are extremely important because they help save lives.

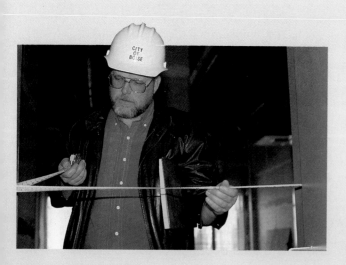

■ *A building inspector must decide if a new building is safe for people to use.*

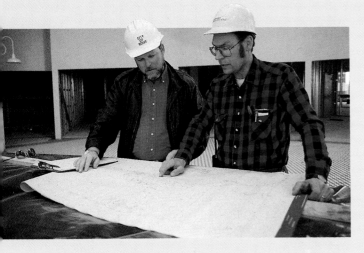

■ *Mr. Hattrick tells a builder what changes need to be made for the building to pass inspection.*

What other specific safety features do you check?

When I inspect buildings, I think of many kinds of safety. I make sure that railings are high enough so that people do not fall over them. I check openings in the railings to make sure they are too narrow for children to fall through or get caught in. I also see to it that people in wheelchairs will be able to get in and out of buildings easily. I do this by making sure that buildings have ramps, elevators, or chair lifts.

I check beneath buildings to make sure there is no standing water. Standing water can cause a variety of problems in a building. It can cause mildew, and it can be a breeding ground for insects and disease. It may even cause the building to sink.

What training is needed to become a building inspector?

Many people work as carpenters before becoming inspectors. Being a carpenter is a good way to learn about construction. People can also take college courses to prepare to be inspectors. Inspectors must be licensed, so they have to pass a state test. I think that any young people interested in becoming inspectors should take courses in science and drafting. Inspectors need to know about drafting to read the blueprints that show the plans for a building.

What suggestions do you give people about being safe in buildings?

First, I suggest that whenever they go into a public building, they notice where the exits are. They should think of two ways to get out of the building in case of fire. Second, students should look at their classrooms and hallways and make sure nothing is blocking windows and doors. They might also want to check which way the school doors open and how wide the hallways are. Then they could compare them to the doors and hallways in their homes. Doing this will give them a better idea of why certain buildings look the way they do. Students should ask their parents or other adult family members about smoke detectors for their homes, and talk to them about ways to get out of the home in case of fire.

> *Learn more about people who keep homes and other buildings safe. Interview a building inspector. Or write for information to Building Officials and Code Administrators International, 4051 West Flossmoor Road, Country Club Hills, IL 60477.*

Main Ideas

- Thinking and acting safely can prevent most accidents.
- Failure to act responsibly often leads to accidents.
- If you know what to do when an accident happens, you may be able to save someone's life.
- Knowing you can perform emergency procedures when an accident happens can build your self-esteem.
- Some basic steps for emergencies apply to most serious injuries.
- Each kind of life-threatening emergency requires its own first-aid procedures.
- Safety in the home involves recognizing hazards and preventing accidents.
- By being safety-conscious and knowing emergency procedures, you show that you take a personal responsibility for your safety and the safety of other people.

Key Words

Write the numbers 1 to 12 in your health notebook or on a separate sheet of paper. After each number, copy the sentence and fill in the missing term. Page numbers in ( ) tell you where to look in the chapter if you need help.

accident (326)
hazards (329)
emergency (331)
first aid (331)
abdominal thrusts (337)
rescue breathing (338)
poison (342)
sprain (344)
strain (345)
fracture (345)
shock (345)
electric shock (349)

1. _____?_____ are possible dangers that can lead to accidents.
2. Any accident that calls for quick action is an _____?_____ .
3. A _____?_____ is any substance that causes a chemical reaction in the body resulting in injury, illness, or death.
4. The immediate care given to a person who is injured or ill is called _____?_____ .
5. The first-aid procedure to stop choking is called _____?_____ .
6. An emergency procedure used when breathing stops is _____?_____ .
7. When a person has a _____?_____ , some ligaments are stretched or torn.
8. When a person has a _____?_____ , he or she has a muscle that is stretched or torn.
9. A break or crack in a bone is a _____?_____ .
10. Direct contact with an electric current is an _____?_____ .
11. The condition in which an accident victim's circulatory system slows down is called _____?_____ .
12. A sudden, unplanned event that can cause a person harm is an _____?_____ .

Remembering What You Learned

Page numbers in ( ) tell you where to look in the chapter if you need help.

1. According to people who study safety, why do most accidents happen? (326)
2. What factors contribute to a person's safety and well-being? (327–328)

354

3. What steps should you follow in handling any emergency? (332–333)

4. What are the most common life-threatening emergencies? (336–342)

5. Why should someone not slap the back of a person who is choking? (336)

6. How do you stop bleeding? (340–341)

7. What should you do if someone swallows a poison? (342–343)

8. What three kinds of injuries do falls often cause? (344–345)

9. What are some common safety hazards in the home that can lead to accidents? (344)

10. How are first-, second-, and third-degree burns different? (347)

11. What should you do first if a person has suffered an electric shock? (350)

Thinking About What You Learned

1. Why are more deaths among people 5 to 14 years old caused by accidents than by all other causes of death combined?

2. What should you do in an emergency if you have not been trained in first-aid procedures?

3. Why is immediate care necessary in life-threatening emergencies?

4. How might taking a dare be a hazard when you are doing an activity such as riding a bicycle?

5. Explain the importance of staying calm in emergency situations.

6. What are two ways in which a plugged-in radio is a hazard in a bathroom?

Writing About What You Learned

1. Write a report comparing safety features that are different in homes and public buildings. You may want to prepare a diagram of each kind of structure to help show the differences.

2. Write a how-to paper on one emergency procedure that has been highlighted in this chapter.

3. Write a persuasive paragraph to argue for or against this sentence: "Some people are just accident-prone." Take a position and explain it. Compare your paragraph with that of a classmate who has the opposite view.

Applying What You Learned

ART

Create an illustrated pamphlet that shows how to prevent falls, burns, or electric shocks. Under each picture, write a safety rule.

MATHEMATICS

Gather information about accidents that happen in the home. Prepare a graph or chart that shows which accidents happen most often. Discuss ways to reduce the number of these accidents.

Modified True or False

Write the numbers 1 to 15 in your health notebook or on a separate sheet of paper. After each number, write *true* or *false* to describe the sentence. If the sentence is false, also write a term that replaces the underlined term and makes the sentence true.

1. An <u>accident</u> is a sudden, unplanned event that can cause a person harm.

2. The amount of time needed to recognize a danger and take action is the <u>reflex</u> time.

3. A person's performance at a skill can be affected by <u>emotions</u>.

4. A loaded gun left around the house is a <u>hazard</u>.

5. <u>Self-confidence</u> can lead to accidents and injuries.

6. A serious situation that requires immediate action is an <u>event</u>.

7. Do not move an <u>injured person</u> unless it is necessary for the person's safety.

8. <u>Poisoning</u> may cause a life-threatening emergency.

9. Choking occurs when the <u>esophagus</u> is blocked.

10. The first-aid procedure to stop choking is the <u>slap on the back</u>.

11. The first step to stop severe bleeding is to keep the victim calm and make sure he or she is <u>lying down</u>.

12. Half of all injuries in the home are caused by <u>burns</u>.

13. A <u>strain</u> is an injury in which a muscle or tendon is stretched or torn.

14. A <u>simple</u> fracture is one in which the bone goes through the skin.

15. Pale, clammy skin and rapid, irregular breathing are signs of <u>shock</u>.

Short Answer

Write the numbers 16 to 23 on your paper. Write a complete sentence to answer each question.

16. What steps should you take to help a person who is in shock?

17. What signs might indicate a simple, or closed, fracture?

18. What happens to the skin in a third-degree burn?

19. What are the emergency procedures for electric shock?

20. Name four factors that contribute to being safe.

21. What are the three basic steps to take in an emergency?

22. What is the proper way to perform abdominal thrusts?

23. What should you do for severe bleeding?

Essay

Write the numbers 24 and 25 on your paper. Write paragraphs with complete sentences to answer each question.

24. Why can safety be described as a state of mind?

25. What steps can be done to help someone who has stopped breathing?

Projects to Do

1. Collect newspaper articles about recent home accidents. Read the stories critically. Determine the cause of each accident. Decide if the way the people reacted in the emergency contributed to their own or other people's injuries.

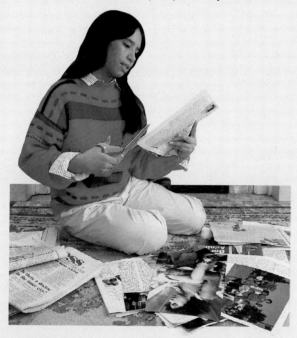

■ *Collect newspaper articles about home accidents.*

2. Call the local chapter of the American Red Cross. Find out about the kinds of health and safety classes that are offered. If possible, sign up for a Red Cross class that is given after school or on weekends.

3. With your family, make a safety inspection of your home. List any safety hazards that might cause falls, burns, or electric shocks. If you discover any real or possible hazards, discuss with your family ways of eliminating these hazards.

Information to Find

1. Adult burn victims need large amounts of protein and other nutrients to grow new skin. Teenage burn victims need even more nutrients. Since many burn patients cannot eat normally, researchers have developed a liquid high-protein formula for these patients' needs. Find out more about nutrition for burn victims.

2. Learn how the Poison Control Center in your area helps people prevent and treat poisonings. Find the center's telephone number, and call to obtain a list of common household poisons.

3. Serious and permanent health problems can result from head injuries. These injuries occur in many diving, motor vehicle, and firearm accidents. In some large cities there are centers where people with head injuries can work to regain their skills. Find out what your community, county, or state has to offer.

Books to Read

Here are some books you can look for in your school library or the public library to find more information about accident prevention, emergency procedures, and home safety.

American Red Cross. *Standard First Aid and Personal Safety.* American Red Cross.

Hubbard, Kate, and Evelyn Berlin. *Help Yourself to Safety.* Charles Franklin Press.

McGee, Eddie. *The Emergency Handbook.* Wanderer.

Santrey, Laurence. *Safety.* Troll Associates.

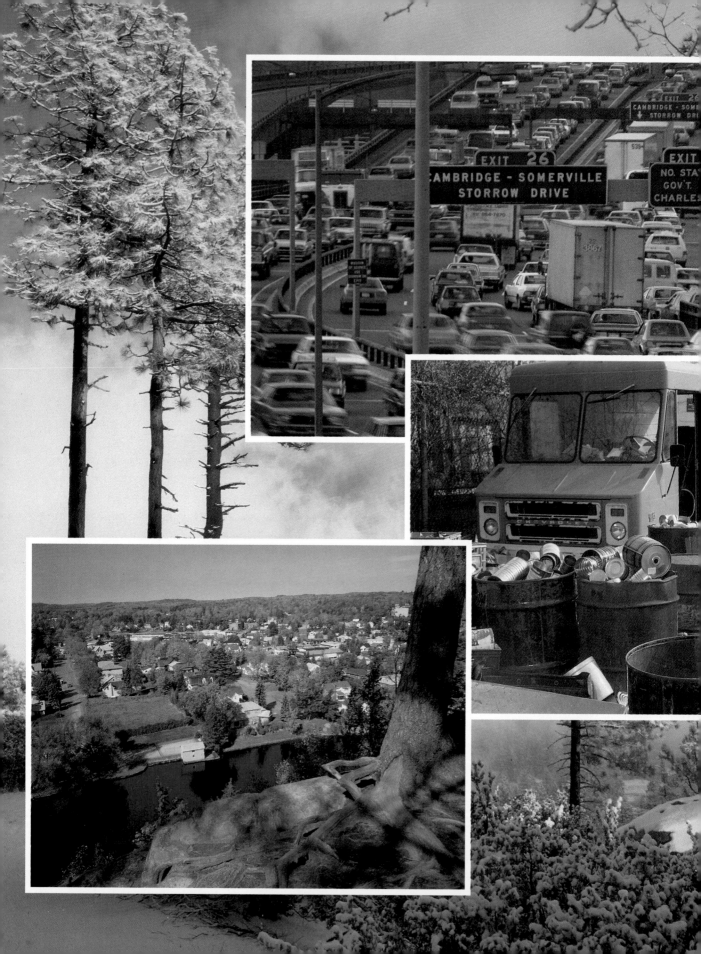

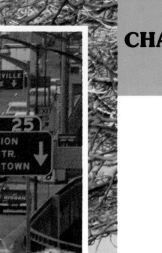

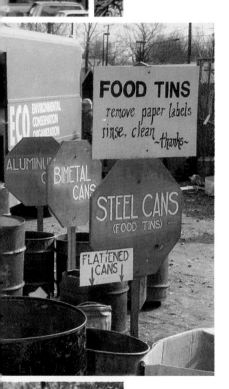

CHAPTER

13

YOUR HEALTH AND YOUR ENVIRONMENT

To stay healthy, you need a clean environment and adequate natural resources. Your wellness depends on clean air and water and on land that is free of harmful substances. In today's world, it is easy to pollute air, water, and land. Pollution can make these natural resources unhealthful. To prevent pollution and maintain good health, people need to manage natural resources wisely. Your future and that of your environment depend on good decision making by leaders and all members of your community, including you.

GETTING READY TO LEARN

Key Questions

- Why is it important to know about environmental health hazards and their causes?
- How can hazards in the environment affect your wellness?
- What can you do to protect community resources?
- Why are community agencies important for the well-being of groups of people?

Main Chapter Sections

1 Air Pollution and Your Health
2 Water Pollution and Your Health
3 Land Pollution and Your Health
4 Community Health Agencies

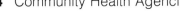

1 Air Pollution and Your Health

pollutants (puh LOOT uhnts), unwanted substances that cause pollution.

carbon monoxide (KAHR buhn • muh NAHK syd), a poisonous gas produced when there is not enough oxygen for a fuel to be burned completely.

Every day of your life, you breathe in about 2,000 gallons (7,570 liters) of air. Although this air sustains your life, it is not always safe to breathe. The air may have **pollutants,** or unwanted substances, in it that can harm your health and damage property.

What Causes Air Pollution?

Air pollution comes from different sources. The air may contain gases from automobile exhausts, power plants, and factories. The air may also contain smoke, soot, and ash. Pollution is very dangerous when several kinds of pollutants combine.

Carbon Monoxide.   When fuels are burned completely, they produce carbon dioxide. When there is not enough oxygen to burn a fuel completely, a poisonous gas called **carbon monoxide** is formed. Carbon monoxide comes chiefly from the exhaust of cars and other motor vehicles. In closed environments, such as restaurants and offices, the burning of fuel or tobacco also makes large amounts of carbon monoxide.

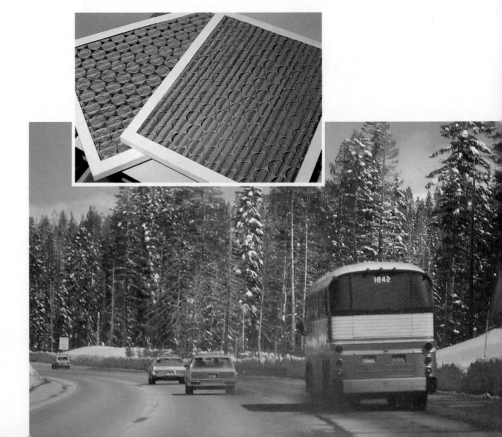

■ Air pollution includes particles large enough to be trapped by filters, as well as invisible pollution, such as carbon monoxide from motor vehicle exhaust.

Carbon monoxide is colorless and odorless. But it is harmful to people because it combines with red blood cells faster than oxygen. It makes the red blood cells less able to carry oxygen that is needed for all body parts to remain healthy.

Hydrocarbons.   Fuels made of hydrogen and carbon are called **hydrocarbons.** Gasoline, diesel fuel, and fuel oil are three examples of hydrocarbons. When these fuels are not burned completely, hydrocarbon gases enter the air. When these gases are inhaled, they become a health risk. They coat the lungs and cause people to develop lung diseases.

hydrocarbons (hy druh KAHR buhnz), fuels and gases made of hydrogen and carbon.

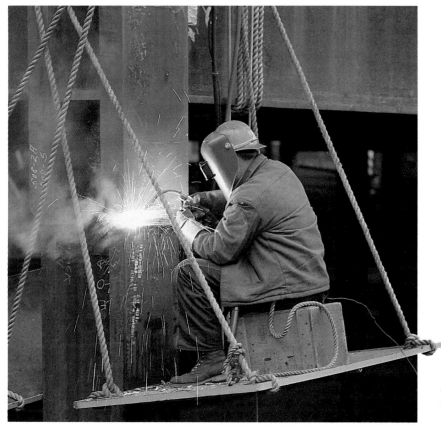

■ *Particulates include fine particles of ash, rock, or metal that get into the air during manufacturing.*

Particulates.   Small bits of solid or liquid matter floating in the air are called **particulates.** Examples are pollen from plants and dust from soil. Ash and smoke are also particulates. Any time something is drilled, sanded, ground, or crushed, particulates are added to the air. Factories add large amounts of particulates to the air in the form of ash, smoke, and soot.

If the air around you is smoky, dusty, or hazy, it likely has particulates in it. When particulates settle on surfaces, they leave a dirty or greasy film. You may have seen this film on buildings, cars, or the leaves of plants.

particulates (puhr TIHK yuh luhts), small bits of solid or liquid matter floating in the air.

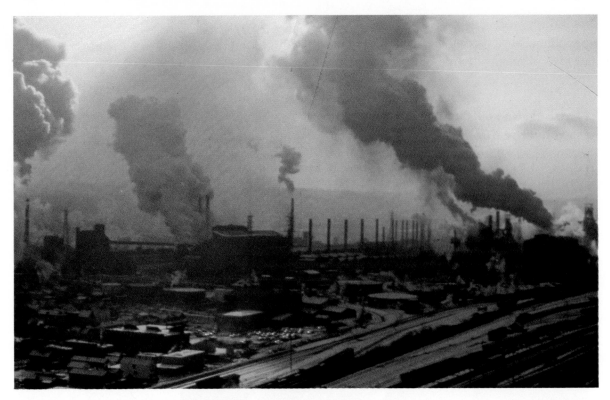

■ *Sulfur oxide and other oxides, which are produced by many factories, combine with moisture in the air to form acid rain.*

sulfur oxides (SUHL fuhr • AHK sydz), gases given off when fuels that contain sulfur are burned.

Sulfur Oxides.   Many fuels have sulfur in them. When these fuels are burned, they form gases called **sulfur oxides.** Sulfur oxides come chiefly from the burning of coal and oil in power plants and factories.

Sulfur oxides have a strong, unpleasant smell. However, the major problem with sulfur oxides is that they mix with water vapor in the atmosphere to form sulfuric acid. This acid then falls with rain, forming **acid rain.** Acid rain damages rivers and lakes, killing fish and plants. Acid rain also kills trees and may destroy entire forests.

acid rain, rain formed when water vapor combines with sulfur oxides in the atmosphere.

Acid rain is hard to control because it may fall hundreds of miles from where the sulfur oxides entered the air. Controlling acid rain calls for the cooperation of many countries, since this form of pollution often crosses national boundaries.

nitrogen oxides (NY truh juhn • AHK sydz), gases formed when certain fuels are burned at high temperatures.

Nitrogen Oxides.   When certain fuels are burned at high temperatures, they form gases called **nitrogen oxides.** Nitrogen oxides are red-brown in color and have a strong, unpleasant odor. They are given off by cars and most other motor vehicles. Nitrogen oxides can add to acid rain by forming nitric acid in the atmosphere.

362

HOW YOU CAN HELP PROTECT THE AIR

- Use public transportation whenever possible. By doing this, you reduce the number of cars on the road and the amount of pollution they make.

- Share rides with others whenever you can. In some major cities, the left-hand lane is reserved for car pools.

- Ride a bicycle or walk when traveling short distances.

- Encourage family members and friends to use cars less by running several errands in a single trip.

- Avoid burning leaves. Use the leaves for fertilizer or ground covering instead.

- Avoid excessive use of electric appliances, furnaces, and air conditioners. When you save energy, the power company can burn less fuel. That means less air pollution in your area.

What Is Smog?

When nitrogen oxides and hydrocarbons in the atmosphere are exposed to sunlight, **smog** forms. Smog is most often found in warm, sunny places where there are many automobiles. Los Angeles and Denver are two cities that have a lot of smog.

The chemical reactions in smog form ozone and other compounds. *Ozone* is a compound made of three oxygen atoms. When ozone is high up in the atmosphere, it helps screen out harmful ultraviolet radiation from the sun. However, in the lower atmosphere, ozone is a harmful gas that can cause health problems.

smog (SMAHG), pollution formed by the combination of nitrogen oxides, hydrocarbons, and sunlight.

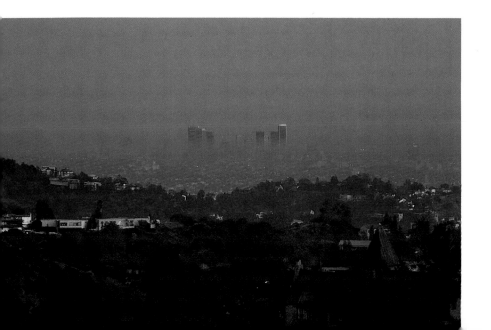

■ *Smog forms over cities such as Los Angeles when pollutants from automobile exhaust react with sunlight.*

What Is a Temperature Inversion?

■ *A temperature inversion often traps pollutants, creating an unhealthful condition.*

Most pollutants enter the air at or near ground level. They most often rise into the atmosphere. Under certain weather conditions, however, pollutants can become trapped near the ground. This situation is called a temperature inversion. A **temperature inversion** happens when a layer of warm air traps a layer of cool air beneath it.

In a temperature inversion, pollutants build up in the trapped air. The amount of pollution can become hazardous to the health of very young, elderly, or chronically ill people. During temperature inversions, people are warned to stay inside and not do heavy work.

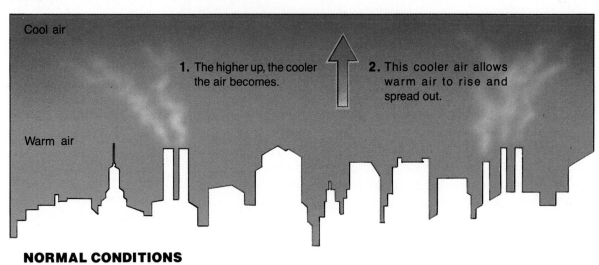

Cool air

1. The higher up, the cooler the air becomes.

2. This cooler air allows warm air to rise and spread out.

Warm air

NORMAL CONDITIONS

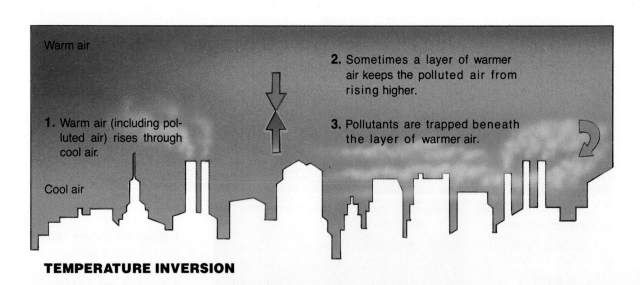

Warm air

2. Sometimes a layer of warmer air keeps the polluted air from rising higher.

1. Warm air (including polluted air) rises through cool air.

3. Pollutants are trapped beneath the layer of warmer air.

Cool air

TEMPERATURE INVERSION

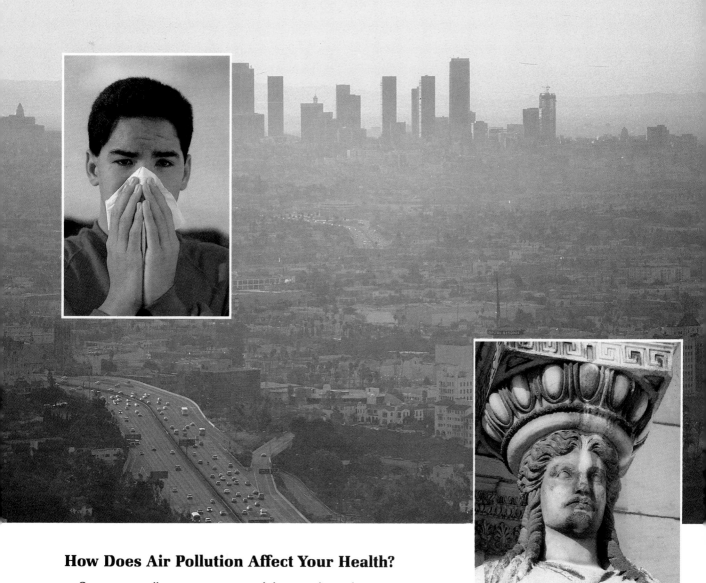

How Does Air Pollution Affect Your Health?

Some air pollutants are powerful enough to damage stone and metal structures. It should not surprise you, then, that air pollutants can damage you, too. Over the years, scientists and physicians have learned a great deal about the effects of certain air pollutants on health.

Air pollutants affect your eyes, respiratory system, and skin. People who often breathe polluted air can have eye irritation, frequent colds and respiratory infections. Some people have more problems with allergies.

Breathing air with high levels of carbon monoxide can affect your ability to think clearly and react quickly. Carbon monoxide reduces the amount of oxygen your blood can carry. Your heart and lungs must work harder to get oxygen to your body cells.

■ *Severely polluted air can cause eye irritation and respiratory problems. It can even damage buildings and sculpture.*

365

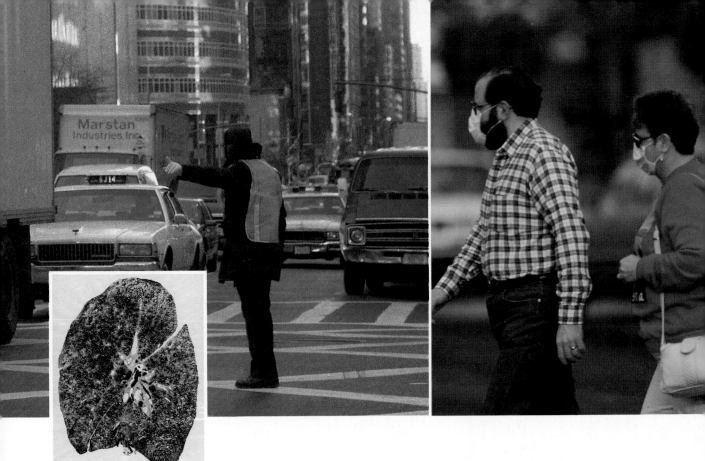

■ *Some people protect themselves from pollution, right. Others are exposed to carbon monoxide and other pollutants, and their lungs are damaged as a result.*

Even breathing small amounts of carbon monoxide can be dangerous. Every year, more people die from carbon monoxide poisoning than from any other poison.

SOME SYMPTOMS OF CARBON MONOXIDE POISONING

- headache
- weakness
- dizziness
- tight feeling across the forehead

- cherry-red skin color
- nausea
- increased pulse rate
- decreased muscle control
- rapid breathing

If you have any of these symptoms in or near a car, or near an indoor heater or a stove, immediately move to a place that has fresh air.

Some kinds of air pollution can harm the lungs. For example, coal miners who breathe in coal dust run the risk of getting lung diseases. Workers who handle asbestos without proper protection also risk lung damage, because asbestos has harmful dust.

People who spend time in heavy traffic and people who work in oil refineries breathe in large amounts of hydrocarbons. Studies show that workers who are exposed to high levels of hydrocarbons run a greater risk of getting lung cancer than people not exposed to high levels of hydrocarbons.

Breathing polluted air that has sulfur dioxide in it can narrow your breathing passages. When this happens, breathing becomes harder. You have a greater chance of getting bronchitis or emphysema. Breathing ozone in smoggy air also makes breathing problems worse and can damage the trachea.

Air pollution can cause the lungs to become stiff; they are not able to expand. Lungs in this condition cannot take in as much oxygen as the body needs from each breath. As a result, the heart must work harder to move the available oxygen all over the body. Over time, this extra work can damage the heart muscle.

Health problems caused by pollution do not go away as soon as a person breathes clean air again. Studies show that it takes a person almost the same amount of time to get well as it took to develop the lung problems. In some cases, the damage caused by air pollution lasts throughout a person's life and cannot be cured.

MYTH AND FACT

Myth: Crystal-clear air is clean air.

Fact: Crystal-clear air has little particulate matter in it, but it may be polluted in other ways. Air that looks clean can be full of deadly carbon monoxide and other harmful gases.

STOP REVIEW
SECTION 1

REMEMBER?

1. What are three air pollutants?
2. How does a temperature inversion trap pollutants?
3. How does carbon monoxide affect a person's health?
4. What health problems are caused by air pollution?

THINK!

5. What is the difference between fog and smog?
6. What forms of public transportation are especially helpful to the environment?
7. Give two reasons that communities allow air pollution to exist even though the health dangers are well known.

Health Close-up

Noise Pollution

In the course of your day, you may hear noises from airplanes, automobiles, construction equipment, radios, power tools, and household appliances. Noise can be irritating, and it can affect your health.

Too much noise is called *noise pollution.* Noise pollution is a growing problem that already may affect more people than any other form of pollution.

Noise is measured in decibels. The higher the decibel level, the more intense the noise. Above a certain level of intensity, noise can harm your health. A quiet conversation is about 40 decibels, a harmless level of sound. A loud rock concert is about 110 decibels. This level is dangerous. Exposure to sounds over 85 decibels is harmful, especially if you are exposed for a long time.

Noise damages your hearing by destroying the sensory hair cells in the inner ear. The sensory cells send nerve impulses to the brain. When the sensory cells are damaged, they are less sensitive to sound. The damage can be permanent.

Noise can cause other health problems along with hearing loss. Prolonged exposure to noise has been linked to high blood pressure, heart disease, and ulcers. The stress of continual noise also makes people irritable and tense.

There are three ways noise can be reduced. Machinery, which causes much of the noise pollution, can be redesigned to reduce the noise it makes. Buildings can be constructed using soundproofing materials. Finally, people can protect themselves by wearing ear plugs or ear muffs.

Some communities have passed antinoise laws. Citizens can be fined for operating

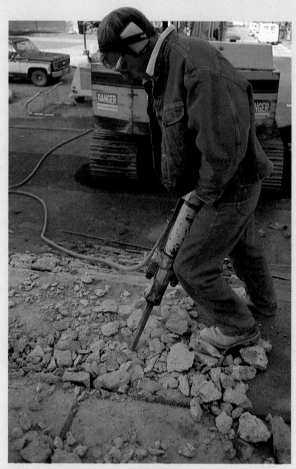

■ *Protection against noise pollution is needed to prevent hearing loss.*

noisy cars, radios, or stereos. Keeping noise to a minimum adds to a healthful environment.

Thinking Beyond

1. How can you protect your hearing when you use power tools or lawn mowers?
2. Why is avoiding loud music a wise habit for a young person?

2 Water Pollution and Your Health

When you look at a map of the world, you may think there is more water than could ever be needed. But only 3 percent of all the water in the world is fresh water. The rest is salt water. People must have fresh water for drinking, farming, manufacturing, and preparing food. Because the supplies of fresh water are limited, fresh water must be used over and over again. For this reason, the water must be kept as clean and pure as possible.

Today, much of our fresh water is not pure. Harmful substances are found in lakes, rivers, and other fresh water. These substances pollute the water, making it dirty and unhealthful to use.

KEY WORDS

sediment
sewage
soluble wastes
thermal pollution

What Causes Water Pollution?

Water pollution has many different causes. Some water pollutants are wastes that are carelessly dumped into rivers, lakes, and oceans. Other pollutants enter the water in the ground. Still other pollutants get into water from polluted air.

■ *Only a small percentage of the water on Earth is fresh water, and much of that is being polluted by careless dumping of wastes.*

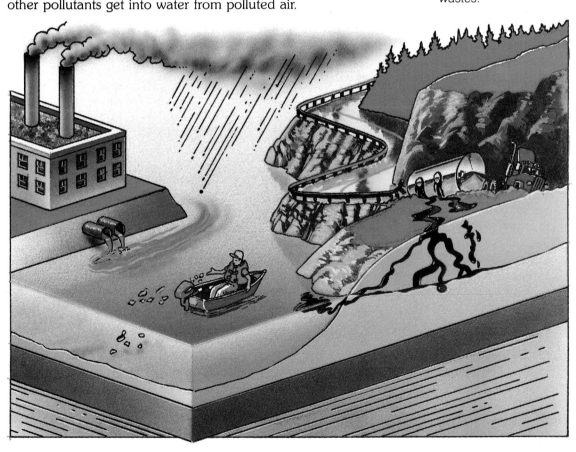

369

sediment (SEHD uh muhnt), solid matter that settles from water.

sewage (soo ihj), human waste.

Sediment. Water contains many different kinds of matter. Solid matter that settles from water is called **sediment.** Bits of soil and sand that are washed by rain into rivers, streams, and lakes can form sediment. Animal wastes and bits of plant matter can also form sediment after they enter the water. Sediment can affect water in many ways. It can make water unfit for drinking, bathing, and recreation. It can also damage or destroy plants and animals that live in the water.

Sewage, or human waste, can produce large amounts of sediment. Major health hazards can develop if untreated sewage enters water supplies. Untreated sewage has billions of microbes, many of which cause disease. Most communities treat sewage to remove solid materials and kill harmful microbes. After sewage is treated, it is often dumped into rivers, lakes, and oceans. However, even treated sewage has chemicals that can pollute water.

REAL-LIFE
SKILL

Selecting Low-Phosphate Detergents

Detergents that are low in phosphates cause less water pollution than detergents that are high in phosphates.
Go to a nearby grocery store, and look at the labels on the detergents.
List the names of detergents that are low in phosphates or that contain no phosphates.

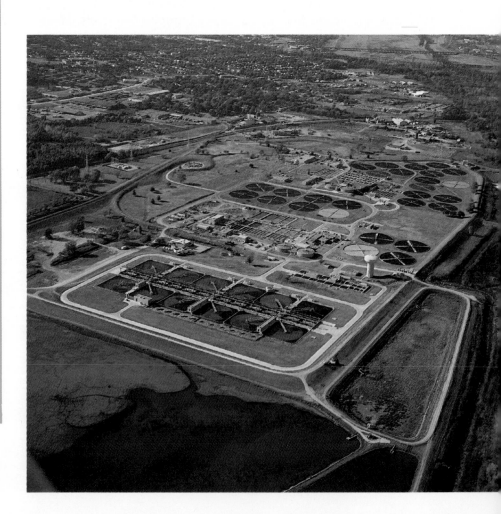

■ Even after sewage is treated, it still contains chemicals that can pollute water.

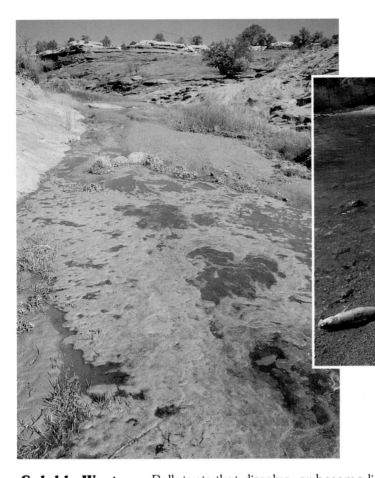

Soluble Wastes. Pollutants that dissolve, or become liquid, when they enter water are called **soluble wastes.** Soluble wastes can come from homes, factories, farms, and mines. For example, many homes and factories use detergents that have soluble wastes called *phosphates* in them. When phosphates are dumped into a lake or river, they upset the balance of plant and animal life. Phosphates make water plants grow rapidly, but the plants slowly die and decay. This decay lowers the level of oxygen in the water. In many cases, the level of oxygen becomes so low that the water cannot support life. When this happens, the water has an unpleasant odor and may have poisons from the decaying plants and animals in it.

Chemical fertilizers can also cause water pollution. Fertilizers help make crops and lawns grow. However, they also drain into water supplies through storm sewers and drainage ditches. In the water, fertilizers have the same effects as phosphates.

Heat. In some factories and energy plants, water cools the machinery. Cool water is pumped from a lake or river and sent around the machinery, where it gets warm. Then the water is put

soluble wastes (SAHL yuh buhl • WAYSTS), pollutants that dissolve when they enter water.

371

thermal pollution (THUR muhl • puh LOO shuhn), the warming of a naturally cooler water supply.

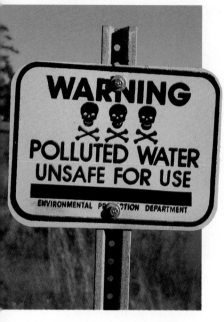

■ Many recreational areas and public water supplies have been closed because of pollution.

back into the water supply, making it warmer than it was. This warming of the water is called **thermal pollution.**

Thermal pollution, although not widespread, can greatly affect the quality of water. The warm water changes the normal conditions of the environment. Some life forms that cannot adapt to warm water die.

How Does Water Pollution Affect Your Health?

Water pollution can affect your health in several ways. Untreated sewage is the chief source of pathogens in water. You cannot see these pathogens, yet they can cause dysentery, typhoid fever, cholera, hepatitis A, and other diseases. The pathogens enter your body if you drink polluted water. They also get into the bodies of fish or shellfish, such as clams and oysters. You can become ill if you eat them.

Polluted water can also have any number of hazardous chemicals in it, such as lead and mercury from factories. Many of these substances are dangerous and can even cause death.

Some chemicals in water affect the body very quickly. Other chemicals affect the body slowly. The damage these cause may not show up for several years. Some chemicals, such as mercury, damage the nervous system. Other chemicals can harm the liver, heart, brain, and kidneys.

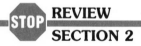 **REVIEW**
SECTION 2

REMEMBER?

1. What effect do phosphates have on the quality of water?
2. Why would eating shellfish that lived in contaminated water be dangerous to your health?
3. What is thermal pollution?

THINK!

4. People do not drink water from the ocean. Why, then, is pollution of ocean water a problem?
5. Why is sewage treatment important for farm wastes as well as human wastes?

3   Land Pollution and Your Health

Land provides people with basic resources. It provides soil for growing crops, and it provides raw materials for making buildings and the many goods people use. In the past, the resources of the earth seemed so abundant that few people thought about using them wisely. Land was often misused and resources were wasted. Today the demand for many of the earth's resources is at an all-time high. This demand for resources puts a great strain on the environment.

KEY WORDS

soil erosion
pesticides
herbicides
sanitary landfill
nuclear wastes

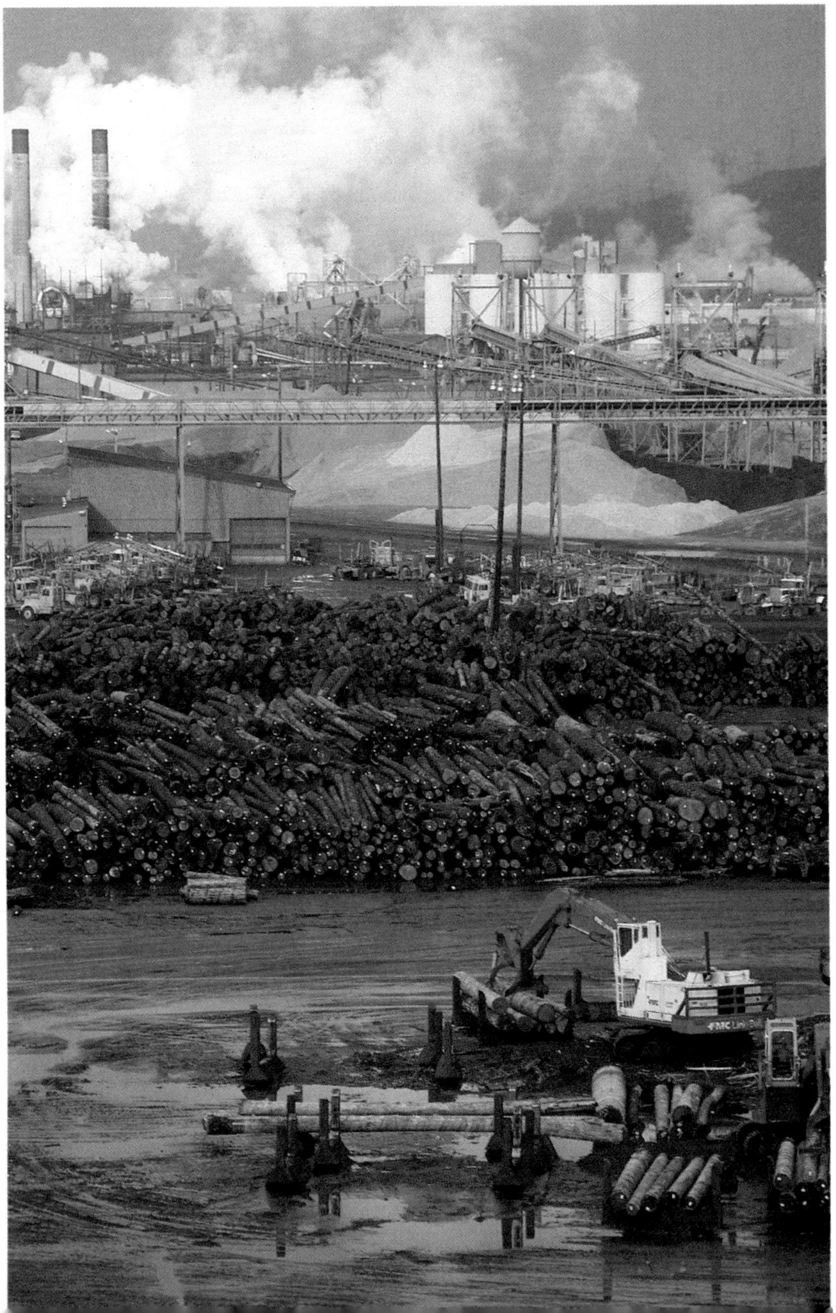

■ *Some natural resources are being used up faster than they can be replaced.*

373

What Causes Land Pollution?

Land is damaged when people take the resources they need from it without thinking about the consequences. In the United States, thousands of acres of land have been harmed by poor mining practices and excessive cutting of trees for lumber. Accidents with hazardous wastes, chemicals, and radioactive materials have also damaged the land.

■ *Much open land has been replaced by urban areas or destroyed to get the mineral resources under the soil.*

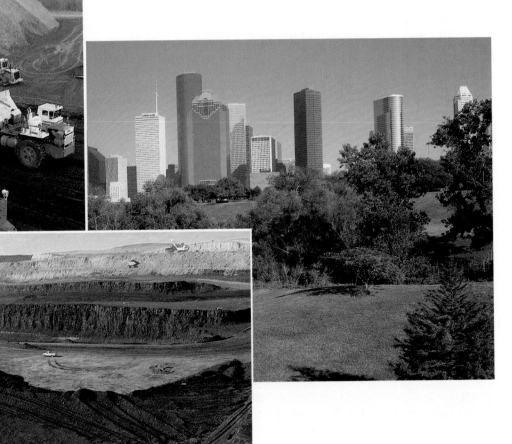

Overbuilding. In many cities and towns, much of the land has been covered with roads, buildings, and parking lots. There is not much space for grass, trees, and other plants. Without planted areas in communities, the quality of the environment suffers.

"Green space," such as parks and other areas with plants, helps make the community a more pleasant place in which to live. It also helps lower noise pollution, makes oxygen, and moderates the temperature of the community. Careful planning can guarantee enough green space in a community to provide beauty, improve air quality, and lower noise.

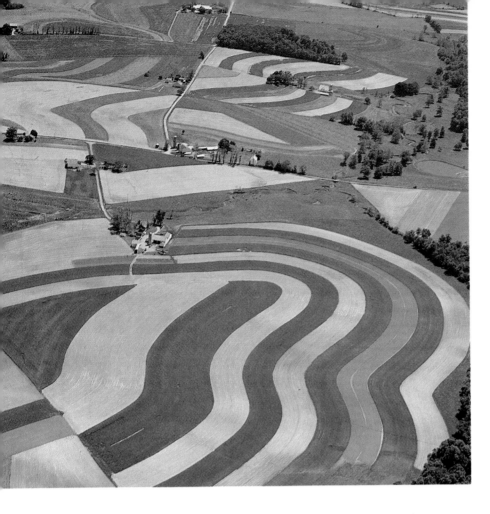

■ *Planting a variety of crops and contour plowing are effective ways of preventing soil erosion.*

Soil Erosion. Topsoil, the top layer of soil, holds most of the materials plants need for growth. Topsoil most often is held in place by the roots of plants. But plant life cannot help if the land is overgrazed, if it is plowed and not quickly replanted, or if too many trees are cut down. Then the topsoil can be washed away by water or blown away by wind. This wearing away of the topsoil is called **soil erosion.** Land that has undergone soil erosion does not support the growth of many plants.

One way to reduce soil erosion is called *contour plowing.* This means rows for crops are plowed across the normal flow of water. Each row acts like a dam to keep water from washing soil down the slope. Another way to reduce erosion is to keep fields planted for most of the year. Planting many kinds of crops also puts nutrients back into the soil.

Pesticides and Herbicides. To improve the growth of crops and trees, scientists have made chemicals that kill insects and other pests. These chemicals are called **pesticides.** Farmers also use chemicals to destroy weeds and other plants that hurt the growth of crops. These chemicals are called **herbicides.**

soil erosion (SOYL • ih ROH zhuhn), blowing or washing away of the earth's topsoil.

pesticides (PEHS tuh sydz), chemicals that are used to kill insects and other pests.

herbicides (UR buh sydz), chemicals that are used to kill unwanted plants.

375

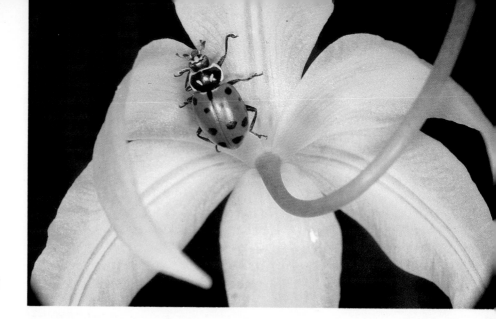

■ *Natural predators can sometimes be used in place of insecticides to kill insect pests.*

Using too many pesticides and herbicides can damage the environment. Rain can wash the chemicals into the soil and into the groundwater. There they can remain for a long time. People and animals that drink water with these chemicals in it may be harmed.

Scientists are searching for ways to reduce the dangers of pesticides and herbicides. Scientists are trying to find new chemicals that will kill insects and weeds but will become harmless by the time they reach the groundwater. In certain cases, it has been found that pesticides do not need to be used at all. Harmless animals or insects are brought into the area. They eat the pests that damage the crops. Ladybugs, lizards, toads, and nonpoisonous snakes and spiders have been used to control pests. These "natural pesticides" reduce the need for chemicals that can be harmful.

Solid Wastes. Solid wastes include trash, garbage, and other wastes from communities and industries. In the United States, each person makes about 5 pounds (2.3 kilograms) of trash and garbage each day. With about 250 million people making so much, it becomes a major problem. If thrown away carelessly, solid wastes can damage the land as well as hurt people's health.

One careless method of disposal is to put solid wastes in open areas of land called *dumps.* Open dumps are often dirty, and they may have a bad smell. They act as breeding grounds for insects, rats, and other pests. Many of these pests can spread disease. Water that comes from dumps can pollute groundwater and nearby streams and lakes.

Another careless disposal method is to dump solid wastes into the ocean. This removes the garbage from sight but damages the ocean environment. The garbage often kills or injures ocean organisms.

Some communities dispose of their solid wastes more carefully in sanitary landfills. A **sanitary landfill** is a place where solid wastes are buried with a layer of clay around the wastes on all sides. The clay helps keep rainwater from washing through the garbage. The garbage that is dumped each day is covered by clay and soil. This layer keeps rats and insects away.

Sanitary landfills are an effective way of dealing with solid wastes. They can also be used as new land for industry and even parks. However, many communities are running out of good places for sanitary landfills.

sanitary landfill (SAN uh tehr ee • LAND fihl), a location where solid wastes are buried with a layer of clay between layers of wastes.

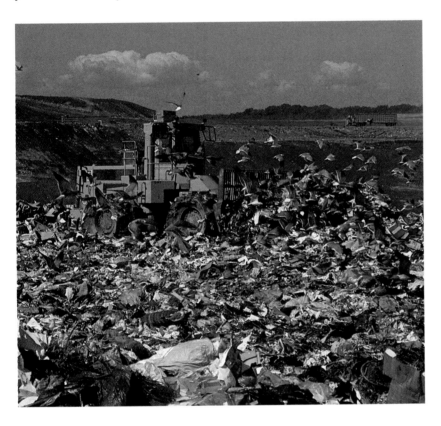

■ In a sanitary landfill, wastes are buried each day under a layer of soil. This keeps away groundwater contamination and eliminates many insects and rodents.

Another, but more costly, method of waste disposal is called *incineration*. Wastes are burned in large furnaces. The ashes take up little space and can be used as landfill or as fertilizer. Burning the wastes, however, can cause air pollution in the form of particulates and poisonous gases. Costly equipment is used to screen the exhaust from the furnaces to cut down on air pollution.

As communities grow, the problems of waste disposal become greater. There is not always enough land suitable for dumping sites. And many modern products, such as plastics, do not decay. They will remain in the environment for a long time. They can become hazards to wildlife if not disposed of correctly.

SOME WAYS TO PROTECT LAND FROM POLLUTION

- Recycle, or reuse, aluminum cans, glass bottles, newspapers, cardboard boxes, and magazines.
- Return soft-drink bottles and cans to the store, or take them to a recycling center.
- Use fewer paper and plastic products.
- Plant flowers, grass, and shrubs to improve the environment.
- Use grass cuttings, leaves, and spoiled fruit and vegetables to fertilize gardens.
- Avoid using chemical pesticides and herbicides.
- Set out bird-feeding equipment to encourage birds to stay in your area to eat unwanted insect pests.

FOR THE CURIOUS

Many hazardous chemicals are sold in stores. Chemicals such as cleaners, pesticides, and motor oils are easy to buy. However, they can cause serious environmental damage when disposed of improperly. Some communities have collection stations where potentially dangerous chemicals can be dropped off for safe disposal.

What Are Hazardous Wastes?

Every year, technology helps people improve their lives and solve many problems. However, technology has created problems of its own. One of these is the making of hazardous wastes. *Hazardous wastes* are dangerous substances given off during certain industrial processes, such as making electricity with nuclear energy.

Nuclear Wastes. Nuclear energy plants use the energy in radioactive elements to make electricity. Like any other way to make electricity, this method has both advantages and disadvantages. On the plus side, nuclear energy plants are very efficient and run very cheaply. On the negative side, they are very complex and costly to build and often cause thermal pollution. Nuclear energy plants also use radioactive fuel that is

378

very dangerous. Radioactive fuel is dangerous both during and after its use. In fact, some of the radioactive materials used in nuclear energy plants can be health hazards for thousands of years.

Used fuel and other radioactive materials from nuclear energy plants are called **nuclear wastes.** If not disposed of properly, these wastes will cause great environmental damage. They are also very poisonous.

nuclear wastes (NOO klee uhr • WAYSTS), used fuel and other radioactive materials from nuclear energy plants.

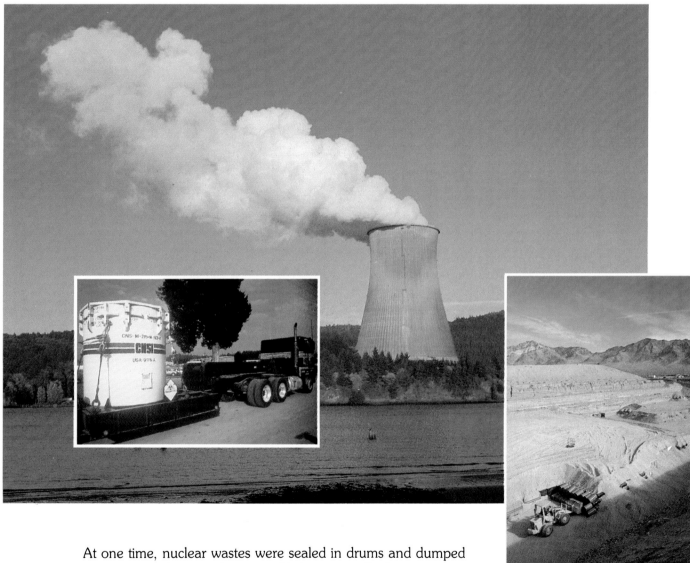

At one time, nuclear wastes were sealed in drums and dumped in the ocean. However, drums are likely to leak. Radioactive materials are a major health risk for a very long time. They must be disposed of in a carefully planned manner. Scientists, politicians, and health officials study proposed methods and possible places for storage. Then special procedures are followed in transporting the wastes to the sites.

■ The wastes of nuclear power plants are transported in sealed containers to specially prepared dumping sites.

Chemical Wastes. When some goods are manufactured, chemicals are given off that are very dangerous. Such chemicals have often been mishandled. They have caused great environmental and health problems. For example, at Love Canal, New York, a chemical company buried large amounts of chemical wastes in what was then an empty field. Later, however, a housing development was built there. In the late 1970s, the buried chemicals were found to be seeping to the surface and making people ill. Because of the number of people and the severity of the illnesses, the people had to leave the area.

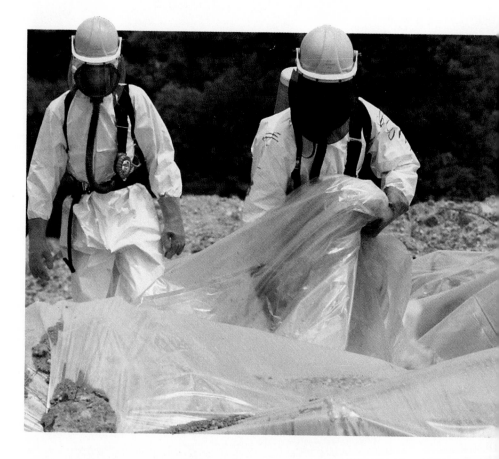

■ *Many areas have been polluted by toxic chemical wastes. Special protective clothing is needed when handling these wastes.*

How Does Land Pollution Affect Your Health?

Land pollution can contaminate large areas of land and make them unfit for animals and people. Polluted land, such as dump sites, can cause water pollution in nearby streams and even in groundwater. Many wells across the United States have been polluted by chemicals entering the water. The chemicals have come from landfills, from chemical dumps, and from leaking gasoline tanks at gas stations.

Even small amounts of nuclear wastes can cause severe health problems. Exposure to certain amounts of radiation can cause cancer and birth defects.

Some radioactive pollution happens naturally. For example, a colorless, odorless gas called *radon* is formed by the breakdown of uranium in the soil. Radon can enter homes. It has been connected to lung cancer in persons who do not smoke tobacco.

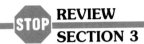

REVIEW
SECTION 3

REMEMBER?

1. How can parks help improve the environment of a city?
2. How can pesticides and herbicides affect the environment?
3. What is a sanitary landfill?
4. Why are nuclear wastes so dangerous?

THINK!

5. How can offshore dumping of garbage affect people?
6. Would you want a nuclear energy plant in your community? Explain your answer.

Making Wellness Choices

John has allergies and a slight case of asthma. He is thinking about taking a job as a stock clerk at an auto parts store. The job is just what he wants, and the pay is good. However, he would have to work in an area where people smoke heavily. The smoke makes the environment unhealthful. John's allergies would be aggravated at this job, and it would be harder for him to breathe.

 What should John do? Explain your wellness choice.

4 Community Health Agencies

Your community has services that add to the health of its residents. You may already know about vaccination programs and testing for certain diseases. Your community health department also works to protect your health in other ways.

By supporting community programs with taxes and fees, members of the community help maintain the wellness of themselves and others. As a member of your community, you should know about the health services that are offered.

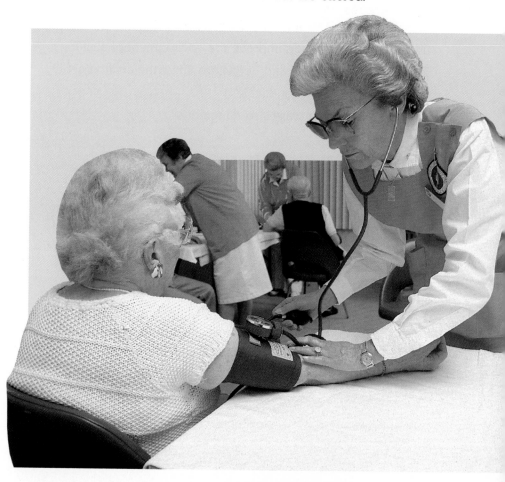

■ In many communities, volunteers help with health screenings, such as blood-pressure tests.

What Are Environmental Health Services?

Many health problems are caused by pathogens that are present in food, water, and waste materials. One task of your health department is to make sure that the food and water are safe. The health department also makes sure that solid wastes are treated to keep them from spreading disease.

To make sure food is safe, the health department checks places where food is prepared for sale. The health department checks restaurants, school cafeterias, and other places where food is prepared or packaged for sale. The health department also makes sure that milk and other dairy products are prepared under clean and proper conditions.

Restaurant Inspections. Every restaurant needs a permit from the health department before it can serve food. After a permit is issued, the health department checks restaurants periodically. It makes sure health standards are kept. Dishes, glasses, tools, floors, and other surfaces must be clean. It makes sure restaurants are free of insects and other animals that can spread disease. Food must be properly handled and stored. Restrooms must be clean and equipped for hand washing.

If a restaurant fails an inspection, the owners of the restaurant are asked to make corrections. If the corrections do not solve the problems, the health department can close the place.

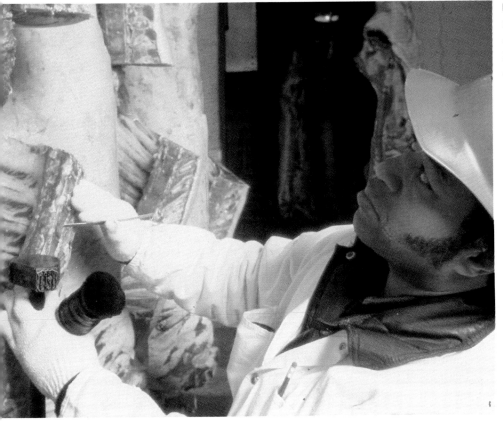

■ Restaurants and food-processing plants are inspected to ensure that they maintain standards of cleanliness.

Dairy Inspections. If milk is not carefully treated, pathogens can grow in it. People who drink such milk may become ill. For this reason, environmental health workers check all the steps used in preparing milk for the consumer. The health workers check dairy farms to see that the cows are free of disease. They make sure that milking procedures meet health department standards. They also make sure the milk is free of bacteria. In a process called *pasteurization,* milk is heated to a temperature of 161 degrees Fahrenheit (72 degrees Celsius) for 15 seconds. Pasteurization kills disease-causing bacteria.

After pasteurization, milk is packaged and shipped to stores. The health department makes sure the milk is kept cold enough during shipping so that no other microbes start to grow in it.

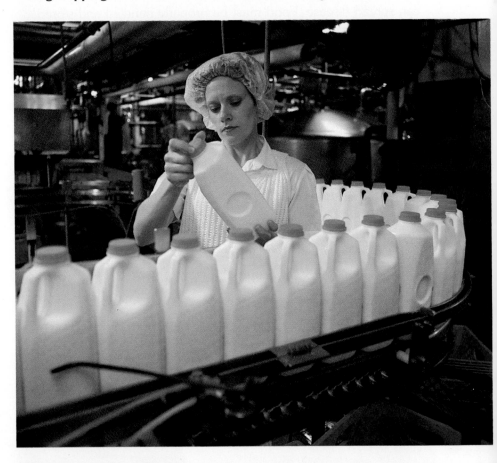

■ Milk is pasteurized to kill any pathogens in it. Then it is kept cold to prevent spoilage.

Water-Quality Control. In most communities, the tap water you drink is pure because of the work of your health department. Communities often get their water from places that can become polluted. Health workers regularly test drinking water to find out if it has harmful bacteria or chemicals in it. If the workers find anything, they can have the water turned off until it is treated and proven safe.

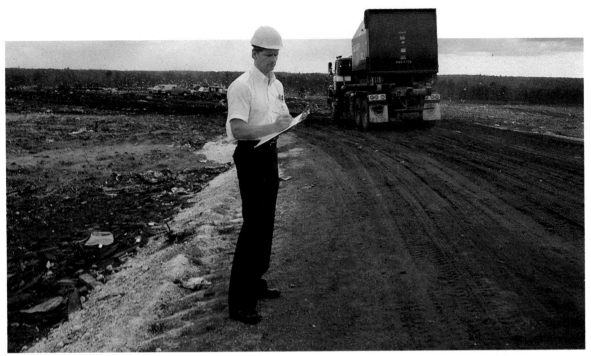

Solid-Waste Control. Communities make large amounts of solid wastes. Improper disposal of these wastes can cause pathogens to grow. The wastes may also attract insects and other unwanted pests. For these reasons, the health department often watches over the disposal of solid wastes.

In some cases, landfills can cause water pollution. Rainwater can soak through the wastes and then enter the water. To prevent this water pollution, health workers check landfill sites. They make sure that wastes are buried at a safe distance from the water.

■ *Health inspectors check landfills to be sure that groundwater is not being contaminated by runoff from buried wastes.*

KINDS OF HEALTH AGENCIES

- Government health agencies have been created by law and are supported with public funds. Some are federal agencies, such as the Food and Drug Administration (FDA). Other government health agencies are your state health department and your local city or county health department.

- Voluntary health agencies receive public donations to work on special health problems. Examples are the American Heart Association, the American Cancer Society, and the American Red Cross.

- Professional health agencies are groups of health workers who pay dues to maintain their professional organizations. Examples are the American Medical Association and the American Dental Association. There are also smaller, state and local professional groups.

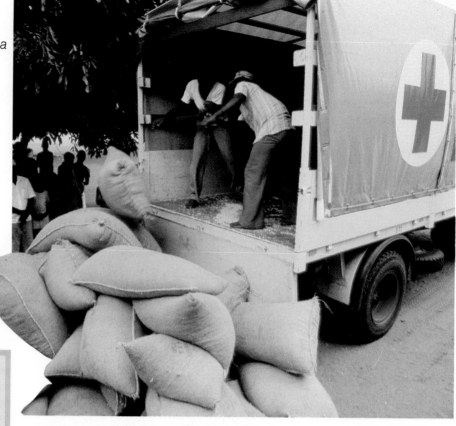

■ *Many agencies, such as the Red Cross, cooperate with communities to maintain a healthful environment.*

Why Is Cooperation Needed for a Healthful Environment?

Most people think chiefly about the environment in and around their own community. Many positive things can be done to work on health and pollution problems on a community level. But these problems go beyond communities. The pollution of one community can affect other communities. The pollution of one country can affect other countries. Pollution has no political boundaries.

Environmental problems need the cooperation of all countries. Acid rain, for example, is a major pollution problem that affects many countries. Much of the acid rain that is destroying Canadian forests forms in the United States.

Overpopulation and famine also cause environmental problems. In times of famine, the wealthy countries of the world often offer help to less wealthy countries. This help includes food, medical supplies, machinery, and training for the places that are in trouble.

The earth has a complex environment that supports many forms of life. It is important that people think about the

386

consequences of their actions to make sure they do not damage the environment. With careful planning, cooperation, and informed decision making, the earth can have a healthful environment for the generations to come.

STOP **REVIEW**
SECTION 4

REMEMBER?

1. What does a local health department do?
2. What is pasteurized milk?
3. Why is acid rain an international problem?

THINK!

4. Government health agencies are expensive to operate. Are they worth the expense? Why or why not?
5. Why should you call the health department if you notice an unsanitary condition in your community?

Thinking About Your Health

Does Your Family Do All It Can to Reduce Pollution?

Much of the pollution that enters the environment comes from ordinary households like yours. Do you and your family carry out all of the following practices? Survey your family's habits, using the following recommendations. These guidelines can help families conserve and protect natural resources.

■ Set the furnace thermostat to no more than 68 degrees Fahrenheit (20 degrees Celsius) in the winter. Set the air conditioner thermostat to no less than 80 degrees Fahrenheit (27 degrees Celsius) in the summer.

■ Conserve water by not letting water run and by taking short showers instead of baths.

■ Save and recycle cans and glass jars.

■ Save and recycle newspapers and other paper goods.

■ Use pesticides carefully and sparingly on the lawn and in the garden.

■ If the oil in the family car is changed at home, take the old oil to a gas station or garage where it can be recycled.

People in Health

An Interview with an Oceanographer

> *Jack Anderson understands the dangers of ocean pollution. He is an oceanographer in Long Beach, California.*

What is an oceanographer?

An oceanographer is a scientist who studies the oceans to understand how they work and how they affect people.

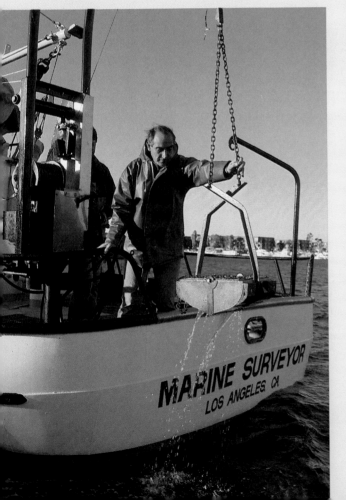

■ *An oceanographer studies the oceans to determine how they affect people.*

How do oceanographers help people?

Oceanographers want the ocean water to be safe for people to swim in, and they want the seafood people eat to be free of chemical poisons. Oceanographers are also concerned about the health of the sea life in the ocean. They look for signs of pollution. They try to solve problems that involve the oceans and the people who live near them.

What kinds of work do you do?

I am the director of the Southern California Coastal Water Research Project. The purpose of this project is to study the effects of ocean pollution on people and sea life along the coast of Southern California. The project covers about 300 miles (480 kilometers) of coastline. Most of the work is done at an ocean depth of about 200 feet (60 meters), but sometimes it is done at almost 1,000 feet (300 meters).

How serious a problem is ocean pollution?

Overall, the oceans are quite healthy. However, some places along the coasts, mostly harbor areas, have problems. Along the west coast of California near Los Angeles, for example, there is a very large amount of DDT in the water. DDT is a powerful chemical once used to kill insects. DDT has bad effects on other life forms, so it was banned from use in the United States in 1972. Even after all these years, there is still a lot of DDT in the coastal waters.

Are you helping to clean up the DDT?

I am involved with trying to solve the DDT problem but not with actually cleaning it up.

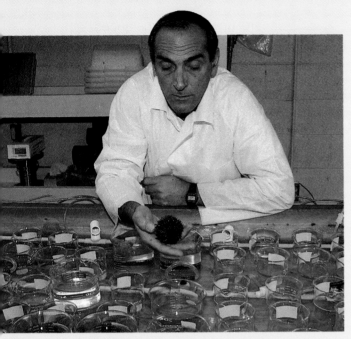

■ *Mr. Anderson studies the effects of chemicals on sea life.*

One of the problems with DDT is that no one knows how to get rid of it. What I do is to study the amounts of DDT in fish. I find the locations of the fish that have the greatest amounts of DDT in their systems.

Do oceanographers spend a lot of time under water?

Many people think that oceanographers spend most of their time exploring underwater like Jacques-Yves Cousteau. This is a great misunderstanding. Actually, oceanographers do very little diving. I often meet young people who know how to scuba dive and think that is all they need to know to be an oceanographer. Frankly, it is much easier to teach a good scientist to be a diver than it is to teach a diver to be a good scientist.

How did you decide to become an oceanographer?

When I was young, I liked going to the beach and the ocean. When I thought about the work I would like to do, I wanted something interesting outdoors or related to the ocean. I also wanted to pursue my interest in science, especially biology. I decided to study marine biology, which deals with the life forms that live in the ocean. After finishing college, I went to work studying the effects of oil pollution on marine life.

What can people do to help save the oceans?

People need to understand that the oceans and the many creatures that live in the oceans are seriously affected by all kinds of pollution. The more that people become aware of the dangers of bad chemicals, the better care they will take to protect the oceans and sea life.

Learn more about oceanographers. If you live near an ocean, interview an oceanographer. Or write for information to the International Oceanographic Foundation, 3979 Rickenbacker Causeway, Miami, FL 33149.

Main Ideas

- Your wellness and the well-being of most life on Earth depend on clean air, water, and land.
- Air pollution is the result of a variety of pollutants that cause health problems from allergic reactions to lung cancer.
- Water pollution is caused by pollutants such as sewage, soluble wastes, and harmful chemicals.
- Land pollution is caused by overbuilding and soil erosion and by pollutants such as pesticides, garbage, and hazardous wastes.
- Your local health department has the responsibility of protecting the health of the people in your community.
- International cooperation is needed to protect the earth's environment.

Key Words

Write the numbers 1 to 10 in your health notebook or on a separate sheet of paper. After each number, copy the sentence and fill in the missing term. Page numbers in ( ) tell you where to look in the chapter if you need help.

pollutants (360)
particulates (361)
acid rain (362)
smog (363)
temperature inversion (364)
sediment (370)

pesticides (375)
herbicides (375)
sanitary landfill (377)
nuclear wastes (379)

1. The combining of sulfur oxides with water vapor in the air produces ___?___.

2. ___?___ are unwanted substances that cause pollution.

3. A ___?___ occurs when a layer of warm air covers and traps a layer of cool air close to the ground.

4. The action of sunlight on nitrogen oxides and hydrocarbons produces ___?___.

5. Small bits of solid or liquid matter floating in the air are called ___?___.

6. A ___?___ is a disposal site where solid waste is covered on all sides by clay.

7. Used fuel and radioactive materials from nuclear energy plants are ___?___.

8. Chemicals used to kill insects are ___?___.

9. Chemicals used to kill unwanted plants are ___?___.

10. Solid matter that settles from water is ___?___.

Write the numbers 11 to 18 on your paper. After each number, write a sentence that defines the term. Page numbers in ( ) tell you where to look in the chapter if you need help.

11. carbon monoxide (360)
12. hydrocarbons (361)
13. sulfur oxides (362)
14. nitrogen oxides (362)
15. sewage (370)
16. soluble wastes (371)
17. thermal pollution (372)
18. soil erosion (375)

Remembering What You Learned

Page numbers in ( ) tell you where to look in the chapter if you need help.

1. What is the effect of air pollution on the environment? (360)

2. How could you be exposed to carbon monoxide without even knowing it? (361)

3. What are some sources of particulates in the air? (361)

4. How does acid rain affect the environment? (362)

5. How does smog form? (363)

6. What are three common forms of air pollution that can damage your lungs? (365–367)

7. What happens when untreated sewage enters a community's water supplies? (370)

8. How do fertilizers used on crops cause water pollution? (371)

9. How does contour plowing reduce soil erosion? (375)

10. How can certain harmless insects be used to reduce the amount of chemical pesticides needed for crops? (376)

11. How does a sanitary landfill prevent rainwater from washing through the buried garbage? (377)

12. What are four environmental health services of a local health department? (383–385)

13. Why is it important that the problem of acid rain be handled on an international level? (386)

Thinking About What You Learned

1. What kind of water pollution, do you think, causes the most problems in your area? Explain.

2. Noise pollution from automobiles and other vehicles is a problem in some communities. How could this problem be reduced?

3. How can your family reduce the amount of garbage it produces that must later be disposed of by the community?

4. Why are so many different health agencies needed to maintain the health of a community?

Writing About What You Learned

1. Write a letter to an imaginary company that is polluting a recreational lake in your community. What solutions would you offer? Give reasons why the company should invest in pollution-reducing equipment.

2. Write a paragraph that evaluates the sentence "Pollution is a necessary result of technology." Use as many examples as possible to make your points.

Applying What You Learned

LANGUAGE ARTS

Select a pollution-related issue, such as whether the advantages of nuclear energy outweigh the problems of nuclear waste disposal. Take a position, and debate the topic with a classmate who takes the opposite position.

Modified True or False

Write the numbers 1 to 15 in your health notebook or on a separate sheet of paper. After each number, write *true* or *false* to describe the sentence. If the sentence is false, also write a term that replaces the underlined term and makes the sentence true.

1. Unwanted substances that can harm your health are <u>pollutants</u>.

2. <u>Smog</u> occurs when a layer of warm air covers a layer of cool air.

3. <u>Carbon monoxide</u> is mainly produced by fuel-burning engines in vehicles and machines.

4. Fuels made of hydrogen and carbon are <u>particulates</u>.

5. <u>Ozone</u> is a compound made of three oxygen atoms.

6. Solid matter that settles from water is called <u>acid rain</u>.

7. <u>Phosphates</u> are soluble wastes from detergents.

8. Adding warm water to a lake or river is <u>temperature inversion</u>.

9. The wearing away of the topsoil is called <u>soil erosion</u>.

10. Effective ways of dealing with solid waste are incineration and <u>dumping</u>.

11. <u>Nuclear wastes</u> are hazardous wastes.

12. <u>Radon</u> gas is a naturally occurring radioactive pollutant.

13. <u>Pasteurization</u> kills disease-causing organisms in milk.

14. <u>Nitric acid</u> is a hydrocarbon.

15. Chemicals that destroy weeds and other unwanted plants are <u>pesticides</u>.

Short Answer

Write the numbers 16 to 23 on your paper. Write a complete sentence to answer each question.

16. What is one way to reduce soil erosion?

17. What are three ways to dispose of solid waste?

18. How is acid rain formed?

19. What is the function of ozone?

20. How do phosphates from detergents pollute the environment?

21. How does clean but warm water harm the natural environment?

22. What kinds of services does a health department provide?

23. What is the source of carbon monoxide pollution?

Essay

Write the numbers 24 and 25 on your paper. Write paragraphs with complete sentences to answer each question.

24. Why should you be concerned about the environments of other countries?

25. What can you do to reduce pollution?

ACTIVITIES FOR HOME OR SCHOOL

Projects to Do

1. Start a family recycling project. Discuss the project with your family, and then take the following steps to ensure success:
   - Locate the community recycling center nearest you.
   - Call the center, and find out what items they accept, how the items should be prepared, and whether the center makes pickups in your neighborhood.
   - Set up a place in your home where used products can be stored. Be sure to rinse out all empty cans and bottles and stack newspapers and magazines neatly.
   - Post a schedule showing when the items should either be delivered to or picked up by the recycling center.

2. Volunteer your services to a community health organization. One way to get started is to call or write your community's volunteer bureau. If your community does not have a bureau, call some organizations directly.

3. Visit a local supermarket. Make a list of all the detergents that contain few or no phosphates. Then check to see which brand of detergent you use at home. If you are currently using a brand that has phosphates, give your family reasons why a different brand should be used.

Information to Find

1. The Environmental Protection Agency (EPA) is a government agency that works to keep the environment clean. Locate the EPA office nearest you, and find out when the agency was formed and what its duties are. Find out what you can do if you see that a business or individual is polluting the environment.

2. The United States government has set aside money for cleaning up areas polluted by hazardous wastes. This fund is called the Superfund. Find out how much money is in the Superfund and how and where the money is being spent.

3. Find information on the careers related to public health and the control of pollution. Select a career that interests you, and find out what skills and education are required. Find out the current career opportunities and the salary range.

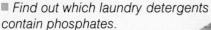

■ *Find out which laundry detergents contain phosphates.*

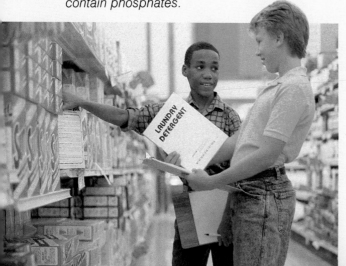

Books to Read

Here are some books you can look for in your school library or the public library to find more information about pollution and managing public resources.

Gay, Kathlyn. *Acid Rain*. Franklin Watts.

Halacy, Dan. *Nuclear Energy*. Franklin Watts.

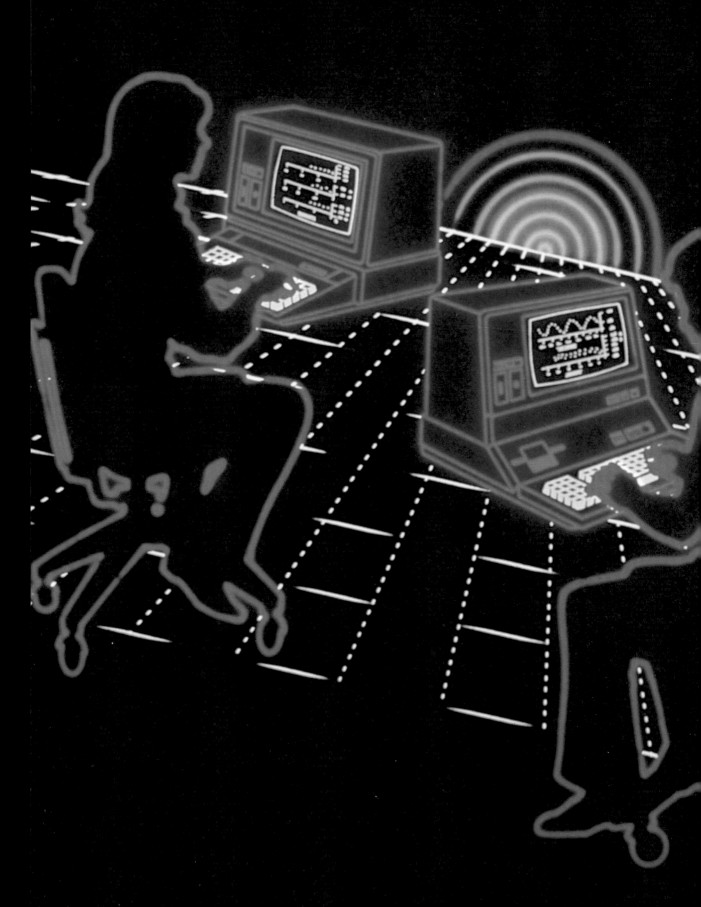

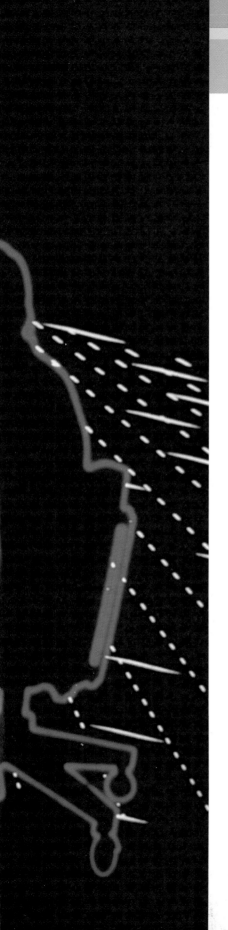

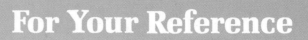

Toll-Free Numbers for Health Information

The following toll-free numbers can provide you with immediate information about health problems or concerns. To call any of these numbers, simply dial 1 and then the number that is listed. Your call will be received by a qualified person who may be able to provide you with the information you need or refer you to someone who can. Do not hesitate to call if you have a question or concern.

General Health	(800) 336-4797		**Headache**	(800) 843-2256
In Maryland	(301) 565-4167			
			Hearing	(800) 222-EARS
AIDS and HIV Infection	(800) 342-AIDS			
In Washington, D.C.	(202) 332-2437		**Learning Disabilities**	(800) ABCD-123
Information in Spanish	(800) 344-SIDA		**(Dyslexia)**	
Auto Safety	(800) 424-9393			
In Washington, D.C.	(202) 366-0123		**Missing Children**	(800) 843-5678
			English and Spanish	
Cancer	(800) 525-3777			
English and Spanish	(800) 4-CANCER		**Pregnancy**	(800) 238-4269
In Alaska	(800) 638-6070			
			Runaway Hotline	(800) 231-6946
Child Abuse	(800) 422-4453			
	(800) 421-0353		**Runaway Switchboard**	(800) 621-4000
Cocaine	(800) COCAINE		**Sexually Transmitted**	(800) 227-8922
			Diseases	
Consumer Product Safety	(800) 638-CPSC			
			Sports and Fitness	(800) 227-3988
Diabetes	(800) 223-1138			
	(800) ADA-DISC		**Teen Crisis (Suicide)**	(800) 621-4000
Drug Abuse	(800) 662-HELP		**Vision Problems**	(800) 232-5463
			In New York	(212) 620-2147
Eating Disorders	(800) 334-8415			

Telephone Etiquette

The following tips will help you communicate effectively when calling any of the numbers listed or when making any other important telephone calls:

■ Before placing a call, spend a few minutes thinking about what you want to say and what you are interested in finding out. You may want to write down your questions on a notepad for ready reference. It is also a good idea to have a notepad and pencil or pen handy for taking notes during the conversation.

■ Select a telephone in a quiet location where you are sure you will not be disturbed.

■ When the party you are calling answers the telephone, give your name immediately: "Hello, my name is Alicia."

■ State the reason you are calling: "I am calling because I would like more information about...."

■ Ask your question or questions. If necessary, refer to your note-pad. After asking a question, be sure to give the person time to answer. Give him or her your undivided attention. If necessary, take notes so you will remember the answer.

■ Upon completing the conversation, thank the person for his or her time and say good-bye in a polite manner.

■ While the information is still fresh in your mind, add to your notes as necessary.

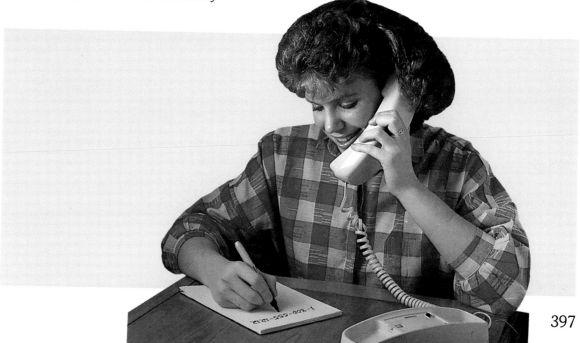

Safety Tips for Baby-sitting

Baby-sitting can be a very rewarding and enjoyable activity. When accepting a job as a baby-sitter, discuss with the parents

- when they expect you to arrive.
- how long they will be away.
- what your responsibilities will be.
- the amount of pay you will receive.
- what arrangements will be made for your transportation to and from home.

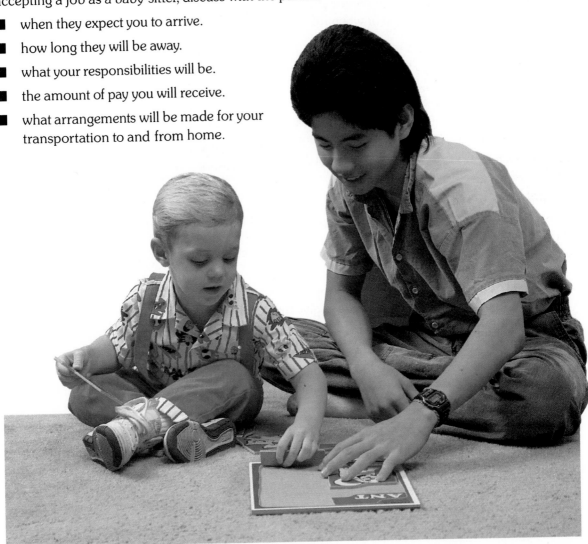

When baby-sitting, your primary concern is for the safety of the children. You are responsible for them, and they depend on you to make safe decisions. The following tips will help you be a successful and safe baby-sitter:

- Arrive for baby-sitting several minutes early so there will be time for the parents to give you important information about the care of their children.

398

- Write down where the parents can be reached.

- Know where emergency telephone numbers, such as those for the fire and police departments and for the children's physician, are located.

- Ask where first-aid supplies and any special medications the children must take are located. Note: You should not give any medications, even children's aspirin or cough syrup, unless specifically directed to do so by either the parents or a physician.

- Ask what and when the children should eat and how the food should be prepared.

- Ask what activities are allowed and preferred before bedtime.

- Ask when the children should go to bed and what the normal routine is for preparing for bed.

Additional Safety Tips

- Never leave an infant alone on a changing table, sofa, or bed.
- Never leave a child at home alone, even for a short time.
- Check children often while they are playing and while they are sleeping.
- Never leave a young child alone in a bathtub.
- Never leave children alone near or in a swimming pool.
- Never let a child play with a plastic bag.
- Keep breakable and dangerous items out of reach of children.
- Know where all the outside doors are and keep them locked.
- Unless the parents have personally given you other instructions, do not unlock the doors for anyone except the parents.
- If the phone rings, take a message in a brief and businesslike manner. Do not tell the caller that you are the baby-sitter or that the parents are out. Simply say that the person asked for is busy now and that you will give him or her the message.
- In case of an accident or illness, depend on parents, neighbors, or emergency personnel instead of trying to handle the situation yourself.

Safety Tips for Being Home Alone

■ Keep the outside doors and windows of your home locked.

■ If someone you do not expect comes to the door, keep the door closed and locked. Ask, "Who is it?" through the closed door. Do not tell the person you are alone. The most you should do is offer to give your parents a message. If the person is selling something, you can simply say, "We're not interested," and nothing more.

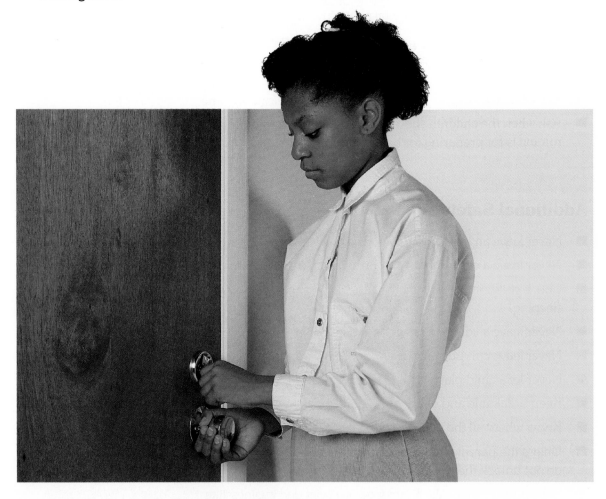

■ If someone calls on the telephone, be polite but do not offer any information. Do not tell the person that you are alone. Say that your parents are busy but you would be glad to take a message.

■ If someone calls who is nasty or mean, hang up immediately. Tell your parents about the call when they get home.

400

- If you suddenly see or smell smoke that has an unknown source, leave the house or apartment immediately. If you live in an apartment, do not take the elevator. Go to a neighbor's house, and call the fire department right away.

- If you have a medical emergency, call 911 or 0 (zero) for the operator. Describe the problem, and give your full name, address, and telephone number. Wait for instructions. Hang up only when told to do so.

- Avoid being bored when you are home alone. Work on a hobby, read books or magazines, do your homework, or clean your room.

- Avoid spending your time alone watching television, unless there is a specific program you and your parents agree you should watch. Do not waste time watching just any program that happens to be on.

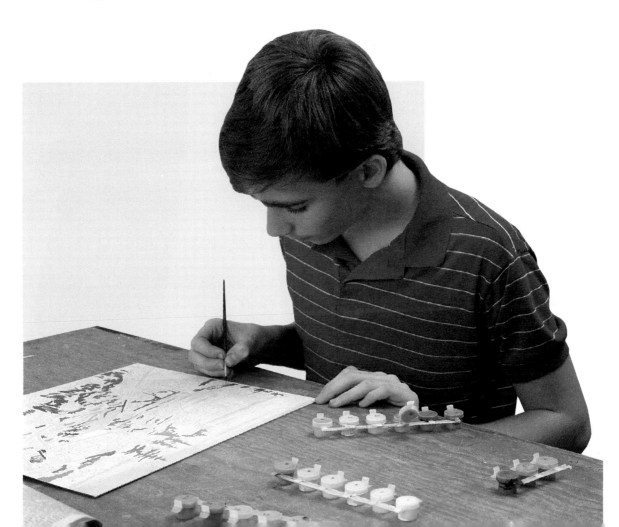

Guidelines for a Healthful Diet

- Eat a variety of healthful foods from the following food groups:
    - Bread, Cereal, Rice, and Pasta Group
    - Vegetable Group
    - Fruit Group
    - Milk, Yogurt, and Cheese Group
    - Meat, Poultry, Fish, Dry Beans, Eggs, and Nuts Group
- Eat few foods that are high in fat content, such as deep-fried foods, butter and other fat-rich dairy products, and red meat.

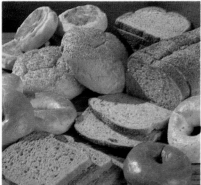 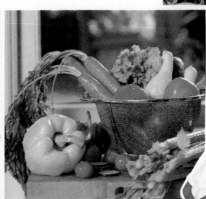

- Eat whole-grain products, vegetables, and fruits. Foods such as whole-grain breads, cereals, potatoes, and fresh vegetables and fruits are high in complex carbohydrates and fiber. Carbohydrates should represent about one-half of your daily calories.
- Achieve and maintain your ideal body weight. You may become overweight by eating more calories than your body uses. You can reduce your weight by eating fewer calories and less fat and by exercising more.
- Limit the amount of sweets that you eat. These foods are high in calories but provide very few nutrients.
- Avoid using additional salt, or sodium, in your diet. Limit your use of the saltshaker, and reduce your intake of foods such as pretzels, salted crackers, dill pickles, and cured or smoked meats.
- Drink plenty of water. Your body needs a ready supply of water to help transport nutrients, eliminate wastes, and regulate body temperature.

402

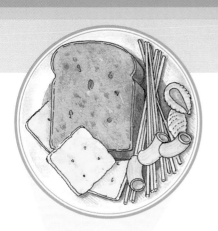
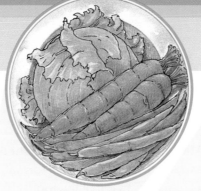
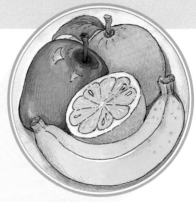

Food Needs of Young People 13 to 19 Years of Age

Food Group	Recommended Daily Amounts	Average Serving
Bread, Cereal, Rice, and Pasta	6– 11 servings	1 slice bread 1 ounce dry cereal 1/2 cup cooked cereal, rice or pasta
Vegetable	3– 5 servings	1 cup raw, leafy vegetables 1/2 cup cooked or chopped raw vegetables 3/4 cup vegetable juice
Fruit	2– 4 servings	1 medium-sized apple, banana, or orange 1/2 cup chopped, cooked, or canned fruit 3/4 cup fruit juice
Milk, Yogurt, and Cheese	2– 3 servings	1 cup milk or yogurt 1 1/2 ounce natural cheese 2 ounces processed cheese
Meat, Poultry, Fish, Dry Beans, Eggs, and Nuts	2– 3 servings	2–3 ounces cooked lean meat, poultry, or fish 1/2 cup cooked dry beans, 1 egg, or 2 tablespoons peanut butter count as 1 ounce lean meat

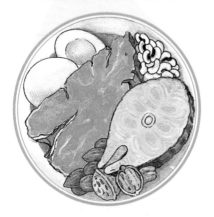
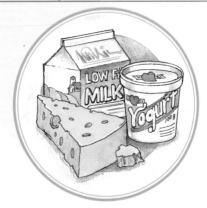

Healthful Snacks

   Your health and growth depend greatly on the foods you eat. Therefore, you should try to eat the most nutritious and healthful foods that you can. This applies whether you are eating a formal meal or just having a snack. Unfortunately, many of the foods that are often eaten as snacks are not very healthful. They contain many calories and few or no nutrients. The foods listed here will help you to "snack smart." These foods are easy to find, nutritious, and taste great!

Crunchies

Apples and pears
Broccoli spears
Carrot and celery sticks
Cauliflower chunks
Green-pepper sticks
Radishes
Unsalted rice cakes
Zucchini slices

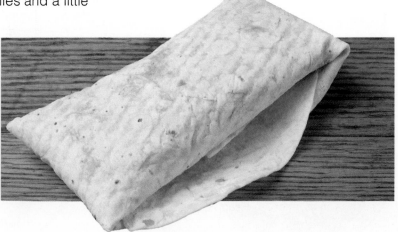

Hot Stuff

Soups: clear soups, homemade vegetable or tomato soup
Cocoa made with nonfat milk
Tortillas topped with green chilies and a little
     grated mozzarella

Munchies

Almonds and walnuts

Bagels

Bread sticks

Popcorn (prepared without butter, margarine, oil, or salt)

Mixture of 2 cups soy nuts, 2 cups raw peanuts roasted in oven, and 1 cup raisins or other dried fruit

Mozzarella (made from part-skim milk)

Unsalted sunflower seeds

Whole-grain breads

Thirst Quenchers

Nonfat milk or buttermilk

Unsweetened juices

Unsweetened fruit juice concentrate mixed with club soda

Sweet Stuff

Baked apple (plain— without sugar or pastry)

Dried fruit

Fresh fruit

Raisins

Thin slice of angel food cake

Unsweetened canned fruit

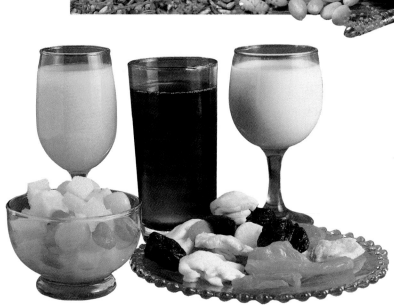

Adapted from *Nutritious Nibbles: A Guide to Healthy Snacking* (Retitled: "Healthful Snacks"). Copyright © 1984 by American Heart Association. Reprinted by permission of American Heart Association.

Nutritional Information on Common Foods

Using the following chart, you can determine the nutritional value of many common foods. The foods are grouped into the following six groups: Meat, Poultry, Fish, Dry Beans, Eggs, and Nuts Group; Fruit Group; Vegetable Group; Milk, Yogurt, and Cheese Group; Bread, Cereal, Rice, and Pasta Group; and Fats, Oils, and Sweets Group. A seventh group is included that provides information about common restaurant foods.

Food	Portion	Food Energy	Protein	Fat Total/ Saturated	Carbo- hydrate	Major Vitamins and/or Minerals
Meat, Poultry Fish, Dry Beans, Eggs, and Nuts Group		Calories	Grams	Grams		Grams
Bologna	2 slices	170	6	16/6	Trace	Iron
Chicken breast, fried	2.8 oz	160	26	5/1.4	1	Phosphorus, Iron, Vitamin A, Vitamin B_2, Niacin
Chicken leg, fried	1.3 oz	90	12	4/1.2	Trace	Phosphorus, Iron, Vitamin B_2, Niacin
Chicken half, broiled	6.2 oz	240	42	7/2.2	0	Phosphorus, Iron, Vitamin A, Vitamin B_2, Niacin
Chicken chow mein, canned	1 cup	95	7	Trace	18	Vitamin A, Vitamin C
Egg, fried in butter	1 egg	85	5	6/2.4	1	Phosphorus, Vitamin A
Egg, hard cooked	1 egg	80	6	6/1.7	1	Phosphorus, Iron, Vitamin A, Vitamin B_2
Fish sticks, breaded	2 sticks	100	10	6/0	4	Phosphorus
Frankfurter	1 frank	170	7	15/5.6	1	Phosphorus, Iron, Vitamin B_2, Niacin
Ground beef, 10% fat	3 oz	185	23	10/4	0	Phosphorus, Iron, Vitamin B_2, Niacin
Ground beef, 21% fat	2.9 oz	235	20	17/7.0	0	Phosphorus, Iron, Vitamin B_2, Niacin
Ham, boiled	1 slice	65	5	5/1.7	0	Vitamin B_1
Peanut butter	1 tbsp	95	4	8/1.5	3	Niacin
Pork chop, broiled	2.7 oz	305	19	25/8.9	0	Phosphorus, Iron, Vitamin B_1, Vitamin B_2, Niacin
Roast beef, lean and fat	3 oz	165	25	7/2.8	0	Phosphorus, Iron, Vitamin B_2, Niacin
Sirloin steak	3 oz	330	20	27/11.3	0	Phosphorus, Iron, Vitamin B_2, Niacin
Salmon, canned	3 oz	120	17	5/.9	0	Calcium, Phosphorus, Vitamin B_2, Niacin
Tuna, canned in oil, drained	3 oz	170	24	7/1.7	0	Phosphorus, Iron, Vitamin A, Niacin
Turkey, roasted	3 slices	160	27	5/1.5	0	Phosphorus, Iron, Vitamin B_2, Niacin

REFERENCE

Food	Portion	Food Energy	Protein	Fat Total/Saturated	Carbohydrate	Major Vitamins and/or Minerals
Fruit Group		Calories	Grams	Grams		Grams
Apples, raw	1 apple	80	Trace	1/0	20	Vitamin A, Vitamin C
Apple juice	1 cup	120	Trace	Trace/0	30	Iron
Bananas	1 banana	100	1	Trace/0	26	Vitamin A, Vitamin C
Fruit cocktail, canned	1 cup	195	1	Trace/0	50	Iron, Vitamin A, Vitamin C
Grapefruit, raw	1/2 fruit	50	1	Trace/0	13	Vitamin A, Vitamin C
Grapes	10 grapes	35	Trace	Trace/0	9	Vitamin A, Vitamin C
Cantaloupe	1/2 fruit	80	2	Trace/0	20	Iron, Vitamin A, Niacin, Vitamin C
Oranges, raw	1 orange	65	1	Trace/0	16	Vitamin A, Vitamin B$_1$, Vitamin C
Orange juice, from frozen concentrate	1 cup	120	2	Trace/0	29	Vitamin A, Vitamin B$_1$, Vitamin C
Peaches, canned with water	1 cup	75	1	Trace/0	20	Vitamin A, Niacin, Vitamin C
Pears, raw	1 pear	100	1	1/0	25	Vitamin C
Pineapple, canned in heavy syrup	1 cup	190	1	Trace/1	49	Vitamin A, Vitamin B$_1$, Vitamin C
Raisins, seedless	1½ oz	40	Trace	Trace/0	11	Iron
Strawberries, raw	1 cup	55	1	1/0	13	Iron, Vitamin A, Vitamin C
Watermelon	1 wedge	110	2	1/0	27	Iron, Vitamin A, Vitamin B$_1$, Vitamin C
Vegetable Group		Calories	Grams	Grams		Grams
Broccoli, cooked	1 cup	40	5	Trace/0	7	Calcium, Phosphorus, Iron, Vitamin A, Vitamin B$_1$, Vitamin B$_2$, Vitamin C
Cabbage, shredded	1 cup	15	1	Trace/0	4	Vitamin A, Vitamin C
Carrots, raw	1 carrot	30	1	Trace/0	7	Vitamin A, Vitamin C
Celery, raw	1 stalk	5	Trace	Trace/0	2	Vitamin A
Corn, canned	1 cup	175	5	1/0	43	Phosphorus, Iron, Vitamin A, Niacin, Vitamin C

407

Food	Portion	Food Energy	Protein	Fat Total/Saturated	Carbo-hydrate	Major Vitamins and/or Minerals
Vegetable Group		Calories	Grams	Grams		Grams
Cucumber slices	6 slices	5	Trace	Trace/0	1	Vitamin A
Green beans	1 cup	30	2	Trace/0	7	Vitamin A, Vitamin C
Lettuce	1 cup	5	Trace	Trace/0	2	Vitamin A
Peas, green, frozen	1 cup	110	8	Trace/0	19	Phosphorus, Iron, Niacin, Vitamin A, Vitamin B_1, Vitamin B_2, Vitamin C
Potatoes, baked	1 potato	145	4	Trace/0	33	Phosphorus, Iron, Vitamin B_1, Niacin, Vitamin C
Potatoes, french fried	10 fries	135	2	7/1.7	18	Niacin, Vitamin C
Potato chips	10 chips	115	1	8/2.1	10	Niacin, Vitamin C
Tomatoes	1 tomato	25	1	Trace/0	6	Vitamin A, Vitamin C
Milk, Yogurt, and Cheese Group		Calories	Grams	Grams		Grams
Cheddar cheese	1 oz	115	7	9/6.1	Trace	Calcium, Phosphorus, Vitamin A
Cottage cheese	1 cup	205	31	4/2.8	8	Calcium, Phosphorus, Vitamin A, Vitamin B_2
Mozzarella cheese, part skim milk	1 oz	80	8	4/3.1	1	Calcium, Phosphorus, Vitamin A
American cheese	1 oz	105	6	9/5.6	Trace	Calcium, Phosphorus, Vitamin A
Swiss cheese	1 oz	95	7	7/4.5	1	Calcium, Phosphorus, Vitamin A
Whole milk	1 cup	150	8	8/5.1	11	Calcium, Phosphorus, Vitamin A, Vitamin B_2
Low-fat milk (2% fat)	1 cup	120	8	5/2.9	12	Calcium, Phosphorus, Vitamin A, Vitamin B_2
Skim milk	1 cup	85	8	Trace/.3	12	Calcium, Phosphorus, Vitamin A, Vitamin B_2
Chocolate milk	1 cup	210	8	8/5.3	26	Calcium, Phosphorus, Vitamin A, Vitamin B_2
Ice cream, hardened	1 cup	270	5	14/8.9	32	Calcium, Phosphorus, Vitamin A, Vitamin B_2
Ice cream, soft serve	1 cup	375	7	23/13.5	38	Calcium, Phosphorus, Vitamin A, Vitamin B_2
Yogurt, fruit flavored	8 oz	320	10	3/1.8	42	Calcium, Phosphorus, Vitamin A, Vitamin B_2
Yogurt, plain	8 oz	145	12	4/2.3	16	Calcium, Phosphorus, Vitamin A, Vitamin B_2

Food	Portion	Food Energy	Protein	Fat Total/ Saturated	Carbo- hydrate	Major Vitamins and/or Minerals
Bread, Cereal Rice and Pasta Group		Calories	Grams	Grams		Grams
Bagels	1 bagel	165	6	2/0.5	28	Iron, Vitamin B_1
Biscuits, from a mix	1 biscuit	90	2	3/0.6	15	Phosphorus
Bread, enriched white	1 slice	70	2	1/0.2	13	Vitamin B_1
Bread, whole-wheat	1 slice	60	3	1/0.1	12	Phosphorus
Oatmeal	1 cup	130	5	2/0.4	23	Phosphorus, Iron, Vitamin B_1
Cornflakes	1 cup	95	2	Trace/0	21	Vitamin A, Vitamin B_1, Vitamin B_2, Vitamin C
Wheat flakes	1 cup	105	3	Trace/0	24	Phosphorus, Vitamin A, Vitamin B_1, Vitamin B_2, Niacin, Vitamin C
Angel food cake	1 piece	135	3	Trace/0	32	Calcium, Phosphorus
Brownies with nuts	1 brownie	95	1	6/1.5	10	Vitamin A
Chocolate chip cookies	4 cookies	205	2	12/3.5	24	Phosphorus, Iron, Vitamin A
Macaroni and cheese	1 cup	430	17	22/8.9	40	Calcium, Phosphorus, Iron, Vitamin A, Vitamin B_1, Vitamin B_2, Niacin
Pancakes, from a mix	1 pan-cake	60	2	2/0.7	9	Vitamin A
Popcorn	1 cup	25	1	Trace/Tr	5	Phosphorus
Rice, instant	1 cup	180	4	Trace/Tr	40	Iron, Niacin
Waffles, from mix	1 waffle	205	7	8/2.8	27	Calcium, Phosphorus, Iron, Vitamin A, Vitamin B_1, Vitamin B_2
Spaghetti, enriched	1 cup	140	5	1/0	32	Iron, Vitamin B_1, Niacin
Fats, Oils, and Sweets Group		Calories	Grams	Grams		Grams
Bacon, broiled or fried	4 slices	170	8	16/5	Trace	Iron, Vitamin B_1, Niacin
Butter	1 tbsp	100	Trace	12/7.2	Trace	Vitamin A
Margarine, stick	1 tbsp	100	Trace	12/2.1	Trace	Vitamin A
Margarine, whipped	1 tbsp	65	Trace	8/4.7	Trace	Vitamin A
Mayonnaise	1 tbsp	100	Trace	11/2.0	Trace	Vitamin A
Sour cream	1 cup	495	7	48/30	10	Calcium, Phosphorus, Vitamin A, Vitamin B_2

Food	Portion	Food Energy	Protein	Fat Total/ Saturated	Carbo- hydrate	Major Vitamins and/or Minerals
Common Restaurant Foods		Calories	Grams	Grams	Grams	
Beef and vegetable stew	1 cup	220	16	11/4.9	15	Phosphorus, Iron, Vitamin A, Vitamin B_1, Vitamin B_2, Niacin, Vitamin C
Potato salad with cooked salad dressing	1 cup	250	7	7/2.0	41	Calcium, Phosphorus, Iron, Vitamin A, Vitamin B_1, Vitamin B_2, Niacin, Vitamin C
Chicken noodle soup	1 cup	55	2	1/0	8	Vitamin A
Spaghetti with meatballs	1 cup	330	19	12/3.3	391	Calcium, Phosphorus, Iron, Vitamin A, Vitamin B_1, Vitamin B_2, Niacin, Vitamin C
Pizza	1 slice	145	6	4/1.7	22	Calcium, Phosphorus, Iron, Vitamin A, Vitamin B_1, Vitamin B_2, Niacin
Cheeseburger	1/4 lb	580	33	34/17	34	Calcium, Phosphorus, Iron, Vitamin A, Vitamin B_1, Vitamin B_2, Niacin
Hamburger	1/4 lb	470	26	26/11	33	Phosphorus, Iron, Vitamin B_1, Vitamin B_2, Niacin
Hot dog	1	190	10	17/6.1	22	Phosphorus, Iron, Vitamin B_1, Vitamin B_2, Niacin, Vitamin C
Bean burrito	1	350	15	11/7	48	Phosphorus, Iron, Vitamin A, Vitamin B_1, Vitamin B_2, Niacin, Vitamin C
Taco	1	370	20	20/11	26	Calcium, Phosphorus, Iron, Vitamin A, Vitamin B_1, Vitamin B_2, Niacin
French fries	regular order	220	3	11/5	26	Calcium, Iron, Vitamin B_1, Vitamin B_2, Vitamin C
Onion rings	1 order	351	5	16/7	32	Vitamin B_1, Iron, Niacin

Food	Portion	Food Energy	Protein	Fat Total/ Saturated	Carbo- hydrate	Major Vitamins and/or Minerals
Common Restaurant Foods		Calories	Grams	Grams	Grams	
Banana split	1	612	12	15/8	101	Phosphorus, Iron, Vitamin A, Vitamin B_1, Vitamin B_2, Niacin, Vitamin C
Coffee (black)	6 oz	3	Trace	Trace	0	No significant nutrients
Milk shake (vanilla)	10 oz	314	10	10/5	50	Calcium, Phosphorus, Vitamin A
Soft drink (cola)	12 oz	145	0	0	37	Phosphorus
Soft drink (fruit flavor)	12 oz	170	0	0	45	Phosphorus

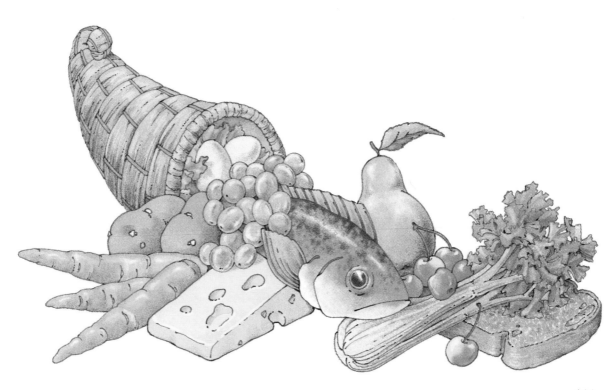

Guidelines for Safe Exercise

REFERENCE

Exercise is a necessary part of a healthful life-style. Exercise can help you tone your muscles and improve your cardiovascular system. Exercise can also help you look and feel your best.

- Start each workout by doing warm-up exercises. First, spend a few minutes stretching your muscles as shown on pages 414 to 416. These exercises will improve your flexibility. Then spend a few minutes gradually working into the main activity of your workout. By taking it slowly, you will gradually increase your heart rate and prepare yourself for vigorous exercise. An adequate warm-up will reduce your chances of injury during the workout and will make the workout less of a strain and more enjoyable.

- Set realistic goals for the workout. Do not try to do too much too fast.

- Stop exercising if pain occurs. Continuing to exercise while in pain may lead to serious injuries.

- Avoid exercising in high-heat situations. If you are not used to the heat, exercise less than your normal amount.

- Drink plenty of fluids, particularly water.

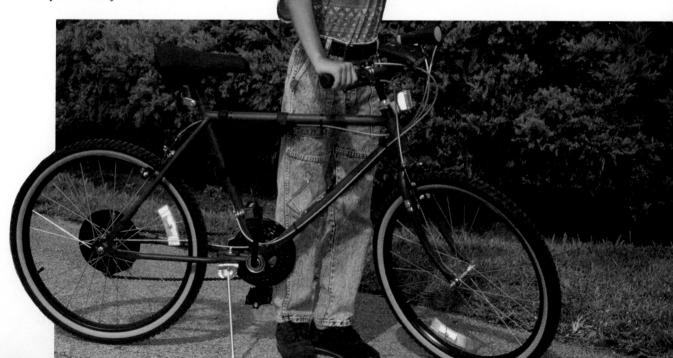

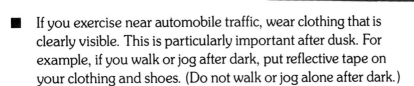

- In cold weather, wear layers of clothing when exercising. That way you can take off a layer at a time as you get warm. Wear a hat when exercising outdoors in cold weather.

- Do not do vigorous exercises immediately before or after a meal. It is best to exercise at least one hour before or two hours after eating.

- Avoid exercising on extremely hard surfaces, such as concrete. Surfaces with more "give," such as grass, dirt, and wooden floors, are easier on the joints of your body. Also avoid exercising on an uneven surface, which may cause you to fall and injure yourself.

- Wear shoes that are comfortable and suited to the type of exercise you are doing. The shoes should provide necessary cushioning and support.

- If you exercise near automobile traffic, wear clothing that is clearly visible. This is particularly important after dusk. For example, if you walk or jog after dark, put reflective tape on your clothing and shoes. (Do not walk or jog alone after dark.)

- At the end of your exercise routine, spend a few minutes doing cool-down exercises. Your cool-down should be the opposite of your warm-up. Gradually decrease the vigor of your workout to slowly decrease your heart rate. Then finish with at least two minutes of flexibility exercises.

- Get plenty of rest and sleep between workouts.

Warm-Up and Cool-Down Exercises

Every workout should begin with warm-up exercises and end with cool-down exercises. Start your warm-up by doing the flexibility exercises shown here. Spend at least two minutes doing these nine exercises. Then spend another few minutes easing into the main activity of your workout. This portion of your workout increases your heart rate gradually. At the end of your warm-up, you will be ready to begin the vigorous portion of your workout. Your muscles will be flexible, and your heart rate will be at a safe level.

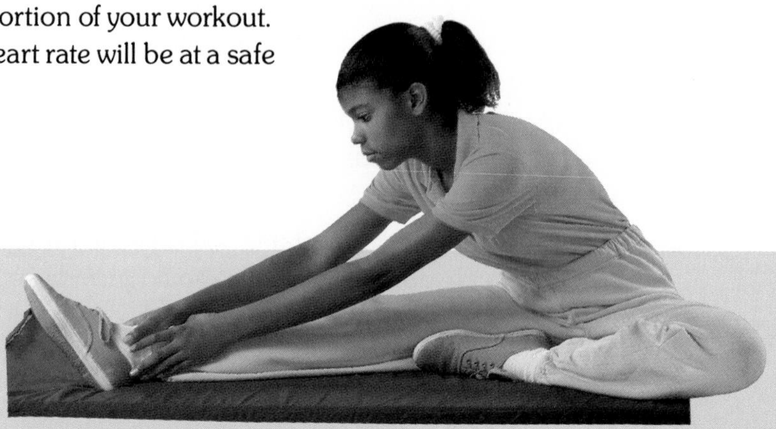

Hurdler's Stretch

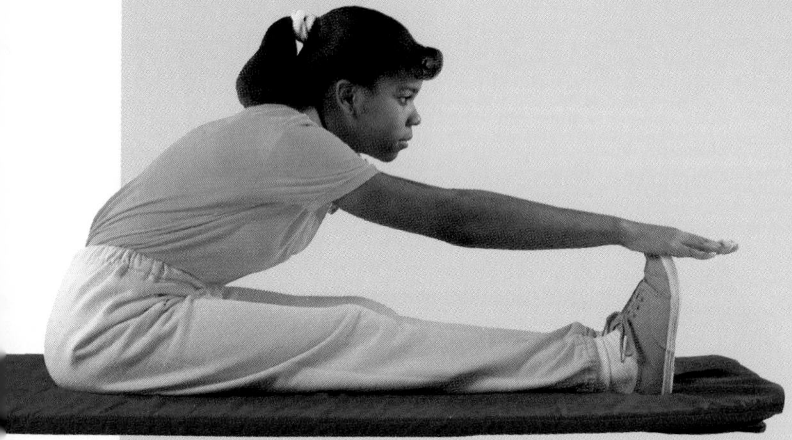

Sit-and-Reach Stretch (Low Back and Hamstring Stretch)

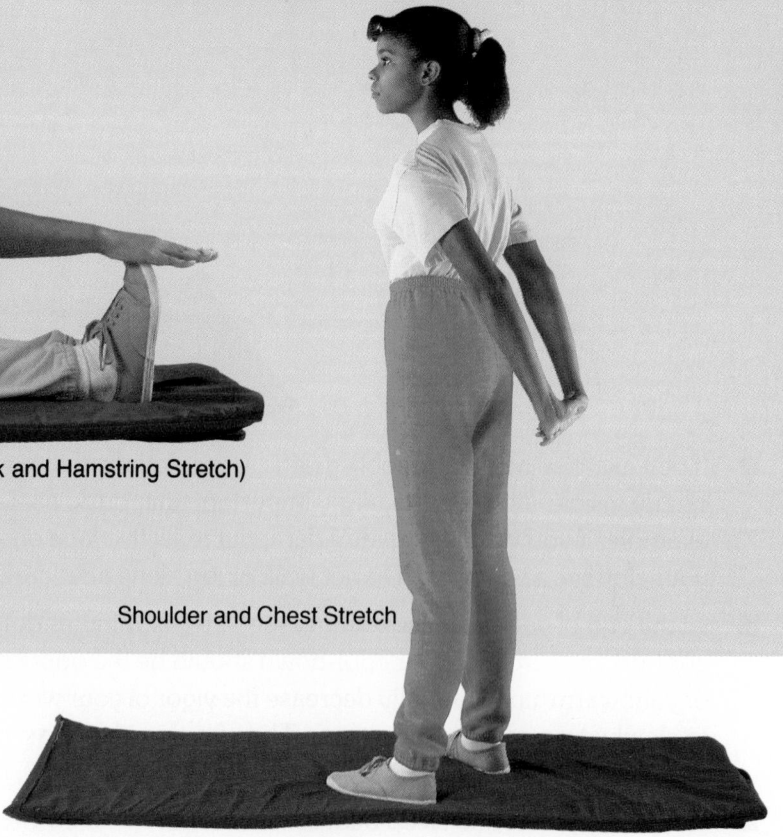

Shoulder and Chest Stretch

414

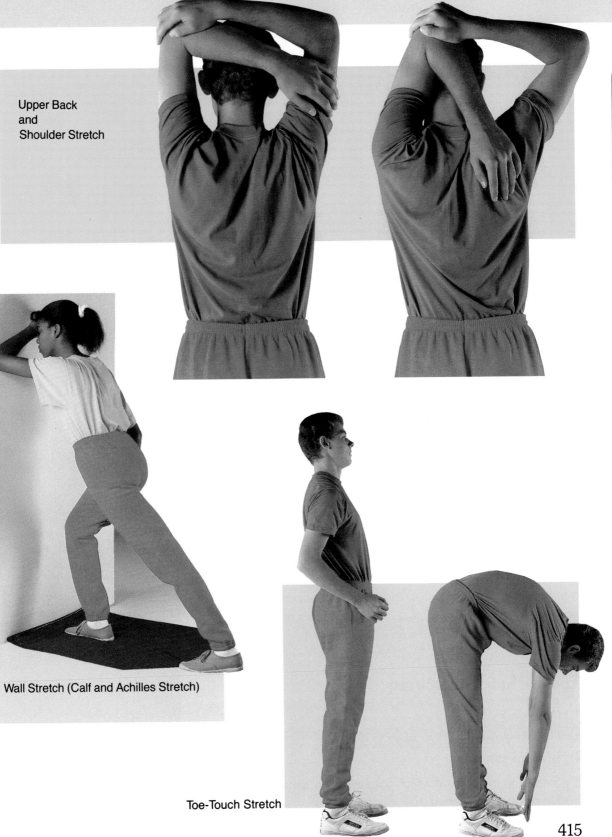

Upper Back
and
Shoulder Stretch

Wall Stretch (Calf and Achilles Stretch)

Toe-Touch Stretch

415

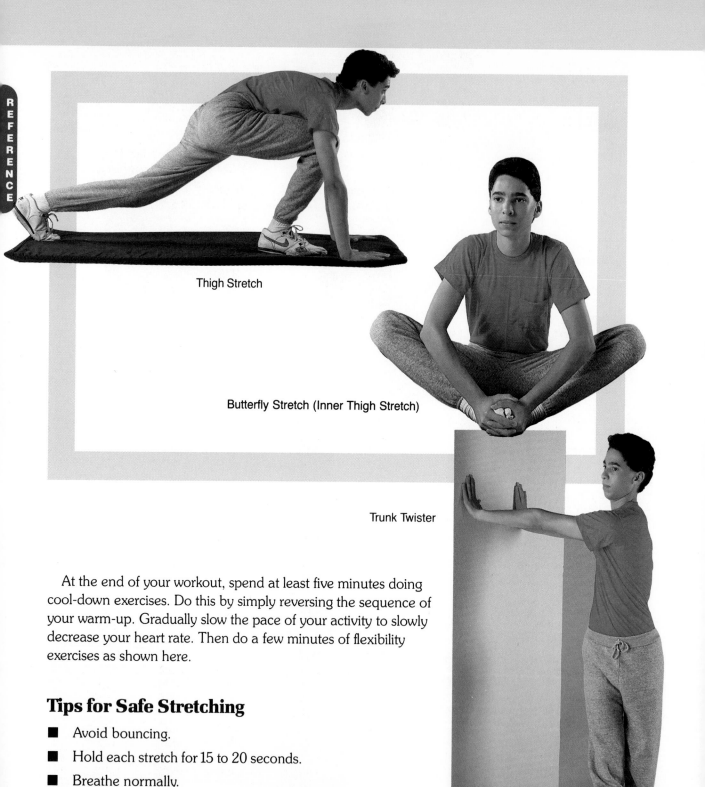

Thigh Stretch

Butterfly Stretch (Inner Thigh Stretch)

Trunk Twister

At the end of your workout, spend at least five minutes doing cool-down exercises. Do this by simply reversing the sequence of your warm-up. Gradually slow the pace of your activity to slowly decrease your heart rate. Then do a few minutes of flexibility exercises as shown here.

Tips for Safe Stretching

- Avoid bouncing.
- Hold each stretch for 15 to 20 seconds.
- Breathe normally.
- Stretch to the point at which you feel a slight pull. Do not stretch so hard that you feel pain.

Benefits of Various Sports and Activities

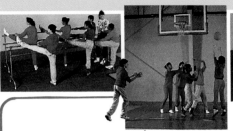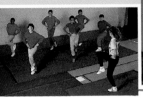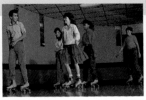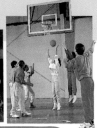

| Activity | Health and Fitness Rating | | | Calories Used per Hour by a Person Weighing: | | |
	Endurance	Strength	Flexibility	77 lbs. (35 kg)	99 lbs. (45 kg)	110 lbs. (50 kg)
Aerobic dancing	High	Low	High	405	480	515
Archery	Low	Low	Low	195	230	245
Badminton	Medium	Low	Low	215	255	277
Backpacking	Medium	High	Low	375	435	470
Baseball*	Low	Low	Low	175	205	220
Basketball*	High	Medium	Medium	345	405	435
Bicycling						
(moderate)	High	Medium	Low	150	175	190
(vigorous)	High	High	Low	410	480	515
Billiards	Low	Low	Low	105	120	130
Bowling	Low	Low	Low	165	195	210
Canoeing	Low	Medium	Low	390	460	490
Fencing	Medium	Low	Medium	185	220	235
Football*	High	High	Medium	520	610	660
Golf	Low	Low	Low	235	275	295
Gymnastics*	Medium	High	High	165	195	210
Handball	High	Medium	Medium	485	565	610
Hockey	High	Medium	Medium	385	455	485
Jogging (5.5 mph)	High	High	Low	405	480	515
Judo/Karate	Low	Medium	Medium	490	575	620
Jumping rope	High	Medium	Low	865	1015	1090
Racquetball	High	Medium	Medium	340	410	450
Skating						
(ice and roller)	Medium	Medium	Low	215	255	275
Skateboarding	Low	Low	Low	150	175	190
Skiing						
(downhill)	Low	Medium	Low	370	435	465
(cross-country)	High	High	Low	435	510	550
Soccer	High	Medium	Medium	375	435	470
Swimming	High	Medium	High	185	220	235
Table tennis	Low	Low	Low	185	220	235
Tennis	Medium	Medium	Low	265	310	335
Volleyball	Medium	Low	Low	215	255	275
Walking (briskly)	High	Low	Low	165	205	225
Watching TV	Low	Low	Low	50	55	60
Waterskiing	Low	Medium	Low	255	305	335
Weight training	Low	High	Low	235	280	300
Wrestling*	Medium	High	High	490	575	620

*Preparing for these and a few other sports often includes special training that increases cardiovascular fitness, strength, and flexibility. The ratings in this chart are based only on the activity identified. The ratings do not account for any specialized training.

Directory of Diseases and Disorders

Diseases	Cause/ Transmission	Symptoms	Treatment/ Prevention
Acne	Bacteria, increased testosterone during puberty	Pimples, whiteheads, and blackheads on skin	Treated and prevented with frequent washing of skin with mild or medicated soap and shampooing of hair; severe cases may require antibiotic, or vitamin A, or other treatment.
Acquired Immunodeficiency Syndrome (AIDS) (HIV infection)	HIV (viral) infection; transmitted by blood-to-blood contact, sexual contact, sharing of hypodermic needles, and contact between pregnant woman and her baby	Extreme fatigue, inability to fight infections, certain cancerous tumors	No treatment available; can be prevented by avoiding contact with virus
Alcoholism	Unknown; possibly due to hereditary and psychological factors	Inability to control drinking of alcohol; all body systems affected	Professional treatment; support groups like Alcoholics Anonymous
Alzheimer's Disease	Unknown; possibly hereditary	Progressive memory loss and confusion	No known treatment or prevention
Anorexia Nervosa (eating disorder)	Psychological factors; usually begins during adolescence	Starvation, malnutrition, hormone imbalance	Treated with hospitalization and psychological counseling
Anemia	Usually due to low number of red blood cells or low amount of hemoglobin	Tiredness, pale color, fast heart rate	Treated with increased dietary iron; medical care for nondiet causes; prevented with an iron-rich diet
Allergy	Exposure to air-borne allergens, such as pollen	Frequent sneezing; runny nose; red, itchy, watery eyes	Treated with antihistamines to prevent or stop attacks
Appendicitis (inflamed appendix)	Unknown; probably caused by obstruction	Nausea, vomiting, fever, severe pain in lower right abdomen	Treated by surgical removal of appendix; no known prevention

418

Diseases	Cause/Transmission	Symptoms	Treatment/Prevention
Asthma	Airway blockage caused by an allergy	Periodic breathing difficulty, cough, wheezing	Treated with medications; no known prevention
Astigmatism	Uneven curvature of cornea, usually present at birth	Distorted vision	Treated with eyeglasses or contact lenses; no known prevention
Atherosclerosis	Thickening of the walls of arteries caused by cholesterol and other fats	Reduced blood flow in arteries, usually to brain and legs; complications include stroke and coronary artery disease	Treated with drugs and surgery; prevented by eating foods high in fiber and low in animal-fats, exercising regularly, and not smoking
Athlete's Foot	Fungal infection spread through contact with wet surfaces	Red, itchy, cracked skin on feet, especially between toes	Treated with antifungal medication; prevented by keeping skin clean and dry
Boils	Bacterial infection	Hard, swollen areas of the skin filled with pus; can affect all layers of skin	Treated with warm soaks for minor infections; more serious infections may require lancing and antibiotics
Bulimia (eating disorder)	Psychological factors; usually begins during adolescence	Excessive eating followed by self-induced vomiting	Treated with special diet and psychological counseling
Cancer	Cancer-causing substances start about 80 percent of cancers; viral infection may be another cause	Symptoms vary with the type and location of the cancer	Treated with chemotherapy, radiation, and surgery; prevented by avoiding cancer-causing substances and sun damage
Cerebral Palsy	Abnormal brain development or brain damage before, at, or after birth	Stiffening and spasms of limbs; distortion of speech, hearing, and vision	Treated with training to help the patient learn to function with the disorder; no known prevention

Diseases	Cause/Transmission	Symptoms	Treatment/Prevention
Chicken Pox	Viral infection; spread by droplets from mouth and nose	Fever, headache, itchy blisters on skin that leave scars if scratched	Treated in severe cases with antihistamine to relieve itching; experimental vaccine may provide prevention
Chlamydia	Microbe; spread by contact (especially sexual contact) with infected person	Eye infection; drainage from reproductive organs	Treated with antibiotics; prevented by avoiding contact with infected person
Chronic Bronchitis	Viral or bacterial infection; may be caused by an allergy to certain substances, such as tobacco smoke	Inflammation of membranes lining bronchi; deep cough with grayish or yellow sputum, breathlessness, wheezing, fever	Treated with rest, cough suppressants, and antibiotics; prevented by avoiding smoke and other allergens
Cold	Viral infection; spread by droplets from mouth and nose	Stuffy or runny nose, sneezing, sore throat, coughing	Treated with extra rest, extra liquids, and non-aspirin medications; no known prevention
Conjunctivitis (pinkeye)	Bacterial infection or viral allergy; spread through contact with contaminated articles	Itchy, reddened lining of eyelids; drainage from eye	Treated with antibiotic or other eyedrops or ointment; prevented by keeping hands clean and not sharing towels and other personal items
Coronary Artery Disease	Reduction or stoppage of flow of blood through coronary arteries	No symptoms in early stages; chest pain, heart attack	Treated and prevented by following a low-cholesterol, low-salt diet, getting regular exercise, and not smoking
Cystic Fibrosis	Hereditary	Weight loss, respiratory infection, cough, fever, malnutrition	Treated with extracts of animal pancreas, daily respiratory therapy, and antibiotics; no known prevention

Diseases	Cause/Transmission	Symptoms	Treatment/Prevention
Diabetes	Heredity, obesity, disorders of pancreas	Sugar in urine; increased sugar in blood; excessive urination, thirst, and hunger; weight loss; itching; coma	Treated with special diet, insulin therapy, or both; no known prevention, except avoidance of obesity
Down Syndrome	Chromosomal disorder	Mental retardation, with typical physical features and often a heart defect	Treated with special training programs
Dysentery	Protozoan or bacterial infection	Severe, often bloody diarrhea, cramps	Treated with antiamoebic medications or antibiotics and replacement of body fluids; prevented by avoiding unsanitary food and water
Epilepsy	Usually unknown; sometimes results from infection or head injury	Periodic convulsive seizures	Treated with drug therapy to control seizures; no known prevention
"Flu"	(see influenza)		
Food Poisoning (botulism, salmonella, shigella, staph)	Bacterial infections from toxins produced by bacteria	Vomiting, stomach cramps, diarrhea, nausea	Treated with medication to relieve vomiting and diarrhea; prevented by avoiding spoiled foods
Gingivitus	Poor dental hygiene	Swollen gums that bleed easily	Treated and prevented by flossing daily and brushing properly
Gonorrhea	Bacterial infection; spread by sexual contact with infected person	Pus discharge from external sex organs; abdominal pain, painful urination; sterility if untreated	Treated with antibiotics; prevented by avoiding sexual contact with infected person
Heart Attack	Blockage of a coronary artery by blood clot	Crushing pain in center of chest, dizziness, shortness of breath, sweating, chills, nausea, fainting, shock, heart failure	Treated with drug therapy, surgery and rest; prevented by following a healthful life style

Diseases	Cause/ Transmission	Symptoms	Treatment/ Prevention
Hepatitis (viral)	Type A spread by food, contact with infected urine and intestinal waste. Type B spread through blood and sexual contact	Enlarged liver; nausea, vomiting; yellow tint to skin and whites of eyes	Treated with bed rest and special diet; Type A is prevented by washing hands before eating; type B is prevented by avoiding blood and sexual contact with infected persons
Herpes Simplex Type 1	Viral infection	Blisters on lips and mouth that are filled with clear liquid and become encrusted	No known treatment or prevention
Herpes Simplex Type 2	Viral infection; spread by sexual contact	Painful blisters on sex organs, fever, headache, tiredness	Treated by cleansing infected areas with soap and water; cannot be cured; prevented by avoiding sexual contact with infected person
Hypertension (high blood pressure)	Heredity, hormonal imbalance, kidney disease, obesity, nicotine, stress	No symptoms unless blood pressure is very high; then headaches, palpitations	Treated and prevented by low-salt diet, reduction of stress, medications to regulate blood pressure, exercise, weight control
Influenza	Viral infection; spread by droplets from mouth and nose	Muscle aches, fever, headache, cough	Treated with extra rest, extra liquids, and non-aspirin medication
Laryngitis	Bacterial or viral infection; irritation from allergy, or overuse of voice	Hoarseness, temporary loss of voice	Treated by resting voice and with medications; prevented by avoiding straining voice
Leukemia	Unknown; possibly caused by certain chemicals and radiation	Weakness, pain in bones, infections, fever, mouth and lip ulcers, tendency to bruise and bleed	Treated with radiation therapy, antileukemic drugs; no known prevention

Diseases	Cause/ Transmission	Symptoms	Treatment/ Prevention
Lyme disease	Microorganisms (bacteria) that are passed to humans from bite of tick	Rash, fever, inflamed knee and ankle joints, headache, memory lapses, depression, poor muscle control	Treated with antibiotics in early stages; prevented by wearing long pants tucked into socks when in wooded areas
Measles (10 day measles)	Virus, spreads by droplets from mouth and nose	Fever, rash, watery eyes, dry cough; can have serious complications	Prevented with vaccine at 15 months of age
Migraine headache	Individual factors cause narrowing and then swelling of arteries that lead to the brain	Severe headache, nausea, visual problems, sensitivity to light and sound	Treated with relaxation in dark room, prescribed medicines; prevented by controlling factors that cause headache
Mononucleosis	Unknown; probably by direct contact such as kissing	Enlarged lymph nodes, fever, enlarged spleen, sore throat, aching joints, weakness	Treated with rest and fluids; prevented by avoiding contact with infected person
Multiple Sclerosis	Unknown; possibly an immune system abnormality	Weakness in limbs, unsteadiness, blurred vision, slurred speech, muscle spasms	Treated with physical therapy and emotional support; no known prevention
Mumps	Viral infection	Swollen salivary glands, fever, feeling of illness, pain when chewing and swallowing	Treated with rest; prevented with vaccine at 15 months of age
Muscular Dystrophy	Unknown; sometimes hereditary	Progressive weakening of muscles until walking and breathing become difficult	Treated with physical therapy to minimize muscle deformities; no known prevention
"Pinkeye"	(see conjunctivitis)		
Pneumonia	Virus or bacteria; usually follows respiratory infection	Cough, fever, chills, shortness of breath, chest pain	Treated with cough medicine, antibiotics, extra liquids

Diseases	Cause/ Transmission	Symptoms	Treatment/ Prevention
Polio	Virus; spread by contact with moisture from mouth and nose	Nerves that send messages to muscles are damaged; any muscle may be affected	Treated with physical therapy; prevented with vaccine (starting in infancy)
Rabies (hydrophobia)	Viral infection; spread through bite of infected animal	Fever, muscle spasms, excessive salivation, paralysis	Treatment with vaccine to produce immunity during incubation period; no known treatment after onset; prevented by avoiding stray and wild animals
Reye's Syndrome	Unknown; has been observed to occur when aspirin is given during viral infections	Inflamed brain tissue, inflamed liver and other abdominal organs, nausea, vomiting, amnesia	Symptoms treated with non-aspirin medications; no known prevention except to avoid treatment with aspirin during viral infections
Rheumatic Fever	May follow streptococcal infection and scarlet fever	Sore throat, inflamed joints, fever, nosebleeds, skin rash; heart tissue affected	Treated with penicillin, salicylate, and cortisone; sometimes prevented by adequate care of strep infection
Ringworm (tinea)	Fungal infection; spread through contact with items that were in contact with infected hair	Bald patches on scalp, ringlike patches on face or body	Treated with fungicide; prevented by avoiding contact with infected items
Rocky Mountain Spotted Fever	Microorganisms (rickettsia) that live inside ticks; spread when tick bites human	Severe headache, high fever, muscle aches, rash, weakness	Treated with antibiotics; prevented by checking for and removing ticks from skin at least every hour while in wooded areas
Scoliosis	Heredity	Spine curves in an S-shape, commonly starting in puberty during growth spurt	Not treated in mild cases; severe cases are treated with braces or surgery; no known prevention, although early detection is important

Diseases	Cause/Transmission	Symptoms	Treatment/Prevention
Sickle Cell Anemia	Heredity	Change in shape of hemoglobin in red blood cells causing pain in joints, blood clots, fatigue	Affected joints treated with rest; extra water to drink; analgesic medicines; no known prevention
Spina bifida	Birth defect; part of spinal cord is left unprotected by bone	Paralysis of muscles controlled by nerves at or below defect in spine	Treated with physical training and therapy; no known prevention
"Strep" throat and scarlet fever	Streptococcus bacteria, spread by droplets from mouth and nose	Sore throat, fever; scarlet fever also includes a bright red rash that starts on the face	Treated with antibiotics; prevented by washing hands often and avoiding contact with infected person
Syphilis	Bacterial infection; usually transmitted through sexual contact	Painless sores on external sex organs, skin rash, swollen lymph nodes; eventual paralysis, senility, and insanity if untreated	Treated with antibiotics; prevented by avoiding sexual contact with infected person
Tetanus	Bacterial infection	Muscle spasm, stiffness of jaw and facial muscles, severe convulsions	Treated with tetanus antitoxin; prevented with vaccine and booster every 10 years
Tonsillitis	Viral or bacterial infection	Swollen tonsils, fever, vomiting, cough	Treated with antibiotics; in severe cases, surgery to remove tonsils and adenoids; no known prevention
Tuberculosis (TB)	Bacterial infection; spread by droplets from mouth and nose	Cough, fever, drenching sweats, rapid weight loss, weakness	Treated with antibiotics; prevented by avoiding contact with infected person
Typhoid	Bacterial infection, usually from contaminated water	High fever, loss of appetite, rose-colored spots on abdomen and chest, bloody diarrhea	Treated with antibiotics, cortisone; prevented with good hygiene; vaccine is also used

425

Measurement Conversion Table

Metric Units	Converting Metric to English	Converting English to Metric
Length		
kilometer (km) = 1,000 meters	1 kilometer = 0.62 mile	1 mile = 1.609 kilometers
meter (m) = 100 centimeters	1 meter = 1.09 yards	1 yard = 0.914 meter
	1 meter = 3.28 feet	1 foot = 0.305 meter
centimeter (cm) = 0.01 meter	1 centimeter = 0.394 inch	1 foot = 30.5 centimeters
millimeter (mm) = 0.001 meter	1 millimeter = 0.039 inch	1 inch = 2.54 centimeters
Mass		
kilogram (kg) = 1,000 grams	1 kilogram = 2.205 pounds	1 pound = 0.454 kilogram
gram (g) = 0.001 kilogram	1 gram = 0.0353 ounce	1 ounce = 28.35 grams
Volume		
kiloliter (kl) = 1,000 liters	1 kiloliter = 264.17 gallons	1 gallon = 3.785 liters
liter (l) = 1,000 milliliters	1 liter = 1.06 quarts	1 quart = 0.946 liter
milliliter (ml) = 0.001 liter	1 milliliter = 0.034 fluidounce	1 pint = 0.47 liter
		1 fluidounce = 29.57 milliliters

Temperature Conversion Scale

The left side of the thermometer is marked off in degrees Fahrenheit (F). To read the corresponding temperature in degrees Celsius (C), look at the right side of the thermometer. For example, 50 degrees Fahrenheit is the same temperature as 10 degrees Celsius. You may also use the formulas below to make conversions.

Conversion of Fahrenheit to Celsius:

degrees Celsius =
$$\text{5/9 (degrees Fahrenheit } - 32)$$

Conversion of Celsius to Fahrenheit:

degrees Fahrenheit =
$$\text{9/5 degrees Celsius } + 32$$

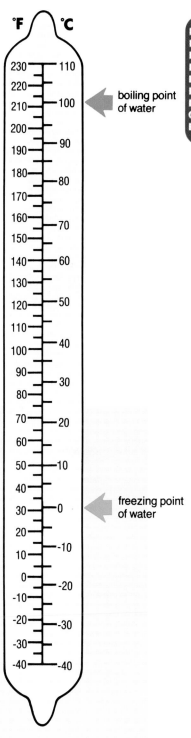

Glossary

PRONUNCIATION KEY

Sound	As In	Phonetic Respelling
a	bat	(BAT)
ah	lock	(LAHK)
	argue	(AHR gyoo)
ai	rare	(RAIR)
aw	law	(LAW)
awr	horn	(HAWRN)
ay	face	(FAYS)
ch	chapel	(CHAP uhl)
ee	eat	(EET)
	feet	(FEET)
	ski	(SKEE)
eh	test	(TEHST)
eye	idea	(eye DEE uh)
ih	bit	(BIHT)
ihng	going	(GOH ihng)
k	card	(KAHRD)
	kite	(KYT)
oh	over	(OH vuhr)
oo	pool	(POOL)
ow	out	(OWT)

Sound	As In	Phonetic Respelling
oy	foil	(FOYL)
s	cell	(SEHL)
	sit	(SIHT)
sh	sheep	(SHEEP)
th	that	(THAT)
th	thin	(THIHN)
u	pull	(PUL)
uh	medal	(MEHD uhl)
	talent	(TAL uhnt)
	pencil	(PEHN suhl)
	onion	(UHN yuhn)
	playful	(PLAY fuhl)
	dull	(DUHL)
uhr	paper	(PAY puhr)
ur	fern	(FURN)
y	ripe	(RYP)
y	yes	(YEHS)
z	bags	(BAGZ)
zh	treasure	(TREHZH uhr)

A

abdominal thrusts (ab DAHM uhn uhl • THRUHSTS), first-aid procedure for helping someone who is choking. (**337**)

accident (AK suh duhnt), sudden, unexpected event that may cause a person harm. (**326**)

acid rain (AS uhd • RAYN), rain formed when water vapor combines with sulfur oxides in the atmosphere. (**362**)

acne (AK nee), skin condition in which sebum becomes infected and pimples are produced. (**106**)

acquired attribute (uh KWYRD • A truh byoot), quality that a person develops as a result of his or her experiences. (**4**)

acquired immunodeficiency syndrome (uh KWYRD • ihm yuh noh dih FIHSH uhn see • SIHN drohm), incurable disease caused by HIV, a virus that attacks the body's immune system; also called AIDS. (**194**)

addiction (uh DIHK shuhn), severe physical and emotional dependence on a drug. (**250**)

adolescence (ad uh LEHS uhns), stage of human growth between childhood and adulthood. (**79**)

advertising (AD vuhr tyz ihng), process of giving consumers information that encourages them to buy a product or service. (**101**)

aerobic exercise (air OH bihk • EHK suhr syz), vigorous exercise that makes the body use large amounts of oxygen for at least 20 minutes. (**159**)

AIDS (AYDZ), acquired immunodeficiency syndrome; incurable disease caused by HIV, a virus that attacks the body's immune system. (**194**)

alcoholic (al kuh HAWL ihk), person who has an emotional and physical dependence on alcohol. (**280**)

alcoholism (AL kuh haw lihz uhm), condition in which a person builds a tolerance to alcohol, resulting in emotional and physical dependence. (**280**)

alternative (awl TUR nuht ihv), option, or one way to solve a problem. (**22**)

alveoli (al VEE uh ly), tiny air sacs in which oxygen and carbon dioxide are exchanged in the lungs. (**55**)

amino acids (uh MEE noh • AS uhdz), building blocks of proteins. (**129**)

ammonia (uh MOH nyuh), harmful substance in tobacco smoke; commonly used in household cleaners. (**302**)

amphetamine (am FEHT uh meen), very powerful stimulant; some are legal and prescribed by physicians, and some are illegal and very dangerous. (**250**)

analgesic (an uhl JEE zihk), medicine that relieves pain. (**222**)

anesthetic (an uhs THEHT ihk), medicine that acts on the nervous system to block or relieve pain. (**221**)

anorexia nervosa (an uh REHK see uh • nuhr VOH suh), serious eating disorder in which a person thinks of himself or herself as being overweight and does not eat enough to stay healthy. (**148**)

antibiotic (ant ih by AHT ihk), medicine that kills certain kinds of bacteria or controls their growth. (**221**)

antibodies (ANT ih bahd eez), substances in the blood that are made by white blood cells; they destroy pathogens and provide immunity to certain diseases. (**199**)

antigen (ANT ih juhn), protein found in microbes that causes white blood cells to make antibodies. (**199**)

antihistamine (ant ih HIHS tuh meen), medicine that relieves the effects of histamines, which can cause itching of the skin or swelling and increased mucus in the respiratory system. (**223**)

antiperspirant (ant ih PUR spuh ruhnt), product that makes the sweat glands produce less perspiration. (**108**)

arsenic (AHRS nihk), strong poison in tobacco smoke; used in weed killers and insecticides. (**302**)

artery (AHRT uh ree), blood vessel that carries blood away from the heart. (**52**)

aspartame (AS pahr taym), low-calorie artificial sweetener. (**151**)

asthma (AZ muh), allergic disease that causes breathing difficulty. (**208**)

atherosclerosis (ath uh roh skluh ROH suhs), condition in which fat builds up on the inner walls of arteries, making the heart work harder to pump the blood through the body; can lead to a heart attack. (**206**)

attribute (A truh byoot), certain quality of a person. (**4**)

autonomic nerves (awt uh NAHM ihk • NURVZ), nerves that send messages to vital organs, such as the heart, without the person's knowledge or control. (**46**)

B

bacteria (bak TIHR ee uh), common single-cell microbes that have various shapes and can reproduce on their own; each microbe of this type is called a bacterium. (**187**)

balanced diet (BAL uhnst • DY uht), combination of food choices from each of the five basic food groups; gives the body the nutrients needed for good health. (**139**)

barbiturates (bahr BIHCH uh ruhts), strong and addictive depressants; some are prescribed by physicians, and some are illegal and extremely dangerous. (**253**)

blood alcohol concentration (BLUHD • AL kuh hawl • kahn suhn TRAY shuhn), measure of the amount of alcohol in a person's blood; abbreviated BAC. (**278**)

body system (BAHD ee • SIHS tuhm), group of organs that work together to do a certain job in the body. (**34**)

brain stem (BRAYN • STEHM), the part of the brain that controls the body's involuntary movements, such as breathing. (**46**)

bronchial tube (BRAHNG kee uhl • TOOB), one of the two tubes through which air passes from the bottom of the trachea to the lungs. (**55**)

bulimia (byoo LIHM ee uh), eating disorder in which a person overeats and then vomits or uses laxatives to get rid of the food. (**148**)

C

caffeine (ka FEEN), natural stimulant found in products such as chocolate, coffee, tea, and most cola drinks. (**250**)

calorie (KAL uh ree), unit of measure for energy the body obtains from food. (**127**)

cannabis (KAN uh buhs), plant from which marijuana and hashish are obtained; also called hemp. (**259**)

capillary (KAP uh lehr ee), smallest type of blood vessel; where nutrients and wastes are exchanged. (**52**)

carbon monoxide (KAHR buhn • muh NAHK syd), poisonous gas produced when there is not enough oxygen for a fuel to be burned completely; present in tobacco smoke. (**302, 360**)

cardiopulmonary resuscitation (KAHRD ee oh PUL muh nehr ee • rih suhs uh TAY shuhn), emergency procedure for helping someone whose heart and breathing have stopped; combines rescue breathing with chest compressions; also called CPR. (**340**)

cardiorespiratory system (KAHRD ee oh RES puh ruh tohr ee • SIHS tuhm), body system that includes both the circulatory and respiratory systems. (**160**)

cartilage (KAHRT uhl ihj), connective tissue that acts as a cushion between bones. (**39**)

cerebellum (sehr uh BEHL uhm), the part of the brain that coordinates the movements of voluntary muscles. (**44**)

cerebrum (suh REE bruhm), the part of the brain that controls emotions, thinking, memory, and sensation. (**44**)

chemotherapy (kee moh THEHR uh pee), cancer treatment in which the patient is given medicines that destroy cancer cells. (**206**)

chewing tobacco (CHOO ihng • tuh BAK oh), smokeless tobacco that is made of ground tobacco leaves and is placed in the mouth. (**311**)

chlamydia (kluh MIHD ee uh), sexually transmitted disease that can damage internal reproductive organs. (**193**)

cholesterol (kuh LEHS tuh rohl), waxy substance found naturally in the blood and in some foods; too much in the blood can clog blood vessels and lead to heart disease. (**128**)

chromosomes (KROH muh sohmz), threadlike structures that are made of DNA and are contained inside the cell nucleus. (**70**)

chronic bronchitis (KRAHN ihk • brahn KYT uhs), disease in which the mucous membranes of the bronchial tubes and the lungs become irritated and infected. (**208**)

chronic disease (KRAHN ihk • dihz EEZ), long-lasting disease, such as diabetes, asthma, or bronchitis. (**202**)

chyme (KYM), partly digested food in the form of a thick liquid in the stomach. (**56**)

cilia (SIHL ee uh), tiny hairs that line the respiratory passages and that sweep mucus containing dirt and dust particles out of the respiratory system. (**54**)

cirrhosis (suh ROH suhs), liver damage that prevents the liver from getting rid of body wastes and doing its other jobs; the leading cause of death among alcoholics. (**282**)

cocaine (koh KAYN), one of the most dangerous illegal stimulants; creates strong feelings that make people emotionally dependent on it. (**251**)

codeine (KOH deen), opiate that is used in some prescription medicines to relieve pain or control dry coughs. (**256**)

communicable disease (kuh MYOO nih kuh buhl • dihz EEZ), illness that can be spread from person to person; caused by microbes. (**186**)

complete protein (kuhm PLEET • PROH teen), a protein that contains all the essential amino acids. (**130**)

complex carbohydrates (KAHM plehks • kahr boh HY drayts), carbohydrates made of many simple carbohydrates that are chemically bound together. (**127**)

compound fracture (KAHM pownd • FRAK chuhr), fracture in which the bone breaks and goes through the skin; also called an open fracture. (**345**)

connective tissue (kuh NEHK tihv • TIHSH oo), tissue that joins, supports, or protects other tissues. (**33**)

consequence (KAHN suh kwehns), result. (**5**)

consumer (kuhn SOO muhr), anyone who buys or uses a product or service. (**98**)

contour plowing (KAHN tur • PLOW ihng), method of planting crops in rows that cross the normal flow of water; reduces soil erosion. (**375**)

coronary heart disease (KAWR uh nehr ee • HAHRT • dihz EEZ), condition in which the heart receives a reduced supply of blood. (**207**)

crack (KRAK), extremely powerful and dangerous illegal drug made by chemically changing cocaine powder into blocks. (**252**)

cyanide (SY uh nyd), deadly poison present in tobacco smoke; can cause severe respiratory problems. **(302)**

D

daughter cells (DAWT uhr • SEHLZ), two new cells that are made by the division of a parent cell. **(70)**

deceptive trade practice (dih SEHP tihv • TRAYD • PRAK tuhs), act of selling a product or service that cannot perform as promised. **(115)**

decision (dih SIHZH uhn), choice that is made after considering different possibilities. **(18)**

decongestant (dee kuhn JEHS tuhnt), medicine that is used to relieve a stuffy nose by shrinking blood vessels in the nasal passages. **(222)**

demineralized bone matrix (dee MIHN ruh lyzd • BOHN • MAY trihks), new bone tissue made by combining powdered bone with certain chemicals. **(43)**

deodorant (dee OHD uh ruhnt), product that controls perspiration odor by stopping the growth of bacteria on the skin. **(108)**

depressant (dih PREHS uhnt), drug that slows down the functioning of the nervous system. **(253)**

depression (dih PREHSH uhn), condition in which a person feels very sad for a long time; can also make a person feel hopeless. **(17)**

dermatologist (duhr muh TAHL uh juhst), physician who treats skin problems. **(107)**

dermis (DUR muhs), layer of skin directly beneath the epidermis. **(106)**

desirable weight (dih ZY ruh buhl • WAYT), person's weight that falls within a range determined to be healthful; depends on the person's age, gender, and frame size. **(145)**

detoxification (dee tahk suh fuh KAY shuhn), a process in which a drug user receives medical care while he or she stops using a drug. **(263)**

digestion (dy JEHS chuhn), process in which food is broken down so it can be used by the cells of the body. **(56)**

digestive juices (dy JEHS tihv • JOOS uhz), liquids made by the body to help digest foods. **(56)**

distillation (dihs tuh LAY shuhn), process in which a liquid is boiled and then its vapor is condensed to a liquid again; makes an alcoholic liquid more concentrated. **(277)**

dominant (DAHM uh nuhnt), describes the stronger member of a pair of genes. **(72)**

dosage (DOH sihj), correct amount of a medicine to take at one time and how often to take it. **(233)**

drug (DRUHG), any substance, other than food and water, that causes a change in the body. **(220)**

dump (DUHMP), open area where solid wastes from a community are disposed of. **(376)**

E

electric shock (ih LEHK trihk • SHAHK), painful jolt caused by direct contact with an electric current. **(349)**

embryo (EHM bree oh), new organism developing from a fertilized cell; in humans, the unborn child during the first three months of development. **(75)**

emergency (ih MUR juhn see), unexpected situation that calls for quick action, as when someone is injured in an accident. **(331)**

emotion (ih MOH shuhn), strong feeling. **(9)**

emotional dependence (ih MOH shuhn uhl • dih PEHN duhns), condition in which a person feels uncomfortable if he or she is not experiencing the effects of a drug. **(246)**

emotional needs (ih MOH shuhn uhl • NEEDZ), requirements a person has for feeling loved and accepted. **(10)**

endocrine gland (EHN duh krihn • GLAND), gland that secretes one or more hormones into the blood. **(47)**

endurance (ihn DUR uhns), ability to perform an activity for a long time without getting too tired to continue. **(161)**

environment (ihn VY ruhn muhnt), combination of people, places, and things that surround a person. **(4)**

epidermis (ehp uh DUR muhs), outer layer of skin. **(106)**

epithelial tissue (ehp uh THEE lee uhl • TIHSH oo), tissue, such as the skin, that covers the outside of a structure; also covers internal body parts such as the heart and stomach. **(33)**

esophagus (ih SAHF uh guhs), muscular tube that leads from the mouth to the stomach. **(56)**

essential amino acids (ih SEHN chuhl • uh MEE noh • AS uhdz), eight amino acids that cannot be made in the body and must come from food. **(129)**

estrogen (EHS truh juhn), hormone made by the ovaries of a female after she reaches puberty; causes the body to change from that of a girl to that of a woman. **(80)**

ethanol (EHTH uh nawl), type of alcohol in alcoholic beverages; made from grains, fruits, and certain other substances that contain sugar. **(276)**

exercise (EHK suhr syz), any activity that makes the body work hard. **(158)**

F

fad diet (FAD • DY uht), diet that promises quick weight loss and is usually popular for only a short time. **(147)**

fatigue (fuh TEEG), tired feeling. **(171)**

fat-soluble vitamins (FAT sahl yuh buhl • VYT uh muhnz), vitamins that dissolve in fats and can be stored in the body. **(131)**

fermentation (fuhr muhn TAY shuhn), chemical process in which sugar molecules are broken down and ethanol is produced. **(276)**

fetal alcohol syndrome (FEET ihl • AL kuh hawl • SIHN drohm), mental and physical problems a baby has because the mother drank alcohol, which interfered with the baby's development. **(283)**

fetus (FEE tuhs), an unborn baby after the second month of development. **(75)**

fever (FEE vuhr), body temperature that is higher than normal. **(198)**

fiber (FY buhr), complex carbohydrate in foods such as bran cereal, whole grains, seeds, and many kinds of fruits and vegetables; cannot be digested but helps the digestive system work as it should. **(127)**

R E F E R E N C E

first aid (FURST • AYD), immediate care that is given to someone who is injured or suddenly ill. (**331**)

first-degree burn (FURST dih GREE • BURN), also called *superficial burn,* burn that damages only the outer layer of skin; causes redness and some swelling. (**347**)

flammable (FLAM uh buhl), catches fire easily. (**346**)

flexibility (flehk suh BIHL uh tee), ability of the movable joints to work freely and smoothly. (**162**)

fluoride (FLUR yd), substance often put in drinking water and toothpaste to help strengthen tooth enamel. (**110**)

formaldehyde (fawr MAL duh hyd), harmful substance in tobacco smoke; used as a disinfectant and as a preservative for dead animals. (**302**)

fracture (FRAK chuhr), break or crack in a bone. (**345**)

fungi (FUHN jy), one of four main types of microbes, which can grow on or inside the body; each organism of this type is called a fungus. (**187**)

G

general anesthetic (JEHN uh ruhl • an uhs THEHT ihk), anesthetic that causes a person to become unconscious so he or she cannot feel pain; used for major surgery. (**222**)

genes (JEENZ), small bits, or units, of hereditary information. (**72**)

glucose (GLOO kohs), blood sugar, or sugar that is carried by the blood to the cells where energy is needed. (**127**)

glycogen (GLY kuh juhn), form of glucose that is stored in the muscles and liver for later use. (**127**)

gonorrhea (gahn uh REE uh), sexually transmitted disease caused by certain bacteria. (**193**)

growth plate (GROHTH • PLAYT), layer of bone cells that divide to produce new bone tissue. (**38**)

H

hallucinogen (huh LOOS uhn uh juhn), drug that changes the way a person senses the world. (**258**)

hangover (HANG oh vuhr), illness a person feels as the body rids itself of alcohol. (**280**)

hashish (HASH eesh), illegal drug made from the sticky juice of cannabis flowers. (**259**)

hazard (HAZ uhrd), person's behavior or environmental condition that is not safe. (**329**)

hazardous wastes (HAZ uhrd uhs • WAYSTS), dangerous substances given off during certain industrial processes, including the production of electricity from nuclear energy. (**378**)

heart attack (HAHRT • uh TAK), condition in which the flow of blood to the heart is reduced or cut off, causing the heart to stop beating. (**207**)

heat exhaustion (HEET • ihg ZAWS chuhn), illness that occurs when the body loses too much fluid because of sweating. (**169**)

herbicide (UR buh syd), chemical that is used to kill unwanted plants. (**375**)

heredity (huh REHD uht ee), total of all the traits a person receives from his or her parents; the passing of characteristics from parents to their children. (**3**)

heroin (HEHR uh wuhn), the most dangerous and life-threatening opiate; it is illegal and can lead to tolerance and strong emotional and physical dependence. (**255**)

herpes simplex type 2 (HUHR peez • SIHM plehks • TYP • TOO), incurable sexually transmitted disease caused by a virus; produces painful blisters and sores where the virus entered the body. (**193**)

histamines (HIHS tuh meenz), chemicals the body makes during allergic reactions; may cause itchy hives or may cause swelling and increased mucus in the respiratory system. (**223**)

hormone (HAWR mohn), one of the chemicals produced by endocrine glands; controls the functioning of body organs. (**47**)

human carrier (HYOO muhn • KAR ee uhr), person who has a disease-causing microbe and can spread it without becoming ill. (**188**)

human immunodeficiency virus (HYOO muhn • ihm yuh noh dih FIHSH uhn see • VY ruhs), virus that causes AIDS; also called HIV. (**194**)

hydrocarbons (hy druh KAHR buhnz), fuels and gases made of hydrogen and carbon. (**361**)

hypertension (HY puhr tehn chuhn), high blood pressure. (**206**)

I

immovable joints (ihm OO vuh buhl • JOYNTS), joints in which the bones fit together too tightly to move. (**38**)

immunity (ihm YOO nuht ee), condition in which the body has resistance against the pathogen for a certain disease. (**199**)

incineration (ihn sihn uh RAY shuhn), method of disposing of solid wastes by burning them. (**377**)

incomplete protein (ihn kuhm PLEET • PROH teen), a protein that does not have all of the essential amino acids. (**130**)

inhalant (ihn HAY luhnt), chemical whose vapors produce druglike effects when inhaled. (**261**)

inherited trait (ihn HEHR uh tehd • TRAYT), characteristic a person receives from his or her parents. (**3**)

inner defenses (IHN uhr • dih FEHNS uhs), parts inside the body, such as white blood cells, that fight pathogens. (**198**)

insulin (IHN suh luhn), hormone that lets blood sugar enter the cells of the body; made by the pancreas. (**209**)

intellectual needs (int uhl EHK chuhl • NEEDS), requirements a person has that help him or her maintain a healthy mind. (**10**)

435

intoxicated (ihn TAHK suh kayt uhd), in a condition in which one's physical and mental abilities are severely affected as a result of drinking alcohol. **(279)**

intramuscular (ihn truh MUHS kyuh luhr), describes injections of medicines into muscles. **(228)**

intravenous (ihn truh VEE nuhs), describes injections of medicines into the circulatory system. **(228)**

involuntary muscles (ihn VAHL uhn tehr ee • MUHS uhlz), muscles that work without a person's control; they make some of the body's inner organs work. **(40)**

irradiation (ihr ayd ee AY shuhn), process of exposing food to low levels of radiation for a short time to help keep the food fresh. **(151)**

isopropyl alcohol (eye suh PROH puhl • AL kuh hawl), type of alcohol that is used as a disinfectant; also called rubbing alcohol. **(276)**

J

joint (JOYNT), place where two bones connect. **(38)**

K

kwashiorkor (kwahsh ee AWR kuhr), serious form of malnutrition in infants and children; caused by a deficiency of protein; affects skin color, growth, and mental ability. **(143)**

L

license (LYS uhns), permit that allows certain activities to be carried out; given to a health care professional only after he or she meets basic qualifications. **(102)**

ligament (LIHG uh muhnt), strong band of connective tissue that holds bones together at movable joints. **(39)**

local anesthetic (LOH kuhl • an uhs THEHT ihk), anesthetic that prevents a person from feeling pain in only a portion of the body; used for minor surgery. **(222)**

LSD (ehl ehs DEE), illegal drug that is the most powerful known hallucinogen. **(258)**

lymph (LIHMF), tissue fluid that collects wastes from cells and passes through lymph vessels. **(52)**

lymph node (LIHMF • NOHD), lump of tissue, located in a lymph vessel, that traps and destroys disease-causing microbes. **(52)**

lymph vessel (LIHMF • VEHS uhl), vessel, located next to a vein, that collects tissue fluid, or lymph. **(52)**

lymphatic system (lihm FAT ihk • SIHS tuhm), part of the circulatory system; helps destroy pathogens in the body. **(198)**

M

macrominerals (mak roh MIHN uh ruhlz), minerals that the body needs in large amounts to stay healthy. **(133)**

mainstream smoke (MAYN streem • SMOHK), smoke that is exhaled by a smoker. **(304)**

malnutrition (mal noo TRIHSH uhn), condition in which the body does not get all the nutrients it needs to be healthy.   (**142**)

marijuana (mair uh WAHN uh), illegal drug made from the dried leaves and flowers of the cannabis, or hemp, plant.   (**259**)

maturity (muh TUR uht ee), state of being fully developed.   (**79**)

medical insurance (MEHD ih kuhl • ihn SHUR uhns), plan that can be purchased to help pay a person's medical expenses; helps protect a person from large medical expenses that he or she cannot afford.   (**116**)

medicine (MEHD uh suhn), drug that is used to treat or cure a health problem.   (**220**)

meiosis (my OH suhs), cell division that forms reproductive cells.   (**71**)

mescaline (MEHS kuh luhn), dangerous hallucinogen made from the peyote cactus.   (**258**)

methadone (MEHTH uh dohn), narcotic that is used to help cure heroin addiction.   (**256**)

methyl alcohol (MEHTH uhl • AL kuh hawl), poisonous type of alcohol that is made from wood materials and is used in paints and wood-finishing products.   (**276**)

microbe (MY krohb), tiny organism.   (**186**)

mitosis (my TOH suhs), cell division in which two cells identical to the original are formed.   (**70**)

morphine (MAWR feen), strong, highly addictive opiate that is used as a pain reliever when no other pain reliever is strong enough.   (**255**)

motor nerves (MOH tuhr • NURVZ), nerves that carry messages to muscles.   (**44**)

movable joints (MOO vuh buhl • JOYNTS), joints of the skeleton that allow bone movement.   (**38**)

mucous membrane (MYOO kuhs • MEHM brayn), layer of skin cells inside the nose, mouth, and throat that produce mucus.   (**197**)

mucus (MYOO kuhs), thick, sticky substance that lines the body's nasal passages, trachea, and bronchial tubes; traps dust and dirt.   (**54**)

multiple sclerosis (MUHL tuh puhl • skluh ROH suhs), noncommunicable disease that destroys the coverings on the nerves of the brain and spinal cord; reduces muscle control because messages from the brain do not reach the proper muscles.   (**210**)

muscle fiber (MUHS uhl • FY buhr), bundle of long muscle cells.   (**161**)

muscle tissue (MUHS uhl • TIHSH oo), tissue made up of muscle cells, which contract to move parts of the body.   (**33**)

muscular dystrophy (MUHS kyuh luhr • DIHS truh fee), inherited disease that causes the body's muscles to weaken slowly.   (**211**)

N

narcotic (nahr KAHT ihk), drug that reduces the brain's ability to recognize pain.   (**254**)

needs (NEEDZ), requirements that a person must meet or satisfy for good health. **(10)**

negative stress (NEHG uht ihv • STREHS), type of stress that makes a person feel tense, pressured, unhappy, and out of control. **(15)**

neonatal (nee oh NAYT uhl), relating to newborn babies. **(62)**

nerve tissue (NURV • TIHSH OO), tissue made up of nerve cells, which carry information in the body. **(34)**

neurological diseases (nur uh LAHJ ih kuhl • dihz EEZ uhz), diseases of the nervous system, which affect the brain, nerves, or both. **(210)**

nicotine (NIHK uh teen), stimulant drug present in tobacco products. **(250, 301)**

nitrogen oxides (NY truh juhn • AHK sydz), gases formed when certain fuels are burned at high temperatures. **(362)**

noise pollution (NOYZ • puh LOO shun), loud sounds that affect people's health. **(368)**

noncommunicable disease (nahn kuh MYOO nih kuh buhl • dihz EEZ), disease that cannot be passed from person to person; is not caused by pathogens. **(202)**

nuclear wastes (NOO klee uhr • WAYSTS), spent fuel and other radioactive materials from nuclear energy plants. **(379)**

nucleus (NOO klee uhs), the part of the cell that controls the cell's activities. **(70)**

nutrient density (NOO tree uhnt • DEHN suht ee), amount of nutrients a food contains compared to its calories. **(141)**

nutritional deficiency (nu TRIHSH uhn uhl • dih FIHSH uhn see), condition in which a person is not getting enough of one or more nutrients to maintain good health. **(143)**

O

opiates (OH pee uhts), drugs that are made from opium and that cause dullness and inaction. **(255)**

opium (OH pee uhm), highly addictive narcotic obtained from the poppy plant. **(254)**

organ (AWR guhn), body part made up of different kinds of tissues that work together to carry out a body function. **(34)**

Osgood-Schlatter's disease (ahs guhd SHLAT uhrz • dihz EEZ), disease in which a lump grows under one or both knees of a young person; causes knee swelling and soreness. **(67)**

osteoporosis (ahs tee oh puh ROH suhs), disease that causes bones to become thin and brittle. **(43)**

OTC medicine (OH tee see • MEHD uh suhn), over-the-counter medicine; medicine that does not require a prescription and is considered safe if used responsibly and according to directions. **(222)**

outer defenses (OWT uhr • dih FEHNS uhz), portions of the body, such as the skin, that help keep pathogens from entering the body. **(197)**

outpatient (OWT pay shuhnt), person who receives medical treatment at a hospital but does not need to be admitted to stay there. **(237)**

ovary (OHV uh ree), female reproductive organ. **(48)**

overdose (OH vuhr dohs), amount of medicine that is greater than the recommended dosage and can cause harm or even death. **(233)**

ovum (OH vuhm), female reproductive cell. **(71)**

oxidation (ahk suh DAY shuhn), process by which cells use nutrients and oxygen to release energy, water, and carbon dioxide. **(33)**

ozone (OH zohn), compound that is found in the air and is made up of three oxygen atoms; in the upper atmosphere, ozone is helpful, but in the lower atmosphere, it is a pollutant. **(363)**

P

parent cell (PAIR uhnt • SEHL), cell that produces two new cells by dividing. **(70)**

particulates (puhr TIHK yuh luhts), small bits of solid or liquid matter floating in the air. **(361)**

pasteurization (pas chuh ruh ZAY shuhn), process in which milk is heated for a short period of time in order to kill disease-causing bacteria. **(384)**

pathogen (PATH uh juhn), microbe that can cause disease. **(187)**

pathology (puh THAHL uh jee), study of the nature of diseases. **(212)**

PCP (pee see PEE), dangerous and illegal hallucinogen. **(259)**

peer (PIHR), person who is the same age or in the same class as another person. **(6)**

peer pressure (PIHR • PREHSH uhr), influence on a person by other people who is about the same age or in the same class. **(6)**

personality (puhrs uhn AL uht ee), sum of all a person's traits; qualities that make a person different from every other person. **(2)**

personality trait (puhrs uhn AL uht ee • TRAYT), characteristic that contributes to the way a person thinks, feels, and acts. **(3)**

pesticide (PEHS tuh syd), chemical that is used to kill insects or other pests. **(375)**

physical dependence (FIHZ ih kuhl • dih PEHN duhns), condition in which a person's body becomes accustomed to the presence of a drug and cannot function normally without it. **(246)**

physical fitness (FIHZ ih kuhl • FIHT nuhs), condition in which each of the systems of the body works properly. **(158)**

physical needs (FIHZ ih kuhl • NEEDZ), requirements for maintaining a healthy body. **(10)**

physical trait (FIHZ ih kuhl • TRAYT), characteristic that contributes to the shape and appearance of a person's body. **(3)**

pituitary gland (pih TOO uh tehr ee • GLAND), endocrine gland that makes several hormones; controls other endocrine glands and directs the growth and development of the body. **(47)**

plasma (PLAZ muh), liquid part of the blood. **(49)**

platelets (PLAYT luhts), tiny parts of cells in the blood that help the blood thicken, or clot, when a person gets a cut or wound. **(51)**

poison (POYZ uhn), substance that in the body, causes a chemical reaction resulting in injury, illness, or death. **(342)**

pollutant (puh LOOT uhnt), unwanted substance that harms the environment. **(360)**

pores (PAWRZ), small openings from which sweat passes out through the skin. **(60)**

REFERENCE

439

positive stress (PAHZ uht ihv • STREHS), type of stress that makes life more challenging and enjoyable. **(15)**

posture (PAHS chuhr), how a person holds his or her body while sitting, standing, and walking. **(163)**

prescription (prih SKRIHP shuhn), order given by a physician or other qualified doctor for medicine. **(220)**

proof (PROOF), number that expresses the amount of ethanol in liquor; equals twice the percentage of ethanol. **(277)**

protozoa (proht uh ZOH uh), single-cell microbes that must have water to live; some types can cause disease; each microbe of this type is called a protozoan. **(187)**

psilocybin (sy luh SY buhn), dangerous and illegal hallucinogen made from a certain kind of mushroom. **(259)**

puberty (PYOO buhrt ee), time at the start of adolescence when rapid changes take place in the body that lead to physical maturity. **(79)**

Q

quack (KWAK), person who pretends to be a health professional. **(114)**

R

radon (RAY dahn), colorless, odorless, radioactive gas is produced naturally from the breakdown of uranium in the soil. **(381)**

reaction time (ree AK shuhn • TYM), time it takes for a person to recognize a danger and take action. **(328)**

recessive (rih SEHS ihv), describes the weaker member of a pair of genes. **(72)**

reflex (REE flehks), muscle response, such as shivering, that is not controlled by the brain. **(46)**

rescue breathing (REHS kyoo • BREETH ihng), emergency procedure used when a person cannot breathe; method of breathing air into a person's lungs. **(338)**

respiratory conditions (REHS puh ruh tohr ee • kuhn DIHSH uhnz), diseases of the lungs and bronchial tubes that make it hard to breathe and that affect the supply of oxygen to the body. **(207)**

role model (ROHL • MAHD uhl), person whose behavior is copied by others. **(5)**

S

sanitary landfill (SAN uh tehr ee • LAND fihl), location where solid wastes are buried with a layer of clay between layers of waste. **(377)**

saturated fat (SACH uh rayt uhd • FAT), fat that is usually solid at room temperature. **(128)**

sebaceous gland (sih BAY shuhs • GLAND), oil gland that is attached to each hair follicle in the dermis. **(106)**

sebum (SEE buhm), oil produced by the sebaceous glands to help keep skin soft and moist. **(106)**

second-degree burn (SEHK uhnd dih GREE • BURN), also called *partial-thickness burn*, very painful burn that causes the skin to turn red, swell, and blister. **(347)**

sediment (SEHD uh muhnt), solid matter that settles from water.   (**370**)

self-concept (sehlf KAHN sehpt), how a person sees himself or herself.   (**7**)

self-esteem (sehl fuh STEEM), good feeling a person has about himself or herself; feeling of worth.   (**10**)

sensory nerves (SEHN suhr ee • NURVZ), nerves that carry information from sense organs to the brain.   (**44**)

serving (SUR vihng), for one food, the amount a person would be likely to eat during a meal.   (**136**)

sewage (SOO ihj), human waste.   (**370**)

sexually transmitted disease (SEHKSH uh wuhl ee • tranz MIHT uhd • dihz EEZ), communicable disease spread by intimate body contact with a person who has the disease; also called STD.   (**193**)

shock (SHAHK), dangerous condition in which the circulatory system slows down and fails to provide a normal blood flow; often occurs when a person suffers a serious injury.   (**345**)

side effect (SYD • ih FEHKT), unwanted or unnecessary reaction a person may have to a medicine.   (**228**)

sidestream smoke (SYD streem • SMOHK), tobacco smoke that goes directly into the air, such as smoke from the burning end of a cigarette.   (**304**)

simple carbohydrates (SIHM puhl • kahr boh HY drayts), types of sugars found in milk, fruits, vegetables, and sweets; are digested easily and supply quick energy.   (**127**)

simple fracture (SIHM puhl • FRAK chuhr), fracture in which a bone breaks but does not go through the skin; also called a closed fracture.   (**345**)

smog (SMAHG), pollution formed by the combination of nitrogen oxides, hydrocarbons, and sunlight.   (**363**)

smokeless tobacco (SMOH kluhs • tuh BAK oh), tobacco that is chewed, held in the mouth for a while, or sniffed.   (**311**)

smoker's cough (SMOH kuhrs • KAWF), cough that many smokers get when the tar from cigarette smoke damages the cilia in the bronchial tubes.   (**308**)

snuff (SNUHF), type of smokeless tobacco that is sniffed into the nose.   (**311**)

social needs (SOH shuhl • NEEDZ), requirements a person has for associating with other people.   (**10**)

soil erosion (SOYL • ih ROH zhuhn), blowing or washing away of the earth's topsoil.   (**375**)

soluble wastes (SAHL yuh buhl • WAYSTS), pollutants that dissolve, or become liquid, when they enter water.   (**371**)

solvent (SAHL vuhnt), liquid that gives off fumes causing druglike effects if the fumes are inhaled.   (**261**)

sperm cell (SPUHRM • SEHL), male reproductive cell.   (**71**)

sprain (SPRAYN), injury in which the ligaments connecting the bones at a joint are stretched or torn.   (**344**)

starch (STAHRCH), complex carbohydrate in foods such as potatoes, rice, corn, and noodles.   (**127**)

stimulant (STIHM yuh luhnt), drug that speeds up the functioning of the nervous system, which in turn speeds up other body systems.   (**249**)

strain (STRAYN), injury in which a muscle or tendon is stretched or torn. **(345)**

strength (STREHNGTH), amount of force muscles can apply. **(161)**

stress (STREHS), response of the body to physical or emotional pressure. **(15)**

stroke (STROHK), condition in which an artery to the brain is blocked, causing brain cells to die because they do not get enough oxygen. **(207)**

subcutaneous tissue (suhb kyoo TAY nee uhs • TIHSH oo), layer of skin directly beneath the dermis. **(106)**

suicide (SOO uh syd), act of killing oneself. **(17)**

sulfur oxides (SUHL fuhr • AHK sydz), gases given off when fuels that contain sulfur are burned. **(362)**

sweat glands (SWEHT • GLANDZ), tiny glands that allow excess water and some cell wastes to pass from the body through the skin. **(59)**

syphilis (SIHF luhs), sexually transmitted disease caused by certain bacteria. **(193)**

T

tar (TAHR), sticky brown substance that is produced when tobacco is burned; contains most of the cancer-causing chemicals in tobacco smoke. **(301)**

target heart rate (TAHR guht • HAHRT • RAYT), rate at which a person's heart must beat to ensure that the cardiorespiratory system is working hard enough to make itself stronger. **(160)**

temperament (TEHM pruh muhnt), personality trait that is the general way a person reacts to people and to situations. **(3)**

temperature inversion (TEHM pruh chuhr • in VUR zhuhn), weather condition in which a warm layer of air traps a cooler layer of air near the ground. **(364)**

tendon (TEHN duhn), tissue that connects muscle to bone. **(40)**

testes (TEHS teez), male reproductive organs, each of which is called a testis. **(48)**

testosterone (teh STAHS tuh rohn), hormone made by the testes of a male when he reaches puberty; causes the body to change from that of a boy to that of a man. **(81)**

thermal pollution (THUR muhl • puh LOO shuhn), heating of a naturally cool body of water; may cause harm to the plant and animal life living in the water. **(372)**

third-degree burn (THURD dih GREE • BURN), also called *full-thickness burn*, most severe type of burn; damages several layers of skin and can disrupt the way the whole body functions. **(347)**

tissue fluid (TIHSH oo • FLOO uhd), plasma that passes through the walls of capillaries, bathes body cells, and collects wastes. **(52)**

toddler (TAHD luhr), child who is no longer an infant but is less than about two-and-a-half years. **(77)**

tolerance (TAHL uh ruhns), adjustment of the body to a certain dosage of a drug, causing the person to feel less effect from that dosage. **(245)**

R
E
F
E
R
E
N
C
E

toxin (TAHK suhn), poison made by certain kinds of microbes; can cause disease. **(200)**

toxoid (TAHK soyd), toxin that has been treated so that it does not produce illness; used in a vaccine that causes antibodies to be made against the toxin. **(201)**

trace minerals (TRAYS • MIHN uh ruhlz), minerals that the body needs in small amounts each day for good health. **(133)**

trachea (TRAY kee uh), windpipe, or the air passage between the throat and lungs. **(54)**

trait (TRAYT), characteristic that helps identify what a person is like. **(2)**

U

unit price (YOO nuht • PRYS), price per piece or per unit of weight. **(141)**

unsaturated fat (uhn SACH uh rayt uhd • FAT), fat that is usually liquid at room temperature. **(128)**

ureter (YUR uht uhr), tube through which urine flows from a kidney to the urinary bladder. **(61)**

urethra (yu REE thruh), tube through which urine leaves the body from the urinary bladder. **(61)**

urination (yur uh NAY shuhn), process in which urine is passed out of the body. **(61)**

urine (YUR uhn), liquid waste that has been filtered from the blood by the kidneys. **(60)**

V

vaccine (vak SEEN), substance that gives a person immunity to a disease; causes the body to produce antibodies but does not make the person ill. **(200)**

vein (VAYN), blood vessel that carries blood back toward the heart. **(52)**

virus (VY ruhs), tiny disease-causing microbe that can reproduce only within living cells. **(187)**

voluntary muscles (VAHL uhn tehr ee • MUHS uhlz), muscles that a person can control. **(40)**

W

water-soluble vitamins (WAWT uhr SAHL yuh buhl • VYT uh muhnz), vitamins that dissolve in water in the body; can be stored in only small amounts by the body. **(131)**

wellness (WEHL nuhs), high level of physical, intellectual, social, and emotional health. **(8)**

withdrawal (wihth DRAWL), stopping the supply of a drug on which a person is physically dependent; usually produces painful physical reactions to its absence. **(246)**

REFERENCE

445

REFERENCE

REFERENCE

REFERENCE

CREDITS

Harcourt Brace & Company Photographs

KEY: (t) top, (b) bottom, (l) left, (r) right, (c) center.

Pages vi(t), Eric Camden; vi(b), Charlie Burton; vii(t), Charlie Burton; vii(b), Eric Camden; viii(t), Rob Downey; viii(b), Jerry White; ix(t), Earl Kogler; ix(b), Charlie Burton; x(t), David Phillips; x(b), Rodney Jones; xi(t), Bob Thomason; xi(b), Earl Kogler; xiii(b), Bob Thomason; xiv(t), Eric Camden; xiv(b), Darrell Sampson; xv(t), James F. Green; xv(c), Leonard Lessin; xv(b), Michael Sullivan; xvi(t), Jerry White; xvi(c), Beverly Brosius; xvi(b), Henebry Photography; xvii(t), Jerry White; xvii(c), Earl Kogler; xvii(b), Annette Stahl; xviii–1(background), Jerry White; xviii–1(background inset), Jerry White; xviii–1(tr), Annette Stahl; xviii–1(bl), Eric Camden; xviii–1(br), Rob Downey; 2, Eric Camden; 3(l), Eric Camden; 3(r), Eric Camden; 4(tl), Eric Camden; 4(r), Eric Camden; 4(bl), Eric Camden; 5, Charlie Burton; 6(t), Annette Stahl; 6(b), Annette Stahl; 7, Steve Ruehle; 8, Bob Thomason; 9(l), Joy Glenn; 9(c), Joy Glenn; 9(r), Joy Glenn; 10(tl), Gary Hofheimer; 10(tr), Henebry Photography; 10(bl), Bob Thomason; 10(br), Henebry Photography; 12(l), Charlie Burton; 12(r) Charlie Burton; 13, Henebry Photography; 14, Charlie Burton; 17(t), Charlie Burton; 17(b), Charlie Burton; 18, Charlie Burton; 19, Bob Thomason; 20(tr), Earl Kogler; 20(l), Earl Kogler; 20(cr), Earl Kogler; 20(br), Earl Kogler; 21, Earl Kogler; 22(tl), Annette Stahl; 22(r), Annette Stahl; 24, Michael Sullivan; 25, Michael Sullivan; 29, Charlie Burton; 30–31(background), Jerry White; 33(t), Charlie Burton; 35, Joy Glenn; 36, Charlie Burton; 40, Charlie Burton; 62, James F. Green; 63, James F. Green; 68–69(background), Jerry White; 68–69(br), Charlie Burton; 74(l), Dan Peha; 74(r), Dan Peha; 76(l), Earl Kogler; 79, Greg Leary; 83(t), Bob Thomason; 84(tr), Earl Kogler; 86, Charlie Burton; 87, Charlie Burton; 88, Eric Camden; 89, Wiley & Flynn; 90, Jim West; 91, Jim West; 95, Richard Haynes; 96–97(background), Jerry White; 96–97(cr), Eric Camden; 99, Eric Camden; 100(t), Eric Camden; 100(b), Eric Camden; 101, Charlie Burton; 102, Beverly Brosius; 103, Wiley & Flynn; 104(l), Charlie Burton; 104(r), Charlie Burton; 105, Charlie Burton; 107, Charlie Burton; 109(t), Charlie Burton; 109(b), Terry McMenamy; 110(tl), Jery White; 110(tc), Jerry White; 110(tr), Jerry White; 110(bl), Jerry White; 110(bc), Jerry White; 110(br), Jerry White; 112, Rodney Jones; 113, Eric Camden; 118, Leonard Lessin; 119, Leonard Lessin; 123, Charlie Burton; 124–125(background), Jerry White; 126(t), Annette Stahl; 126(b), Annette Stahl; 127(l), Henebry Photography; 127(r), Annette Stahl; 128, Charlie Burton; 129, Rob Downey; 130(t), Annette Stahl; 130(c), Annette Stahl; 130(b), Annette Stahl; 133, Bob Thomason; 135, Henebry Photography; 137(l), Jerry White; 137(c), Jerry White; 137(b), Jerry White; 139, Jerry White; 140, Charlie Burton; 141(l), Earl Kogler; 141(r), Earl Kogler; 142, Rob Downey; 145, Eric Camden; 148(l), Earl Kogler; 148(r), Earl Kogler; 149, Earl Kogler; 150, Darrell Sampson; 151, Darrell Sampson; 155, Richard Haynes; 156–157(background), Jerry White; 159(t), Charlie Burton; 160, Charlie Burton; 161(l), Jeff Blanton; 161(r), Jeff Blanton; 163(tl), Jeff Blanton; 163(tr), Jeff Blanton; 163(bl), Charlie Burton; 163(bc), Charlie Burton; 163(br), Charlie Burton; 164, Julie Fletcher; 165(l), Dan Peha; 165(r), Darrell Sampson; 166, Jerry White; 167, Charlie Burton; 169, Charlie Burton; 171(l), Bob Thomason; 171(r), Bob Thomason; 172, Charlie Burton; 174, Charlie Burton; 176, Charlie Burton; 178, Bruce McAllister; 179, Bruce McAllister; 183, Charlie Burton; 184–185(background), Jerry White; 184–185(cr), Beverly Brosius; 186(b), Jerry White; 189(l), Annette Stahl; 192, Jerry White; 193, Eric Camden; 197(l), Dave Repp; 197(r), Brian M. Christopher; 203(b), Joy Glenn; 204, Joy Glenn; 208(tl), Earl Kogler; 208(tr), Earl Kogler; 210, Rodney Jones; 212, Alan Whitman; 213, Alan Whitman; 217, Earl Kogler; 218–219(background), Jerry White; 220, Charlie Burton; 220(inset), Charlie Burton; 222, Charlie Burton; 223, Terry McMenamy; 224(t), David Phillips; 224(b), David Phillips; 226, David Phillips; 227(l), Bob Thomason; 227(r), Bob Thomason; 228(l), David Phillips; 228(r), David Phillips; 229(t), Charlie Burton; 229(b), Terry McMenamy; 231(t), Charlie Burton; 231(r), Charlie Burton; 232, Terry McMenamy; 233(t), David Phillips; 233(b), Terry McMenamy; 234, Charlie Burton; 236, Bruce McAllister; 237, Bruce McAllister; 241, David Phillips; 242–243(background), Jerry White; 242–243(tr), Annette Stahl; 245(t), Julie Fletcher; 245(b), David Phillips; 250(l), David Phillips; 250(r), Terry McMenamy; 252, Charlie Burton; 253(l), Charlie Burton; 253(r), Bob Thomason; 255(b), Charlie Burton; 256, Maria Paraskevas; 261, David Phillips; 262, David Phillips; 263, Steve Ruehle; 265, Eric Camden; 268, Lucian Niemeyer; 269, Lucian Niemeyer; 273, David Phillips; 274–275(background), Jerry White; 276(tr), Bob Thomason; 276(b), Charlie Burton; 277, David Phillips; 280, Terry McMenamy; 281, Terry McMenamy; 285, Charlie Burton; 286, Charlie Burton; 287, Rodney Jones; 288, Beverly Brosius; 289, David Phillips; 290, David Phillips; 291, Beverly Brosius; 292, Brent Jones; 293, Brent Jones; 297, David Phillips; 298–299(background), Annette Stahl; 301, Beverly Brosius; 303(l), Beverly Brosius; 303(r), Beverly Brosius; 304(l), Charlie Burton; 304(r), Beverly Brosius; 306, Beverly Brosius; 307(l), Leonard Lessin; 307(r), Leonard Lessin; 308(r), Bob Thomason; 311(c), Charlie Burton; 314, Beverly Brosius; 315, Beverly Brosius; 316, Julie Fletcher; 318, Keith Glasgow; 319, Keith Glasgow; 323, Jerry White; 324–325(background), Jim Shea; 324–325(tl), Earl Kogler; 324–325(tr), Maria Paraskevas; 326(l), Henebry Photography; 326(r), Earl Kogler; 327(l), Gary Hofheimer; 327(b), Earl Kogler; 328(t), Earl Kogler; 328(b), Bill Knight; 330(tl), Earl Kogler; 330(tr), Earl Kogler; 331, Earl Kogler; 332, Rob Downey; 333(l), Dan Peha; 335(t), Earl Kogler; 335(b), Earl Kogler; 336, Rob Downey; 337(tl), Rob Downey; 337(tc), Rob Downey; 337(tr), Rob Downey; 337(b), Rob Downey; 338(t), Rob Downey; 338(bl), Rob Downey; 338(br), Rob Downey; 339(l), Rob Downey; 339(c), Rob Downey; 339(r), Eric Camden; 341, Earl Kogler; 342, Steve Ruehle; 345(l), Dan Peha; 346(tl), Rob Downey; 346(tr), Rob Downey; 346(c), Rob Downey; 346(b), Earl Kogler; 348(l), Gary Hofheimer; 348(r), Gary Hofheimer; 349(t), Eric Camden; 349(b), Eric Camden; 350, Eric Camden; 352, David R. Frazier; 353, David R. Frazier; 357, Richard Haynes; 365(inset), Julie Fletcher; 366(l), Leonard Lessin; 372, Julie Fletcher; 379(br), Dan Peha; 382, Rodney Jones; 384, Wiley & Flynn; 385, Wiley & Flynn; 388, Albert Moldvay; 389, Albert Moldvay; 393, Earl Kogler; 397–411, Terry Sinclair; 412, Maria Paraskevas; 413–417, Terry Sinclair.

All Other Photographs

Pages ii–iii(background), Ken Lax; ii–iii(inset), John P. Kelly/The Image Bank; xii(t), Frank P. Flavin; xii(b), H. Armstrong Roberts, Inc.; xiii(t), Peter A. Simon/Phototake; xviii(t), Linda K. Moore/Rainbow; xviii–1(tl), Dave Stock; 15, Billy Grimes; 30–31(tl), Collignon-Jarosz Ltd.; 30–31(tr), Howard Sochurek/The Stock Market; 30–31(c), James Stevenson, SPL/Photo Researchers; 30–31(br), Buzz Soard; 32(t), Scott Barrow/Superstock; 32(b), Jeanetta Ho; 33(b), Alfred LammeCamera M.D. Studios; 43, Courtesy of Warner-Lambert Co.; 49(l), Grant Heilman Photography; 49(c), Nina Lampen/Phototake; 49(r), G. Musil/Visuals Unlimited; 52, Biophoto Assoc., Science Source/Photo Researchers; 60, Runk, Schoenberger/Grant Heilman Photography; 67, Charles R. Drew, M.D. (1904–1950) by Betsy Graves Reyneau/ American Red Cross; 68–69(tl), Peter Fronk/Tony Stone Images; 68–69(tr), Philippe Plailly, SPL/Photo Researchers; 68–69(bc), Yoav/ Phototake; 70(tl), Arthur M. Siegelman; 70(tr), Arthur M. Siegelman; 70(bl), Arthur M. Siegelman; 70(br), Arthur M. Siegelman; 71, D.W. Fawcett/Photo Researchers; 72(t), Martin Dohrn, SPL/Photo Researchers; 72(b), Comstock; 73(l), Myrlene Ferguson/PhotoEdit; 73(r), Billy Grimes; 75(l), Photri; 75(r), James Stevenson, SPL/Photo Researchers; 76(r), MacDonald Photography/Third Coast Stock Source; 77(tl), Comstock; 77(tr), John Moss; 77(bl), Sally Myers; 77(br), Michael Siluk; 78(t), Alan Carey/The Image Works; 78(b), Chris Gaines/BMA-The Photo Source; 82(tl), Barbara Alper/Stock, Boston; 82(cl), Wayne Floyd/Unicorn Stock Photos; 82(cr), Gabe Palmer/The Stock Market; 82(tr), Barbara Kirk/The Stock Market; 82(bl), Steve Bourgeois/Unicorn Stock Photos; 83(b), Suzanne L. Murphy; 84(tl), Cesar Paredes/The Stock Market; 84(bl), Bob Daemmrich; 84(br), Linda K. Moore/Rainbow; 85(tl), George Glod/Superstock; 85(tc), Myrleen Ferguson/PhotoEdit; 85(tr), Bob Daemmrich; 85(bl), Carol Simowitz; 85(br), Robert Llewellyn/Superstock; 96–97(tl), Bob Daemmrich; 96–97(tr), Larry Mulvehill/PhotoBank; 96–97(br), D. Degnan/H. Armstrong Roberts, Inc.; 115, Rick Browne/Stock, Boston; 117, Bob Daemmrich; 124–125(tl), Tom Myers; 124–125(cl), Tom Raymond/ Fresh Air Photographics; 124–125(cr), Bob Daemmrich/The Image Works; 124–125(bl), M. Saunders/Miller Comstock; 124–125(br), Anne Gardon/Reflexion; 144(t), Hugues De Latude/Sygma; 144(b), Dr. Frank Rodriguez/PhotoEdit; 156–157(tl), Anne Gardon/Reflexion; 156–157(tr), S. Naiman/Reflexion; 156–157(cr), Todd Powell/Light Images; 156–157(b), Bob Daemmrich/The Image Works; 158, Tom Myers; 159(b), Kent & Donna Dannen; 162(l), Allen B. Smith/Tom Stack & Assoc.; 162(r), Tom McCarthy/The Stock Market; 168(l), Tony Freeman/PhotoEdit; 168(r), Tom Myers; 170, Bob Firth; 173(tl), Richard Cash/PhotoEdit; 173(tr), Richard Cash/PhotoEdit; 173(bl), Richard Cash/PhotoEdit; 173(br), Richard Cash/PhotoEdit; 174(inset), Steve Lissau/Rainbow; 175, "Human Sleep Stages" from The Sleep Disorders by Peter Hauri. Copyright © 1982 The Upjohn Company,